Local Food Environments

Local Food Environments
Food Access in America

Second Edition

Kimberly B. Morland, Yael M. Lehmann,
and Allison E. Karpyn

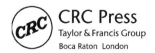

CRC Press
Taylor & Francis Group
Boca Raton London

CRC Press is an imprint of the
Taylor & Francis Group, an **informa** business

Second edition published 2022
by CRC Press
6000 Broken Sound Parkway NW, Suite 300, Boca Raton, FL 33487–2742

and by CRC Press
2 Park Square, Milton Park, Abingdon, Oxon, OX14 4RN

CRC Press is an imprint of Taylor & Francis Group, LLC

© 2022 Taylor & Francis Group, LLC

First edition published by CRC Press 2015

Library of Congress Cataloging-in-Publication Data
Names: Morland, Kimberly B., author. | Lehmann, Yael M., author. | Karpyn, Allison E., author.
Title: Local food environments : food access in America / Kimberly B. Morland, Yael M. Lehmann, and Allison E. Karpn.
Description: Second edition. | Boca Raton : CRC Press, 2022. | Revision of: Local food environments / edited by Kimberly B. Morland. 2015. | Includes bibliographical references. | Summary: "Local Food Environments: Food Access in America, Second Edition, presents four sections of information on (1) disparities between local food environments in the United States; (2) effect of restricted local food environments on dietary intake; (3) interventions to local food environment and their impact on communities; and (d) macro-level influence on the development of local food environments. All chapters include learning objectives and study questions. Equips learners with the tools necessary to design and implement effective interventions within their area's local food environment. Focuses on local food environment disparities and dietary intake. Discusses macro-level Influences on local food environments including U.S. federal and local policies affecting land-use; food production and of course food retailing"—Provided by publisher.
Identifiers: LCCN 2021049762 (print) | LCCN 2021049763 (ebook) | ISBN 9780367465070 (hardback) | ISBN 9780367464967 (paperback) | ISBN 9781003029151 (ebook)
Subjects: LCSH: Diet—United States. | Diet—Canada. | Local foods—Health aspects—United States. | Food supply—United States. | Nutrition policy—United States.
Classification: LCC TX360.U6 L63 2022 (print) | LCC TX360.U6 (ebook) | DDC 363.8/5610973—dc23/eng/20211117
LC record available at https://lccn.loc.gov/2021049762
LC ebook record available at https://lccn.loc.gov/2021049763

ISBN: 978-0-367-46507-0 (hbk)
ISBN: 978-0-367-46496-7 (pbk)
ISBN: 978-1-003-02915-1 (ebk)

DOI: 10.1201/9781003029151

Typeset in Optima
by Apex CoVantage, LLC

Contents

SECTION I   The Food System

SECTION II   State Food Environment Initiatives

SECTION III   Food Store Implementation and Evaluation

Preface

It is our belief that all communities deserve access to basic, high-quality resources and services such as education, health care, transportation, housing, banking, and grocery stores. This book focuses on local food environments, defined as 'the physical, social, economic, cultural, and political factors that impact the accessibility, availability, and adequacy of food within a community or region',[1] with a particular focus on the placement of food stores. For years, public health experts have recognized that equity in access to health care is a key determinant of health and that the inequities in the system have led to disparities. Similarly, as evidenced by work of the NAACP and *Brown v. Board of Education*, efforts to establish equal access to education are recognized as a fundamental pillar of a just society. Yet, unlike these resources that are universally accepted as essential for well-being, some experts have questioned if equal access to healthy food matters and whether programs such as the Healthy Food Financing Initiative (HFFI) work to establish the needed food retail businesses in underserved communities. Within this second edition, *Local Food Environments: Food Access in America* has expanded its scope, placing food store access into the context of other systems impacted by economically underserved communities such as housing, health care, and education. The focus has shifted from the first edition to reflect what government leaders have identified as parallels between these systems and a common solution: to draw private investment into these communities.

The term *underserved* has a long history as a government designation for communities facing structural barriers that prevent them from accessing services such as health care, transportation, education, banking, and high-quality food stores. As defined in the Biden administration's Executive Order *On Advancing Racial Equity and Support for Underserved Communities Through the Federal Government*, the term *underserved communities* refers to 'populations sharing a particular characteristic, as well as geographic communities, that have been systematically denied a full opportunity to participate in aspects of economic, social, and civic life'.[2] Communities identified as underserved by various government agencies at the federal, state, or local level may then qualify for additional government support and funding. Many banks and community development financial institutions (CDFIs) use the term *underserved* interchangeably with the terms *unbanked* or *underbanked*, to reflect individuals who are not adequately served by traditional banking institutions. In fact, in order to receive certification from the U.S. Treasury, CDFIs must prove they are 'dedicated to serving market niches that are often underserved by traditional financial institutions'.[3] When advocating for government support, the term historically has been useful for healthy food access advocates.

Government agencies have utilized existing programs for underserved areas (e.g., the New Markets Tax Credit) and infrastructures (e.g., CDFIs) to provide the capital investment necessary to draw experienced food store operators to communities in need. Since publishing the first edition in 2015, healthy food financing initiatives have flourished across the United States, thereby laying the groundwork with resources for new food store business ventures. Initially, healthy food financing programs were promoted at the state level, where grant funds were channeled through local CDFIs, which then matched the state support with private investment dollars from traditional banks and private foundations. The first healthy-food financing program, created in 2004 in Pennsylvania, became a model for the country, thanks to the visionary leadership of Jeremy Nowak of Reinvestment Fund, Congressman Dwight Evans, and Duane Perry, founder of The Food Trust. States across America have followed the lead of Pennsylvania by adopting similar food financing initiatives. The origination, program planning, and funded business ventures for five states are detailed in Chapters 4 to 8.

CDFIs and other government programs are a response to the consistent history of racism and discrimination within traditional U.S. banks, which has negatively impacted investment, Black home ownership, and business opportunities in many American neighborhoods. This pervasive practice of redlining is documented in Chapter 3, with specific examples in the state initiative chapters. The second edition aims to connect the history of racism and discrimination in the banking industry to the larger food system. We have added the agricultural practices of early colonies' dependence on African and African American slave labor in Chapter 1 and connected it to the migration of Black southerners to northern states after emancipation laws were passed, to describe how underinvested areas originated in the United States. (Chapters 4 to 8). In addition, this second edition elaborates on factors that have influenced the current agricultural system and how policies that have supported 'get big or get out' agriculture have trickled down to the food retail portion of our food system (Chapter 2).

The Food Trust, Reinvestment Fund, PolicyLink, and Congressman Evans worked with Sam Kass, who served as President Barack Obama's Senior Advisor for Nutrition Policy and as the Executive Director for First Lady Michelle Obama's Let's Move! campaign, and many others, to create the federal HFFI in 2010, with a mission to bring grocery stores and other healthy food retailers to underserved urban and rural communities across America. As former First Lady Michelle Obama stated at an event in Philadelphia on February 19, 2010:

> So it's because of this example, [the Pennsylvania FFFI], that as part of 'Let's Move', we created this Healthy Food Financing Initiative that's modeled on what's been going on here. And as Secretary Geithner said, with a modest initial investment of about $400 million a year, we're going to use that money to leverage hundreds of millions more from private and nonprofit sectors to bring grocery stores and other healthy food retailers to underserved communities all across this country. If you can do it here, we can do it around the country. And our goal is ambitious.[4]

Today healthy-food financing programs are flourishing primarily as federal programs. Federal funds for these programs are transferred to local CDFIs and community development corporations from three federal agencies: the Department of Treasury, Department of Agriculture, and the Department of Health and Human Services. These agencies have utilized existing government programs that aim to revitalize areas by attracting private investment. The federal programs, policies, and infrastructures that have been drawn upon to launch the federal HFFI are discussed in Chapter 3.

Now with the Biden administration, there began a new growing momentum and federal support to advance a just and equitable food system in the United States as part of a larger social and racial justice agenda by the administration. Healthy-food financing programs remain a component of President Biden's work, more than fifteen years since the first program in Pennsylvania, as a means to address long-term structural racism in our economy. Vice President Kamala Harris, a long-time champion of CDFIs, secured $12 billion in federal funding to aid the mission-driven work of CDFIs while still a senator in December 2020.[5] As Vice President, she met with Janet Yellen, United States Secretary of Treasury who announced through Twitter:

> The importance of CDFIs was one of the first subjects @VP raised with me, . . . & it's exactly the right place to focus our attention. Because the questions who can access credit and capital and who can't, are at the root of many long term structural problems in our economy.[6]

It is an exciting time to be involved in the continuing work of creating social change. The many HFFI programs that have been supported with state funds are listed in Chapters 4 to 8 and those supported with federal funds are listed in Chapter 12. The simple opening of a new food store or improving the variety of healthy food options in an existing one will decrease food access disparities in the United States. But as researchers and advocates of food equity, we also believe there is value in understanding how specific food retailing changes affect underserved communities. We urge other researchers and advocates to move away from documenting disparities and towards evaluating programs that make changes to local food environments. Throughout this book, there is a call for public-private partnerships acknowledging that food retailing is a corporate owned component of our food system. In Chapters 9–12, we describe program planning and evaluation, starting with identifying key stakeholders such as food retailers, community members, researchers, and government personnel that are positioned to solve food access problems within a given community. We also recognize that one solution will not solve local food environment disparities for every community. Therefore, in Chapters 11 and 12, we borrow implementation science methods used in health care, which is rooted in this viewpoint, to recommend program evaluation strategies aimed to gain lessons learned from each HFFI project. We hope that this book can serve as a resource to students, community organizers, policymakers and others working to increase access to affordable, healthy food in this country.

Kimberly B. Morland
Yael M. Lehmann
Allison E. Karpyn

REFERENCES

1. Rideout K, Mah CL, Minaber L. *Food Environments: An Introduction for Public Health and Practice*. National Collaborating Center for Environmental Health; December 2015.
2. White House. Executive Order on Advancing Equity and Support for Underserved Communities through the Federal Government. January 20, 2021; www.whitehouse.gov/briefing-room/presidential-actions/2021/01/20/executive-order-advancing-racial-equity-and-support-for-underserved-communities-through-the-federal-government/.
3. U.S. Department of Treasury. CDFI Certification: Your Gateway to the CDFI Community. www.cdfifund.gov/sites/cdfi/files/documents/cdfi_program_fact_sheet_certification_updatedjan2016.pdf.
4. The White House. Remarks by the First Lady at Fresh Food Financing Initiative. *Press Release*. February 19, 2010; https://obamawhitehouse.archives.gov/the-press-office/remarks-first-lady-fresh-food-financing-initiative.
5. Office of Mark R. Warner-Press Release: Warner, Booker, Harris Applaud Passage of Bill to Make a Record Investment in Low-Income and Minority Communities. December 22, 2020; www.warner.senate.gov/public/index.cfm/2020/12/warner-booker-harris-applaud-passage-of-bill-to-make-a-record-investment-in-low-income-and-minority-communities.
6. Secretary Janet Yellen. Importance of CDFIs. June 15, 2021; https://twitter.com/SecYellen/status/1404942768485584901.

Acknowledgments

In revising this book, we have benefited greatly from discussions and interactions with many trusted and pioneering agencies and their staff, grocery retailers, researchers, practitioners, policymakers, state and city employees, community residents, and other professionals in the field. Since the early phases of the development of the second edition, the support from Alicia Papanek, a predoctoral candidate within the College of Agriculture and Life Sciences at the University of Florida, has been extremely valuable. We appreciate her contributions, as a student in her early stage of local food environment research and advocacy, in understanding important nuances to local and federal funding outcomes, her thorough and thoughtful reviews of chapters always complete with insightful comments and important edits, as well as her visionary talent in creating the cover of the text.

Further we would like to recognize The Food Trust for its pioneering work in the field. Staff members including Duane Perry, Sandy Sherman, Hannah Burton, John Weidman, Brian Lang, Caroline Harries, Miriam Manon, Dierdre Church, Eugene Kim, Tracey Giang, James Johnson-Piett, and Julia Koprak contributed to the design and operation of fresh food financing programs nationally; without their dedicated efforts the content of this text would not be possible. We also thank Caroline Harries, Julia Koprak, Brian Lang, and John Weidman for their feedback on the text, as well as comments based on their experiences.

The Reinvestment Fund too is responsible for much of the work described in this text, and as a leading Community Development Financial Institution that has pioneered Fresh Food Financing as a viable mechanism of support. The work of Jeremy Nowak, Patricia Smith, Donald Hinkle Brown, Ira Goldstein, Christina Szczepanski, Lance Loethen, and Molly Hartman among others to lay the groundwork for, and operate the Pennsylvania and Healthy Food Financing Initiatives, enabled other cities and states to replicate the work, and, in so doing, to be more effective and efficient in their own financing program operations.

We would also like to recognize Alex B. Hill, for his contributions to the Michigan Chapter and his thoughtful and deeply considerate input about the current work being undertaken in Detroit. We would also like to thank Corrine Munoz-Plaza for providing her knowledge and experience of qualitative methods to the book in the context of mixed methods within implementation science. Finally, we are indebted to the people that were interviewed and have shared their thoughts and experiences interacting with the U.S. food system including Jeremy Peaches, former Delaware Secretary of Agriculture, Ed Kee, Bill Green, Reco Owens, Greg Silverman, and Julia Koprak, as well as Congressman Evans, Sam Kass, and Robert Lawrence for their endorsements of the book's content.

We are also grateful to other voices in the book from: Spencertorry Brown, Tracie McMillan, Michelle Obama, Jeff Brown, Pastor Johnson, Anita Chappell, Angela Glover Blackwell, Risa Lavizzo-Mourey, Burnell Colton, Doris Burbank, Claude Brown, Debra Young, Marcus Garvey, Nicholas D'Agostino, Ruben Diez, Joe Doleh, Kimberly Latimer-Nelligan, Charles Walker, James Hooks, Malik Yakini, Dara Cooper, Sara Fleming, Dave Pagel, Steve Fernandez, the East New York community and Co-op members, the North Carolina Environmental Justice Network members, as well as the authors who contributed to the first edition of this book.

Finally, we the authors recognize the many active residents and pioneering food retailers and entrepreneurs who have spoken up about the need and taken action to enable equal access to affordable nutritious food. Their voice and story are the heartbeat of this text.

About the Authors

Kimberly B. Morland, PhD, MPH, is an epidemiologist who has focused her career on food environment disparities in the United States. She is a forerunner in the public health arena of local food environment research, having published a seminal manuscript titled the 'Contextual Effects of Local Food Environments: The Atherosclerosis Risk in Communities Study' in the *American Journal of Public Health* in 2002. While The Food Trust was advancing state policies for capital spending to support new grocery store ventures, Morland was building partnerships with underserved communities in New York City to gain National Institutes of Health (NIH) funding for a new food store while developing a parallel tract to support communities in need of grocery stores. While aiming to shine a light on this public health disparity, she has published numerous NIH-funded manuscripts on local food environments, served on national and local review panels on this topic, and has received national media coverage for her work. Morland recognized the need for the first edition of *Local Food Environments: Food Access in America*, which describes the academic research on food environments. She initiated this second edition, which details the many public-private partnerships and immense government support that has been gained for local food environment work over the past decade. Currently, she is advancing her work through the Public Health Research Institute of Southern California and teaching at the California State University at Los Angeles. She teaches research methods to undergraduate and graduate students in Public Health and Nutritional Sciences and has started a new graduate course called *Food Environments and Nutrition*, where she hopes to engage and prepare emerging researchers and advocates to join the mission to decrease disparities in food access in the United States. Morland earned her bachelor's in psychology from the University of California at Berkeley (UCB) and master's degree in epidemiology and biostatistics at the School of Public Health at UCB. Finally, she earned her PhD in environmental epidemiology from the University of North Carolina at Chapel Hill where she began her inquiry about local food environments in the United States.

Yael M. Lehmann, MSW, has dedicated her twenty-plus year career to increasing access to affordable, nutritious food for all Americans. After working with the agency for five years, Lehmann became Executive Director of The Food Trust in 2006 where she led its pioneering work until 2018. With her leadership, The Food Trust, originally a small nonprofit of less than ten employees, grew to over 100 staff members. Together with colleagues and stakeholders, Lehmann stewarded the campaign of equal access to food stores in Philadelphia, which gained support from the Robert Wood Johnson Foundation and Congressman Evans to implement the Fresh Food Financing Initiative. Her guidance also deepened partnerships with other organizations such as the Reinvestment Fund and gained the attention of the former First Lady Michelle Obama, who described the work accomplished by The Food Trust during her tenure as being a 'remarkable success' for increasing the availability of fresh fruits and vegetables in schools and reducing by 50% the number of students becoming overweight and modeled the national effort, the Healthy Food Financing Initiative (HFFI), after the Fresh Food Financing Initiative. She is an advocate and speaker on national food access issues, having been quoted in publications such as the *New York Times* and *Washington Post*, and has been interviewed on *PBS NewsHour*, BillMoyers.com, CNN, and *Good Morning America*, among other media outlets. She received several leadership awards, including the Urban Leadership Award from the Penn Institute for Urban Research. After her tenure at The Food Trust, Lehmann served as Executive Director: Mid-Atlantic Region, for the Common Market, a nonprofit that delivers 'local food for the common good'. In response to the COVID-19 pandemic, the Common Market provided approximately one million produce boxes sourced from local farms to food insecure families in New York City, Philadelphia, New Jersey, Baltimore, and Washington, DC. Now serving as the Executive Director of SevaTruck, a non-profit serving fresh, nutritious meals to local communities using food trucks, Lehmann continues to utilizes her experience to work to support the movement of fair and accessible fresh food for all Americans. Lehmann received her bachelor's degree from the University of California at Berkeley and a master's from the University of Pennsylvania's School of Social Policy and Practice. She received additional executive education in nonprofit management at Harvard Business School. Lehmann is a Fellow of the third class of the Health Innovators Fellowship and a member of the Aspen Global Leadership Network.

Allison E. Karpyn, PhD, is a world-recognized food access researcher who has dedicated her career to understanding the impacts of policy efforts to address gaps in food access. Karpyn worked alongside Yael Lehmann for nearly twelve years at The Food Trust, as Director of Research, Evaluation, and Consulting. Her work brings to the field, and to this edition of the text, a rare perspective on the history of food environment research in combination with advocacy, that has guided the current public policies for improving food access. As one of only a handful of social science researchers who has worked to study the food environment issue since the early 2000s and who was on-site and present for much of the day-to-day decision-making leading to programs such as the Fresh Food Financing Initiative, Karpyn tells the story of how economic development, retail, and food systems connect to address inequities and systems of inequality. Today, Karpyn works as Co-Director of the University of Delaware's Center for Research in Education and Social Policy (CRESP) and serves as Associate Professor in the Department of the Human Development and Family Sciences. Karpyn is a Fulbright Scholar and in her twenty years of practice has published widely in journals including *Pediatrics*, *Preventive Medicine*, and *Health Affairs* on program evaluation methods; topics related to hunger, obesity, school food, supermarket access, food insecurity, and healthy corner stores; and strategies to develop and maintain farmer's markets in low-income areas. Karpyn earned her bachelor's degree in public health at Johns Hopkins University and her doctorate in policy research evaluation and measurement at the University of Pennsylvania. She resides in Pennsylvania together with her husband and their four children.

Section I

The Food System

This section of the book introduces the United States Food System to readers, explaining the process by which food products are grown, transported, and sold in the United States. Readers are provided with historical events and federal policies that have shaped the current food system, aiming to educate readers about the food supply chain, beginning with production and ending with retail, to appreciate the many factors that determine the foods Americans eat. Chapter 1 begins with food production, relating the historical events and policies that are drivers for the types of foods that are currently, and have in the past, been produced on American farms and ranches. The evolution of industrialized food production is described in relation to the current efficiency of food production, food prices, and profitability. This section is intended to prepare readers for the second section of the book, which describes state and city public policies that have aided food retailers to be successful in underserved areas of the United States. Therefore, Chapter 2 focuses on how food retail operators remain profitable in the United States and the disparities in access to supermarkets in low-income, predominately Black and other American neighborhoods. Finally, Chapter 3 describes new and existing federal U.S. policies and programs that have been used to support food retailers to conduct business in underserved areas, including the Healthy Food Financing Initiative.

DOI: 10.1201/9781003029151-1

1 Agriculture Production

CONTENTS

INTRODUCTION

Food is an essential element necessary for human survival. When eaten, whole foods are broken down into nutrients, which are then used in the human body to support immune response, physical mobility, cognitive function, and all other aspects that make the human body function efficiently. However, food is also a commodity. A commodity is a raw material that can be bought or sold. As a commodity, food is produced, processed, and sold as any other raw material, such as petroleum or coal. As a raw material, the United States has aimed to protect this resource with food policies that have historically focused on agriculture (the production of foods); nutrition (human consumption) and sales/trade (economics). These policies are rooted within the historical and existing national and international commercial structures that produce, process, trade, and sell foods for human consumption.

The United States food system is composed of stages whereby food is produced, prepared, and sold for human consumption and described simply in Figure 1.1. The food system can be described on a global or local level for the purpose of characterizing the many networks worldwide involved in the production and sale of food products, or the supply chain of a single food product grown in a specific location; hence there are many visual and written descriptions of the food system.[1-4] For the purpose of this book, a simplified version of the system is provided that focuses on stages of the food system that produce profitability along the food supply chain, including growing and harvesting food, processing food, food distribution, food retail, and finally human food purchases/consumption. The focus of this book mainly targets

DOI: 10.1201/9781003029151-2

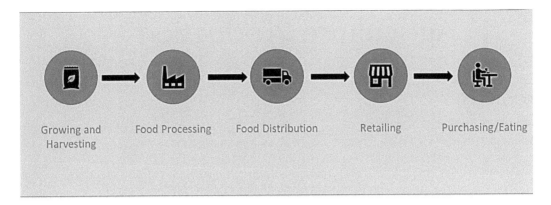

FIGURE 1.1   Components of the U.S. Food System

one component of the food system, food retail. However, the foods available for retail are determined by the components of the food system that precede it. Hence, the overarching objective of this chapter is for readers to gain an understanding of how the agriculture system works in the United States and appreciate how this is the first component of the food system and instrumental in determining the types of foods that are available in food stores across America. The chapter has been organized into three sections so that readers can understand: (a) the historical events and public policies that are the foundations of our current agriculture production system; (b) how the current industrialized monoculture system has developed; and (c) the impacts that the industrialized food production system has on small farms, farmworkers, and local communities as well as foods produced and the environment.

U.S. AGRICULTURE PRODUCTION: HISTORY AND POLICIES

Food production in the United States begins in the 1600s with the colonization of the new world.[5] The English expansion to North America was during a time when food was scarce in England, and many agricultural workers were unemployed. King James of England, Ireland, and Scotland gave the southern portion of what is now the United States to the Virginia Company, which settled Jamestown, Virginia, in 1607; however, it took nine years for colonists to learn from the Native Americans how to grow any agriculture products such as tobacco. The northern half of the Atlantic coastline was given to the Plymouth Company, and the Plymouth Colony was settled in 1620. A decade later the Massachusetts Bay Company settled the colony of Massachusetts, and the Puritans were taught to fish, farm, and hunt by Native Americans. The Carolina Colony, from south Virginia to Florida, was home to farmers who owned vast estates that produced corn, beef, pork, and other staples. These farmers had close ties to English Colonies in the Caribbean, including the island of Barbados, which used African slave labor in their fields; hence the African slave trade became a prominent feature of Carolina Colony development. By the year 1700, there were approximately 250,000 European and African settlers in North America's thirteen English colonies. Seventy-five years later, at the beginning of the American Revolutionary War, there were 2.5 million residents living in the colonies.[6]

British Colonial Agriculture

As early as the 1600s, United States farmers benefited from agricultural policies that endorsed slave labor and new technologies to support the production of crops and livestock. Agricultural productivity is a theme that has been key to the growth of the agricultural economy in the United States stemming as far back as the British colonies and tobacco farming.[5,7] Central to early tobacco production was African slave labor that began in 1619 when twenty kidnapped African men and women arrived in what is now Virginia and were sold to English colonists. At the time, fieldwork in the colonies was typically conducted by indentured servants from Britain who served four to seven years in exchange for a new life in the colonies.[8] Although these first Africans were treated as indentured servants, their arrival to the British colonies gave rise to the Transatlantic Slave Trade (of which Britain was the largest slave trader in Europe) and in turn supported early U.S. agricultural productivity.[9,10]

In areas that are now the southern states of the United States, and in particular Virginia, tobacco was the most successful cash crop in the early 1600s and fundamental to the colony's economy.[7] However, cultivating tobacco was labor intensive and required the use of slave labor to increase profit margins. Southern colonies adopted new laws to support plantation owners. For example, African slaves on plantations were deemed a commodity of the plantation owner. Under these laws, African slaves were considered chattel: (a) owned forever by the plantation owner; (b) their children were automatically enslaved and owned forever; and (c) any of these enslaved people could be bought and sold. As property of plantation owners, these people could also be mistreated with no recourse.[11] These laws gave way for plantation owners to purchase more African slaves, resulting in increased tobacco production and sales to English and Scottish merchants who then processed the tobacco into consumable products. However, the overproduction of tobacco in the early 1700s, due to decreased sales to Great Britain merchants at the beginning of the American Revolutionary War, led to low tobacco prices. By the late 1700s, tobacco profitability had fallen to such an extent that many farmers began growing food crops and other less labor-intensive agricultural products.[12]

First Industrial Revolution, 1760–1820

During the latter part of this period, Europe and the British colonies were participating in the First Industrial Revolution. This was a time when inventions were being made to better transport raw materials and/or improve the production of agriculture.[13] Expanding on the development of the steam engine, new models were being made to integrate it into agricultural processing and transportation. For example, a rotary motor was added to the steam engine by Matthew Boulton, which revolutionized the processing of flour, cotton, and other agricultural products.[14] The steam engine was also used to power trains and boats to transport agriculture products by land and through new waterways such as the Erie Canal.

Another significant innovation was the development of the cotton gin by Eli Whitney.[15] This machine was invented in 1793 and separated cotton fibers from their seeds, a labor-intensive task that was typically performed by African slaves. This design allowed for a significant increase in agricultural output of cotton and launched the beginning of the textile industry. However, this invention did not shield African slaves from agricultural labor. In fact, the efficiency of the cotton gin, resulted in a need to increase the planting and harvesting of cotton. Like tobacco, cotton is a labor-intensive agricultural cash crop. However, because the plantation owners had the infrastructure in place for producing tobacco (land, labor, and the organizational structure), cotton was exchanged as the primary cash crop by most southern farmers. In fact, by 1820, cotton provided 50% of U.S. agricultural exports and that required the enslavement of 250,000 new Africans who were brought to the United States between 1787 and 1808. By 1820, 95% of all African Americans were enslaved, and by 1860, there were four million African slaves in the United States, 60% of whom worked on cotton plantations.[16]

The U.S. Civil War and the Thirteenth Amendment to the U.S. Constitution

It was 89 years after the United States became independent from Great Britain and after a Civil War that the Thirteenth Amendment was ratified by all States of the Union. This amendment to the U.S. Constitution outlawed chattel slavery and involuntary servitude beginning in 1865.[17] The second section of the amendment gives Congress the power to enforce the Thirteenth Amendment with appropriate legislation. Hence, in addition, the Civil Rights Act of 1866 was written and passed, which made the Christian Black Codes of 1724 illegal.[18] The Black Codes were adopted in southern states a century earlier with the intention of placing restrictions on the freedom of emancipated Black slaves. The Black Codes stated that an emancipated slave had to be in service of a White person, could not go out without a White supervisor, could not speak out, could not own a weapon, and imposed other restrictions to the freedom and liberties of African Americans. In addition, the Fourteenth Amendment to the Constitution was ratified on July 9, 1868, to extend the rights provided in the United States Bill of Rights to former slaves. But up to this point in American history, U.S. agricultural productivity was almost entirely due to the workforce of African and African American slaves.

THE GREAT DEPRESSION AND THE AGRICULTURE ADJUSTMENT ACT

One of the most significant historical events of the past century affecting food production in the United States was the Great Depression in the 1930s. During this time there was a major economic downturn that impacted not only the U.S. food supply but also influenced global agriculture production. During this time 25% of the population was unemployed. The effects were felt both in urban and rural areas since many Americans had migrated to cities in hopes of working in factories, which caused a rural decline.[19]

As part of the New Deal, President Franklin D. Roosevelt (FDR) enacted the Agriculture Adjustment Act, known commonly as the Farm Bill, to serve as an emergency measure to address the falling prices of corn during the Depression.[20] At the time, farmers were producing more corn than they were able to sell, which resulted in extremely low prices and few buyers. To stabilize prices, the Agriculture Adjustment Act of 1933 allowed the federal government to pay subsidies to farmers who restricted agriculture production. By paying farmers to not grow corn it allowed supply and demand to stabilize and eventually for prices of corn to increase. In addition to corn, other crops were targeted for restricting production such as cotton and wheat. These subsidized crops became known as *commodity crops*.

This legislation led to the establishment of the Food Commodities Corporation, which engaged in agricultural exports. Other features of the Agriculture Adjustment Act were the Soil Conservation and Domestic Allotment Act, which encouraged conservation by paying farmers to plant soil-building crops such as alfalfa instead of staple crops (e.g., corn and wheat) to preserve farmland for future generations. The New Deal also included loans to farmers for staple crops to be stored until needed in low yield years. The Agriculture Adjustment Act is renewed every five years, and although the original policy covered corn, cotton, and wheat, the legislation has since added soybeans, barley, oats, rice, other grains, dairy, peanuts, and sugar to the list of commodity crops.[21,22] A more detailed description of the Agriculture Adjustment Act can be found in Chapter 3.

In addition to the subsidies, the surplus of commodity crops is purchased by the U.S. Department of Agriculture (USDA) for distribution to United States nutrition assistance programs such as the National School Lunch program, which was initiated during the War on Poverty. The government's commodity foods programs aim to protect the fall of food prices for farmers by offsetting any overproduction by providing low-cost or free food to Americans who are economically at-risk for food insecurity. Commodity crops are critical ingredients in school meals programs and can be a key driver of what is served. Similarly, in 1939 the Food Stamp program became available, which allowed low-income individuals to buy blue food stamps for purchasing commodity surplus foods at grocery stores.[23] When the program was reinitiated during the Kennedy administration, special food stamps for commodity foods were eliminated from the program; however the Food Stamp Act (P.L. 88–525) of 1964 aimed to find a more effective use of agriculture overproduction to strengthen the U.S. agriculture economy while also decreasing rates of hunger in the United States. Since this time, the Food Stamp Program, now called the Supplemental Nutrition Assistance Program or SNAP, has had revisions such as the elimination of the requirement to purchase the food stamps, establishment of national standards for eligibility, and the use of electronic benefit transfer (EBT) cards. In addition, other programs that are supported by the government purchasing of agricultural overproduction of mostly commodity crops aimed primarily to address hunger are described briefly here:[24]

- *Food Distribution Program on Indian Reservations* provides commodity foods to low-income households, including the elderly living on Indian reservations and to Native American families residing in designated areas near reservations.

- *The Emergency Food Assistance Program (TEFAP)* makes USDA commodity foods available to States, which provide the food to local agencies that they have selected, usually food banks, which in turn, distribute the food to soup kitchens and food pantries that directly serve the public.

- *Child and Adult Care Food Program (CACFP)* provides foods to day care centers, to adults who receive care in nonresidential adult day care centers, and to children residing in homeless shelters and youths participating in eligible after-school care programs.

- *National School Lunch Program (NSLP)* provides cash subsidies and donates USDA commodity food to school districts and independent schools that choose to take part in the lunch program. In return, the organizations must serve lunches that meet federal requirements, and they must offer free or reduced-price lunches to eligible children. School food authorities can also be reimbursed for snacks served to children through age 18 in after-school educational or enrichment programs.

- *School Breakfast Program*, like the NSLP, provides cash subsidies to participating schools that serve breakfast.

- *Special Milk Program* provides milk to participating schools and institutions, which receive reimbursement from the USDA for each half pint of milk served. They must operate their milk programs on a nonprofit basis. They agree to use the federal reimbursement to reduce the selling price of milk to all children.

- *Summer Food Service Program (SFSP)* helps fill the hunger gap during summer when the NSLP and SPP are not available.

- *Women, Infants, and Children (WIC)* provides foods to supplement diets, information on healthy eating, and referrals to health care to low-income women, infants, and children up to age five who are at nutritional risk.

- *Commodity Supplemental Food Program (CSFP)* provides USDA commodity foods to supplement the diet of the same population served by WIC but who are not WIC participants.

CHEAP FOOD POLICIES, 1970s–PRESENT

The overproduction of agriculture products that support the programs described in the previous section were galvanized during the 1970s. During this time, the United States Secretary of Agriculture was Earl Butz, who served under Presidents Richard Nixon and Gerald Ford from 1971 to 1976.[25–27] He was a proponent of greater production and lower food prices for Americans. He spurred a new food production framework to reduce subsidies for restricting production, and instead, argued to allow the free market to operate. The 'Get big or get out' signature slogan of Mr. Butz, has fueled Big Ag, favoring large-scale corporate farming. As this investment in Big Ag and a free market approach to food production was adopted, corporate groups such as the Consultative Group on International Agricultural Research (CGIAR) emerged with funding from the Rockefellers and other groups. What resulted was increased investment by private corporations in new technologies for agriculture production.[28] For example, Norman Borlaug[29] received a Nobel Peace Prize for his innovations in plant breeding. A documentary of Norman Borlaug's contribution to the wheat industry can be seen in a PBS documentary (www.pbs.org/wgbh/americanexperience/films/man-who-tried-to-feed-the-world/#part0). Other groups focused on the development of improved fertilizers and pesticides as well as new methods for irrigation. These investments were the building blocks for a monocultural system of farming which is an agricultural practice of growing a single crop or livestock species instead of growing multiple types of crops and raising animals all on the same farm.[30] The adoption of the monocultural agricultural system has resulted in increased productivity in U.S. agriculture since 1970 which Mr. Butz has argued has kept food prices low for Americans. Earl Butz is recognized for stimulating an agricultural system to support 'Cheap Food'. Other legislation, such as the Agriculture Improvement and Reform (FAIR) Act of 1996, also supported increased production by providing direct payments to commodity crop farmers.[31] Productivity has been as central to the economic growth of U.S. agriculture in the past as it is now. Recent increases in productivity are seen in Figure 1.2 where the United States Department of Agriculture has documented that agricultural productivity has tripled between 1948 and 2017. Most of that productivity has taken place since the early 1970s because of the industrialization of agriculture which is described in the next section.

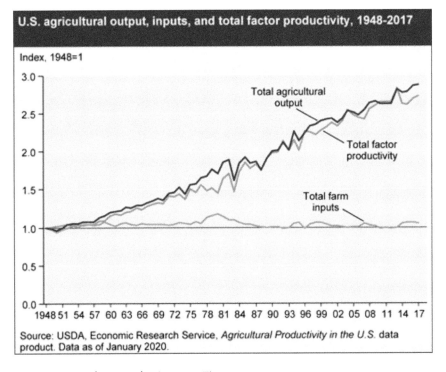

FIGURE 1.2   U.S. Agriculture Production over Time

Farm Systems Reform Act (FSRA)

One of the most recent policies introduced to Congress is the Farm Systems Reform Act by Senator Cory Booker on January 21, 2020, with the support of Senators Elizabeth Warren and Bernie Sanders. The legislation aims to eliminate large, confined animal feeding operations (CAFOs) over the next 20 years and minimize monopolies that are currently in the U.S. food production system. FSRA also aims to provide farmers with the means to be profitable without relying on farm subsidies, which currently cost taxpayers approximately $22 billion per year.[32] Support of the bill continues to grow, and some view it as an opportunity to help smaller farms succeed, regain a younger population of farmers, and even the distribution of wealth within the agriculture industry. Additional benefits would be conservation of U.S. soil while still allowing the same productivity. Opponents argue that there are EPA regulations to CAFOs that control the harmful emissions, whereas other argue that the current industrial agriculture system has many farmers on a treadmill, stuck within a system where the profits from their productivity are marginalized into a larger system.

INDUSTRIALIZATION OF AGRICULTURE

This section of the chapter describes the industrialization of American food production. Industrialization "refers to the organization of agriculture as an in line, quasi-manufacturing process wherein the energy and materials of production are treated as exogenous to the system of biological productivity, and the primary goal is maximum sustained yield of single commodity items."[33]

This form of agriculture has risen since the beginning of the Second Industrial Revolution where production lines were adopted in many types of industries (e.g., automobile), but has accelerated since Cheap Food Policies were adopted fifty years ago. In this section, readers will learn how industrialization has created monoculture systems with changes in farm ownership and labor. Specific examples in the production of corn and hogs are provided.

To understand monoculture systems of food production, one must first understand traditional agricultural systems that have been used in the United States. Traditional agricultural systems are based on producing a diversity of species on smaller farms that are closer in proximity. These traditional farms allow farmers to utilize by-products of production of one product to enhance the production of another. For example, because animal wastes are used to fertilize feed crops, which is then used to grow the next year's livestock, this system results in a feedback loop wherein wastes are recycled on the farm. Furthermore, in pasture-based operations, livestock play an important role in scavenging crop residues that remain in the fields after harvest, reducing insect populations, and conditioning soil by disturbing the ground and depositing manure. Diversity of production not only creates nutrient feedback loops and symbiotic relationships between multiple species, but it also makes agriculture more resistant to periodic problems such as pests, drought, and temperature fluctuations, which usually affect one species more than others. These family farmers support the local economy by purchasing feed, equipment, and supplies from local retailers and spend their profits in their communities. This traditional agricultural system supplies residents with locally sourced foods gained from multiple family farms, allowing supply and demand of food prices to work at the local level.

In contrast, industrial food production has separated traditional farming into compartments where farmers are typically crop or livestock growers and within those agriculture categories is specialization into one species of livestock or crop. The components of farming one species, for instance, is further compartmentalized into growers, finishers, and feed producers, which are typically located many miles away from each other. The adoption of manufacturing principals that were adopted by other U.S. industries during the First and Second industrial revolutions, were placed into the agriculture system, which necessitated large plots of farmland, each specializing in the production of one product to contribute to a larger food system.

The implementation of Mr. Butz's vision for agriculture productivity required the consolidation of farmland and a reorganization of how farms operate in the United States. For example, in 1870 the United States had roughly two million farms that produced food to feed 38 million Americans.[34] The number of farms tripled over the next 60 years to 6.8 million in 1935, then declined after World War II. By 1970, the number of farms in the United States had steadily decreased back to the amount a century before, pushed to produce food for five times as many Americans (205 million). Although the number of farms has decreased, the amount of farmland has not changed since 1935, resulting in larger farms owned by fewer farmers. On average, current farms contain 444 acres of land compared to 155 acres in 1935. There are approximately two million farms currently in operation in the United States, providing food for 329 million Americans. The top ten states for agriculture production are: California, Iowa, Nebraska, Texas, Minnesota, Illinois, Kansas, Wisconsin, North Carolina, and Indiana.[35]

Still today, most U.S. farms are considered small. It is estimated that of the two million farms in the United States, approximately 1,794,000 are small farms (89.7%) and 54,000 are large farms (2.7%). Gross cash farm income was forecasted to be $447 billion in 2020.[34] Based on the projected gross income for the proportion of small farms, the average annual gross income for small U.S. farms in 2020 was projected to be $52,574. By contrast, large farms were expected to gross an average of $3,799,500. The 72-times greater earnings by the large farms suggests the industrialized food production system may not be operating similarly across all types of farms in the United States.

In addition to the consolidation of farms and ranches, the industrialization of the U.S. food system has also impacted other areas of the supply chain necessary for food to be produced efficiently. The industry has become vertically integrated.[36] This means that one company controls the production process from basic inputs to retail sale. For example, livestock producers either own animal production facilities or, more commonly, use contract growers, typically former family farmers, to raise the animals. In the case of hogs, the integrator owns the animals, animal feed, veterinary supplies, trucks, rendering plants, and processing plants. The contract grower owns (and has liability for) the buildings and the waste and must follow the integrator's terms for raising the animals. Most hog producers are unable to remain independent because they cannot get access to processing plants without a contract and integrators control the processing plants. Another example of efficiency relates to the production of plant-based foods. For example, Monsanto specializes in pesticide resistance seeds, and in fact their Roundup resistance soybeans are used in over 90% of all U.S. farms, requiring farmers to purchase new seeds yearly rather than utilizing the yield from the current planting season for the next. When natural cross-pollination occurs (by seeds drifting by wind), which is common, the resulting plants become patented by Monsanto because the new breed has become contaminated with patented traits owned by Monsanto.[37] Furthermore, because Monsanto's seeds are so ubiquitous within commodity crop farming in the United States, traditional crossbreeding conducted by scientists like Mr. Borlaug have become obsolete for these crops because of the domination of Monsanto in that sector of agricultural business. The purchase of crossbred seeds was brought to the Supreme Court in 2013 where Monsanto challenged a farmer for planting crossbred soybean seeds purchased from an independent company. The Supreme Court ruled in favor of Monsanto.[38] The consolidation in the supply chain are nested within the monocultural production systems.

CONSOLIDATION OF FARMS AND RANCHES

The consolidation of U.S. farmland since the 1970s, when the industrialization of the food system began, has been documented by the USDA.[34] Farms are categorized by size, based on the annual gross sales. A small farm earns annual gross cash from farms sales that is less than $350,000, midsized farms ($350,000–$999,999), and large farms earn one million dollars or more per year. In Figure 1.3, the USDA describes the proportion of U.S. farms by size and the

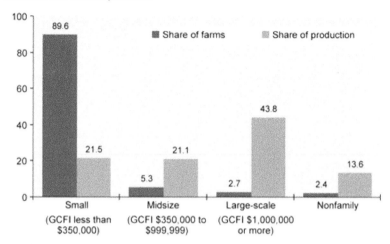

Note: GCFI = annual gross cash farm income before expenses. Nonfamily farms are those where the principal operator and their relatives do not own a majority of the business. Source: USDA, Economic Research Service and National Agricultural Statistics Service, Agricultural Resource Management Survey. Data as of December 2, 2020.

FIGURE 1.3 Gross Cash by Farm Size

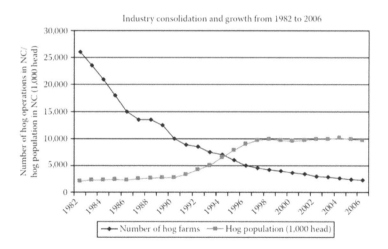

FIGURE 1.4 North Carolina Hog Farm Consolidation

proportion of total productivity attributed to farm size. Of the two million farms in the United States, most of the farms are small (89.7%), earning only a fifth of farm income. In fact, slightly more than half of all U.S. farms are small, with annual farm sales under $10,000. These households rely on off-farm sources of income to meet most of their household needs. By contrast, the large farms earn 45.9% of all farm income, representing less than 3% of all U.S. farms.

In addition to the consolidation of farms and ranches, different agricultural industries have concentrated into specific regions of the United States. For example, between 1970 and 1990, industrial hog operations expanded in North Carolina, causing small- and medium-sized producers to be driven out of business (Figure 1.4).[39] The number of pork producing farms in

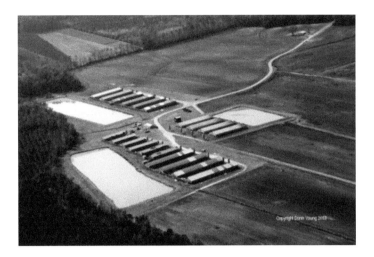

FIGURE 1.5   Components of a CAFO for Hog Production

North Carolina was over 25,000 in 1982 and consolidated to roughly 2,500 by 2006. These 2,500 farms produced roughly 25 million hogs in 2016. North Carolina currently ranks third for hog production behind Iowa and Minnesota, with 9.2 million hogs and pigs in 2020. Unlike the hogs that roam on traditional farms, industrial hogs never touch the ground. Hundreds to thousands of hogs are kept in long buildings referred to as confinements, more commonly known as CAFOs, as previously stated. Figure 1.5 shows the three primary components of an industrial hog operation in North Carolina: (a) the confinements, (b) the waste lagoons, and (c) the spray fields and is also discussed in Dr. Wing's 2013 TEDx Talk. https://www.youtube.com/watch?v=7ZW8-LQftnY.

In addition to the industrialization of animal production since the 1970s, the United States has experienced an explosion of consolidated crop farms and industrialized farming practices to maximize production. For example, only 1% of corn produced in the United States is sweet corn (known as corn on the cob) and edible for humans once harvested. Most corn (99% of Iowa's corn) produced is processed to make other products such as ethanol, livestock feed, or high fructose corn syrup, and this type of corn is called *field corn*. Iowa has approximately 87,500 farms and is known as the Corn State because of its large annual yield of this commodity crop. Hence, Iowa leads other states in the production of ethanol with an average annual yield of 953 million bushels (30% of America's ethanol). Corn ethanol is produced by dry milling kernels into a mash, then combining with enzymes to hydrolyze the starch into simple sugars to be used in products such as beer, wine, distilled spirits, and other products. In addition, nearly 40% of field corn is used as livestock feed. Like hogs, cornfed cattle are confined for 140 to 150 days before reaching a market weight to be slaughtered. Because of the corn-based diet and confinement, these animals are less lean than grass fed cattle who would take several years to reach market weight. The corn feed is cheaper for producers but is also not digestible by cows and inevitably produces acidosis (which would cause death within six months). Most cattle are supplemented with antibiotics to manage the acidosis.

The documentary *King Corn* takes a deeper look at the production of Liberty Lake corn, which is an industrialized corn genetically modified to tolerate crowded cropland (www.youtube.com/watch?v=TWv29KRsQXU). Unlike the farms that grew corn more than fifty years ago, these genetically altered kernels can be planted on an acre of land in less than twenty minutes using industrialized farm equipment. Ian Cheney and Curt Ellis purchased one acre of land in Greene, Iowa, and produced an annual yield of 180 bushels of Liberty Lake corn, gaining $297 when sold. However, this resulted in a net loss of $52.92 once the input costs of seeds, equipment, and herbicides were subtracted from the gross earnings. This net value of the crop was not expected to be profitable by local farmers; rather, the government subsidizes what the local farmers say, 'keeps production at full blast'. Because corn production is so central in raising cattle, a farmer in Greene Iowa states, 'the government subsidizes *Happy Meals* but not the healthy ones'.

INDUSTRIALIZED FARM LABOR

The industrialization of food production has also changed the needs for farm labor. Whereas historically, farms were planted and harvested by family members as well as migrant and slave labor, industrial farm labor is conducted by both the farm owners and hired help.[40] The USDA shows decreased use of both owner and hired labor on farms across the United States between 1950 to the turn of the century (Figure 1.6). In 2000, farms in the United States employed roughly 1.3 million workers. Hired farmworkers make up a small but important proportion of U.S. wage and salary workers (~1%).[40] The costs for labor represents less than 12% of production expenses for all farmers, but that percentage is higher for labor necessary for product grown in greenhouses/nurseries or fruit and tree nut operations, 43% and 39% respectively (Figure 1.7). Jobs range from field crop, nursery, and livestock workers, as well as graders and sorters, agricultural inspectors, supervisors, and hired farm managers. The demographic profiles of the hired farm workforce shows that most have lower education levels, are predominately of Hispanic or Mexican origin, and most are non-U.S. citizens. Hourly wages in

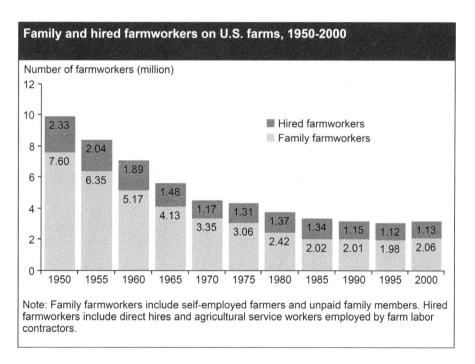

FIGURE 1.6 Trend in U.S. Farmworkers

(From USDA, Economic Research Service using data from USDA, National Agricultural Statistics Service, Farm Labor Survey (FLS). The FLS stopped estimating the number of family farmworkers beginning in 2001. As of 2012, the survey no longer counts contracted agricultural service workers.)

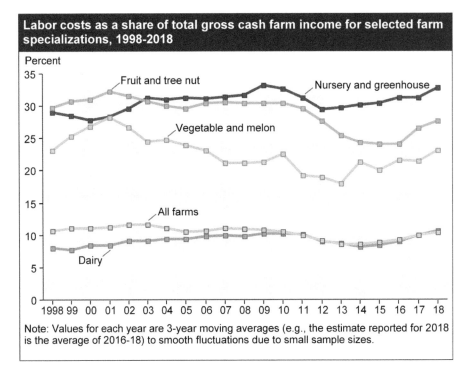

FIGURE 1.7 Trends in Farm Labor Cost by Type of Food Product

(From USDA, Economic Research Service and USDA, National Agricultural Statistics Service, Agricultural Resource Management Surveys, selected years.)

2019 ranged from $13.03 (for graders and sorters) to $14.61 (for equipment operators) and increased by 5% from 2018.[40] Hired managers and supervisors, on average make $24.77 and $21.34 per hour, respectively. However, the Fair Labor Standards Act (FLSA) states that workers do not have to be paid overtime, hand harvesters can be paid at a 'piece rate' and nonlocal minors, 16 years old or younger, are paid at a 'youth minimum wage' of $4.25/hour. Also, farms with less than ten hired farmworkers are exempt from Occupational Safety and Health Administration (OSHA) standards as well as other occupational safety laws.[41]

In addition to hires from the United States, the U.S. has a program to temporarily hire foreign-born workers for a period up to ten months (H-2A Temporary Agriculture Program).[40] Under this program, employers must pay a state-specific minimum wage and provide housing and domestic and international transportation for these employees. This group of hired agricultural workers is dominating the workforce, with just over 48,000 positions certified by the U.S. government in 2005 to nearly 258,000 in 2019. Another group of farm laborers are those that lack legal immigration status to work in the United States. The U.S. Department of Labor's National Agricultural Worker Survey (NAWS) has estimated that this proportion of the workforce has grown over the past several decades, representing 50% of the current hired farmworkers. In the past, it was not uncommon for a farmworker to move from state to state following the harvest to plant seasonal crops. These migrant farmworkers are less common now, with more than 80% of the current hired crop farmworker being classified as 'settled', meaning that they work at a single location within 75 miles of their home. A small proportion (10%) of migrant farmworkers called *shuttlers* cross international borders to get to their worksite.[40]

SOCIAL AND ENVIRONMENTAL COSTS OF INDUSTRIALIZED AGRICULTURE

Industrialized agriculture has increased food production and profitability over the past half century. However, there are repercussions to this form of agriculture that impact small farms, farmworkers, local communities, the environment, and the foods available for retail. This third section aims to introduce these issues.

SMALL FARMS IN THE UNITED STATES

As stated earlier, market consolidation has left owners of smaller farms in compromised positions to remain profitable. The public policies that have supported the monoculture system have left many small farmers with little choice other than accepting the conditions of a vertical integrated system.[31] Although the majority of farms in the United States are small, Jeremy Peaches, a small urban farmer in the Sunnyside neighborhood of Houston, describes how agriculture policies do not support these small farms. Mr. Peaches received formal training in agriculture at Prairie View A&M University and had this to say regarding challenges for owners of smaller farms in the United States:

> For urban farmers, and I'll start there, one challenge in being a farmer is commercial farms vs. the small or medium family farm. The USDA classifies farms by how much they make [revenue] not necessarily by their impact or what they produce. It's [small farmers are] only 1 or 2% out of the whole 100% of farmers in America, of that, it's only 0.3% African American farmers. . . . It's all commercial farms or 2 or 3 large landowners that own all the farms in California, all the farms in the corn belt, so the commercial farm vs. small family farm, we don't have no benefits. I can't get subsidized or programs or USDA backing of funding compared to a commercial farm or a dairy farmer or a commodities farmer. They get so many millions of dollars of breaks per year and some of 'em even get paid not even to farm. But me, as a small family farmer who probably, you know, in a year [is] feeding so many people and you know, make up a lot of the small, local regional food system, we can't get no grants or benefits! You know, Black, White, Hispanic – that don't even matter. So that's number one, America doesn't support the small, local urban, regional farmer, period, in terms of markets. If you're not a commercial commodity producer that the U.S. is helping import and export to other countries or you [are not] on NASDAQ, like, forget about you. And that's the number one thing that's wrong with the food system.[42]

FARMWORKERS

Most of the hired agriculture labor force continues to be predominately a low-income disenfranchised sector of workers who are susceptible to poor working conditions. Current farmworkers are sometimes exposed to chemicals and provided inadequate housing; worksites often lack sanitation. These work conditions affect the mental and physical health of workers and their families.[43] Specific jobs put workers at risk for poor outcomes. For example, acute and repetitive injuries are experienced by workers in livestock processing plants[44–47] and workers in industrial animal confinements are exposed to bioaerosols, ammonia, and hydrogen sulfide,[48] as well as, exchange bacteria and viruses with livestock.[49,50] Although agricultural workers are known to be exposed to these harmful work environments, currently the United States has exempted many agriculture workers from traditional labor laws that protect workers in other industries.[51] For example, this is a particular issue for farmworkers who are likely to be exposed to pesticides either through direct application, 'drift' (indirect exposure by a neighboring farm by wind), or aerial spraying. Acute exposure causes headaches, difficulty breathing, weakness, blurry visions, muscle pain, and twitching.[52] Chronic exposure causes neurological deficits and developmental delays. Overall the prevalence of occupational related disability ranges from 12.3% to 27.1% of this workforce.[53]

In addition to disability, farmworkers are susceptible to biological organisms. For instance, epidemic strains of influenza have emerged from interactions between people, pigs, and poultry in areas where humans are in close contact with their animals. One argument for growing animals in confinement has been that this practice minimizes potential for infectious diseases to be transferred between people and livestock.[54] However, a study of H1N1 swine flu in Iowa found that the odds of having H1N1 antibodies were 55 times higher in swine workers and 28 times higher in their spouses, compared to people who did not live near livestock.[50] Flu virus can be highly infectious and could spread rapidly from high livestock density areas to other populations. There has been concern that the 2010 global pandemic of swine flu originated in Vera Cruz, Mexico, in an area of industrial swine production where the first case was identified.

Due to these concerns, industrial swine facilities, for example, typically use several measures to limit spread of pathogens. This is of economic importance due to the potential for animal mortality. For example, vehicles must have their tires disinfected upon entry, and workers must shower-in, shower-out, and change clothes when they leave confinement buildings. However, bacteria can survive in workers' nasal mucosa,[55] and animal vectors such as rodents and birds, in addition to flies, can carry bacteria off-site.[56] In one study, antibiotic-resistant bacteria were found in the feces of migratory geese that land on swine-waste lagoons.[57] Bacteria resistant to antibiotics that are used in poultry feed have been found in excess behind poultry transport trucks and were carried by flies near poultry operations on Maryland's Eastern Shore.[58] Most recently the United States has witnessed increased risk for the coronavirus among workers in meat processing plants, where over 42,534 meatpacking workers tested positive for the virus in 494 meat plants with 203 deaths.[59] In an executive order dated April 28, 2020, President Trump stated that the closure of some large processing facilities [due to COVID-19 outbreaks]

> threaten the continued functioning of the national meat and poultry supply chain, undermining critical infrastructure during the national emergency. Given the high volume of meat and poultry processed by many facilities, any unnecessary closures can quickly have a large effect on the food supply chain.[60]

This executive order required that these employees return to work.

LOCAL COMMUNITIES

People living near industrial food production are sometimes affected by industrial farming practices. Using North Carolina as an example again, hog operations there house as many as 20,000 pigs each, producing more waste than a city of 60,000 people, but with no sewer treatment plant. Large fans are used to exhaust waste gases and dust from the buildings into the ambient air. Feces, urine, spilled feed, and residues of pesticides drop below slats inside CAFOs and are then flushed into open cesspools, called lagoons. Cesspools are dug into the water tables where rural residents reside, and many of the lagoons have subsurface drains, originally installed to make swampy land arable, thus acting as a conduit for hog waste to reach surface waters. Industrial producers empty these cesspools by spraying the liquid on nearby fields. Although the lagoons have clay or plastic liners that slows the movement of fecal waste into the water table, the spray fields have no barriers to keep the liquid waste from groundwater.

The CAFOs are concentrated heavily in the eastern part of North Carolina known as the Black Belt.[61,62] This region of North Carolina, part of the southern coastal plain, is where agriculture was produced with African and African American slave labor before the Civil War. It is now where the majority of rural Black Americans still reside in North Carolina. Advocacy groups declare that the industrialization of agriculture is an exploitation of Black American communities, citing the fact that ten times as many industrial hog facilities are located in areas with higher proportions of Black Americans compared to White Americans.[62] Rural residents lack connections to municipal water supplies, and instead draw well water, which is susceptible to contamination from CAFO cesspools, for drinking and bathing. In addition, daily spraying of waste produces a foul odor that lingers into the yards and homes of nearby residents. A resident of the Black Belt describes her experience living near CAFOs.[63]

> Lot of my family come and can't stay here. They say, 'God, I can't stand this. How can you live here?' My son has asthma and allergies. . . . He just stays inside. I had a rose garden. . . . Do you see those weeds there? . . . I haven't done it for the past few years. Sometimes it's so unbearable you couldn't even hardly stand it, not even in the house. On a bad day it is not that you can't go outside . . . but the odor determines how long you gonna stay. When the smell [hog odor] get in, you can't get rid of it. I had stuff here in writing saying that the property has gone down 20–30 percent because you are near a hog farm. The water turns everything yellow. If I wash my clothes for a good six weeks in that water, I will have to buy new clothes. . . . I will have to buy new clothes every six weeks. I don't drink the groundwater no more because of the hog farms. . . . Now we have to buy water to drink. It [hog odor] woke me up. And I had to get up. I couldn't sleep. I put the covers up over my face and it didn't do any good.

Eastern North Carolina is also a top producer of turkeys and broiler chickens. Although these producers do not use lagoons and spray fields, the CAFOs contain anywhere from 9,000 to 125,000 birds,[64] depending on the animal sector, and produce the same odor problems for the local community as just described by a resident living near hog CAFOs.

Recently, community groups living near CAFOs in Eastern North Carolina have filed lawsuits against Smithfield, who is a major integrator of hogs. Juries in 2018 and 2019 awarded hog farm neighbors with nearly $550 million in punitive damages. Judges rejected Smithfield's argument that the verdicts are an 'almost existential threat' to North Carolina farmers. One of the judges, Stephanie Thacker, writes in her opinion that Smithfield 'persisted in its chosen farming practices despite its knowledge of the harm to its neighbors, exhibiting wanton or willful disregard of the neighbors' rights to enjoyment of their property'.[65] However, these lawsuits have not protected rural residents of other states from the harmful effects of CAFOs. For instance, the passing of the Missouri Senate Bill 391 in 2019 includes a new definition of groundwater, which has set the stage for an out-of-town company, United Hogs, to raise pigs in CAFOs for one of the largest meat producers in a small farming town of Chillicothe, Missouri.[66]

FOOD AVAILABILITY AND QUALITY

The consolidation of farms has reduced the local availability of foods. In addition, the monocultural system from which most U.S. food products are grown has impacted the quality of foods with the increased the need of antibiotics and food additives for livestock, the use of pesticides, and restriction of grazing.

Local Foods

The concentration of farmland and monocultural systems has impacted the ability of Americans to obtain locally sourced foods. For example, the USDA has documented that in 2012, 163,675 farmers sold an estimated $6.1 billion worth of locally produced foods.[34] This was defined as foods for human consumption sold via direct-to-consumer (e.g., farmers markets, farm stands) as well as intermediate markets (e.g., restaurants, supermarkets, schools). Less than 10% of all U.S. farms sell locally. Moreover, local sales represent less than 2% of agricultural production in the United States and most of the local sales come from the large farms (Figure 1.8).

Local food farms and sales by farm size*

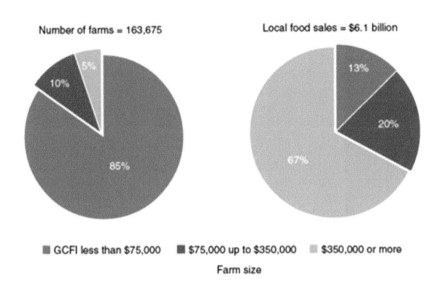

*The share of farms by farm size are based on 2012 Census benchmark counts; the shares of total value of local food sales by farm size are synthetic estimates. GCFI = Gross cash farm income.
Source: USDA, Economic Research Service and National Agricultural Statistics Service, Agricultural Resource Management Survey and USDA, National Agricultural Statistics Service, 2012 Census of Agriculture.

FIGURE 1.8   U.S. Local Farm Sales: 2012

Food Quality

There are several factors involved in the practices of industrial food production that impact the quality of food produced. Several of those factors are described here.

Antibiotics and Food Additives

The majority of antibiotics in the United States are used to promote livestock growth in confined growing facilities, not to treat human disease.[67] Such subtherapeutic administration contributes to the development of antibiotic resistance because bacteria that are susceptible to antibiotics produce fewer offspring than those with genetic resistance. In addition, resistant genes can be transferred directly between bacteria. Antibiotics commonly used to promote livestock growth belong to classes of drugs that are important in medicine; therefore, development of antibiotic resistance in livestock threatens to undermine treatment of human infection. For example, several strains of methicillin-resistant *Staphylococcus aureus*, which is responsible for substantial morbidity and mortality, have been linked to livestock production.[68] *S. aureus* sequence type 398 has been shown to be related to livestock density in the Netherlands.[69]

In addition to antibiotics, additives to animal feed, such as arsenic, is a concern because it is a human carcinogen. Additives containing arsenic are common in poultry feed to improve muscle growth.[70] Land application of animal wastes distributes arsenic onto land, potentially affecting ground and surface water, as well as food crops. Emphasis on renewable energy for electricity production, combined with the large excess of animal waste in high-density livestock production areas like eastern North Carolina, has led to pressures to burn poultry waste for electricity production. This practice produces more air pollution than burning coal, which could result in widespread distribution of arsenic in the environment.[71]

Pesticides

Industrial agriculture relies on pesticides to control insects and weeds from reducing crop production. The use of pesticides has grown over the past fifty years with less than 200 pounds being applied in 1960 to triple that amount by the mid-1970s.[72] The use of pesticides varies by crop and has changed over time. For instance, in 1960 2.74 million pounds of pesticides were used on soybean crops, but by 2008, 111.96 million pounds were used. Five major crops account for 80% of the pesticide use: corn, soybeans, cotton, wheat, and potatoes. The human carcinogenic effects of pesticides have been studied extensively, and the International Agency for Research on Cancer (IARC) regularly conducts hazard assessments along with the U.S. Environmental Protection Agency (EPA) of active ingredients used in pesticides. Two pesticides (arsenical insecticides and 2,3,7,8 Tetrachlorodibenzo-p-dioxin [TCDD]) are classified as 'known carcinogens', whereas other are classified as 'probable human carcinogens'.[73] Pesticides are either directly applied to foods purchased at grocery stores, such as produce, or indirectly applied to crops used to feed livestock. Organochlorine and organophosphorus pesticides are endocrine disruptors and neurotoxic with possible links to cardiovascular, Alzheimer's, and Parkinson's diseases.[74]

Pastured Animals

There is evidence that animals that can roam in pastured farms, instead of grown in CAFOs, produce food that is healthier. For example, researchers compared egg content of specific nutrients of hens raised in pastures compare to caged hens on commercial diets. Authors found that eggs from pasture-raised hens had twice as much vitamin E and long-chain omega 3 fatty acids; 2.5 times more total omega-3 fatty acids; and the ratio of omega-6:omega-3 fatty acids was reduced by half.[75] Other investigators have found similar health benefits for other pasture-raised animals. For instance a greater concentration of vitamin E,[76] polyunsaturated fatty acids in milk,[77] and carotenoids in other dairy products[78] has been documented from animals raised in conditions where they were allowed to roam and consume natural diets.

THE ENVIRONMENT

Finally, the spatial concentration of production requires large-scale transportation throughout the food system from production and processing, and the sale of food products has increased demands for fossil fuels. Large transportation corridors for agricultural products has led to excess local air pollution from ports, rail terminals, road traffic, destruction of housing and community facilities, and reduction of walkability in communities.[79,80] In addition to the long-range transport of crops and livestock, for crops in particular, the monocultural system depletes soil nitrogen and has increased the need for inorganic nitrogenous fertilizers.[33] The absence of manure fertilizer from livestock on monocultural farms requires more chemical fertilizers. This results in large fossil fuel inputs and an increase in levels of reactive nitrogen in the biosphere.[33] Nitrogen pollution presents several health concerns for humans due to the respiratory impacts of air pollution, ingestion of nitrate-contaminated groundwater, and impacts on algal blooms from eutrophication of surface waters. Nitrogen pollution results not only from production of feed grains in the absence of animal manure but also from disposal of animal manure in the absence of adequate capacity for uptake by crops. Dense livestock-producing areas such as eastern North Carolina have large excesses of nitrogen and phosphorus from animal manure, which impact ground and surface waters in those locations and downstream coastal waters.[81] Furthermore, livestock production is a source of environmental methane, which is twenty-five times more potent than carbon dioxide as a greenhouse gas.[36]

Methane's half-life in the atmosphere is less than that of carbon dioxide, but it converts to carbon dioxide.

The food production and refinement of oil, gas, and other petrochemicals impacts nearby communities to create inputs required by industrial agriculture.[82] In agricultural areas, heavy chemical inputs can contaminate groundwater with nitrates and pesticides, which can lead to nutrient runoff and promotes eutrophication of surface waters. Therefore, the burdens of environmental pollution that benefit industrial agribusiness, by helping to keep profits high and prices of industrially produced foods low, are impacted by the local community, while food products reach a global market.

CONCLUSION

The major themes that have been central to the current and historic U.S. Agriculture system have been *productivity, profitability*, and *cheap food*. An abundance of food to prevent famines, store for times of need, or produce excess to keep food prices low, have all been motivators of agricultural productivity. For the American at the grocery store, most sources of protein for example (e.g., pork, chicken, beef, dairy, and eggs) are produced in CAFOs. The social and environmental costs that subsidize the lower prices of foods are not made apparent to the average American who is removed from how crops and livestock are produced. Lower-income Americans have a relatively higher dependence on industrialized foods compared to wealthier Americans who can afford the higher prices of organic and non-GMO produced foods and free-range meats.

The growth and sustainability of the industrialized food system has in some part been justified by an effort to reduce hunger in the United States and worldwide. In fact, the importance of industrial farming that keeps food prices low was emphasized during the Trump administration's U.S. Secretary of Agriculture, Sonny Purdue, in a press briefing. Secretary Purdue states with regard to current challenges in food production for U.S. farmers,

> [T]o produce enough food and agriculture products to meet the needs of growing populations . . . I do not believe we are on track to meet our food needs and develop sustainable farming techniques if we continue to impose policies that stifle innovation. . . . [There is an indication for] a potential doubling of food prices around the world – creating millions of more people in food insecurity.[83]

It was as recently as the 1960s when Congress measured hunger among Americans for the first time.[84] It was reported that some U.S. households were without food for several days a month, some babies were without milk, and severe malnutrition was detected in inner cities. This report led to an expansion of the Food Stamp Program, as well as the initiation of new programs under President Nixon's administration.[85] Further investigations of hunger in the United States and the communities specifically impacted by poverty were conducted in 1983 by the USDA. These studies determined that hunger was continuing to grow and estimated to affect 20 million Americans.[86,87] The direct measurement of hunger used prior to the USDA surveillance was defined as 'painful sensations' associated with inadequate food intake or 'chronically inadequate nutritional intake due to low income status', but these definitions were abandoned.[84] Instead, the USDA began to evaluate hunger in the United States by measuring the food security of households, which is quantified with responses to several questions related to *one's ability to obtain enough safe, nutritious food*. As recently as 2010, it was estimated that 14.5% of American households were food insecure[88]; more recently in 2019, 10.5% of Americans were food insecure at least sometime during the year.[89] Over the past two decades, food insecurity has changed extraordinarily little and instead concern has grown regarding obesity. However, experts believe that hunger may be related to obesity for some people[90,91] because to avoid the experience of hunger when resources are limited, individual's choices are limited to cheaper foods that are often less nutritionally dense. Obesity is thought to be 'an adaptive response when food availability is unreliable'.[84]

While food insecurity is a driving force of policies that support industrialized food production, food security is not often a priority for farmers. As former Delaware State Secretary of Agriculture Kee described:

> The question [was] as a person who has been involved in food production for many years, would you say the business decisions on the production side of the food systems are motivated by addressing issues around food insecurity? And when you say food insecurity, you mean like food deserts and places where it's just hard to attain [food] or you know that you can go down [to] the corner store and buy potato chips and soda, but that's about it. If that's what you're talking about, the answer to your question is I don't know of any farmer that thinks about that when they're planning their crop year. You know they don't say, well maybe I'll have 10% of my watermelon crop or my tomato crop or whatever it is to send into Wilmington or Philadelphia. Having said that though, when organizations like the food bank of Delaware, I don't know if The Food Trust has been down in Delaware much, but a lot of farmers are receptive to helping [because] sometimes they'll have a glut. Sometimes they'll have a tractor trailer load that was sent to New York City and the guy in New York City didn't like it, and it gets kicked back. But even if it's not a kickback load, they are receptive to helping. They may expect, you know, ask for a lower than usual price. But, you know, in the winter and spring, they're really not thinking about food insecurity in Wilmington or Philadelphia.[92]

Secretary Kee's response reveals that current U.S. farmers are not driven by a humanitarian mission to feed the world and reduce hunger like Mr. Borlaug. Rather, they see farming as a business, like any other business. Family farms and corporations aim to produce a product that can be sold for the highest price possible to cover production costs and make a profit. But agribusiness is not parallel to any other U.S. industry. The commodities produced uniquely provide Americans with a basic need. No other industry providing basic needs such as housing and education are completely corporate controlled in the United States.

But growing food is in the fabric of who we are as Americans. In the 1800s, most Americans lived on farms and therefore, were able to produce food for their families.[93] Today, roughly 1% of Americans live on farms. In addition, the pool of Americans with the skills needed for farming is shrinking because farmers are retiring and giving up their farms, while their children are infesting themselves into other U.S. industries. As Americans move away from farms, they also remove themselves away from knowing how the food they eat is produced. Those that are still farming have removed themselves from owning that they are feeding people, and not just their own families, through an industrialized food system, a countless number of other families as well. The decisions of what to plant and how to grow that crop by the farmer in the 1800s would affect his family. But those same decisions made by the farmer in 2020 has a much broader reach. Whether it is an owner of a small, medium, or large farm or ranch, this 1% of Americans determines what foods are available for all Americans. Beyond availability, they also establish the quality and cost of foods.

The rationale to place the United States Food supply in the hands of 1% of Americans is justified by government leaders such as Secretary Perdue, who was concerned that the volume of food produced in the United States will not be sufficient to feed a growing population. The fact is, the United States produces enough food to feed each American over 3500 calories per day, which is 75% more calories per day than what is recommended for a healthy diet (Figure 1.9). This production level is higher than any other nation including Great Britain. Americans also spend a lower proportion of their incomes on these calories compared to other nations, where in the United States, 4.9% of incomes were spent at grocery stores in 2019. Food spending does of course vary by income. Americans with the lowest incomes spend the

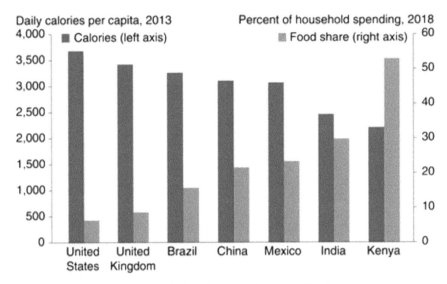

Calorie availability and household spending on food at home as a share of consumption expenditure

Source: Expenditure data from USDA, Economic Research Service using data from Euromonitor International. Calorie data from FAOSTAT.

FIGURE 1.9   Caloric Availability of Food Production and Household Spending on Food by Country

least on groceries; however these food expenditures make up a greater proportion of their incomes (Figure 1.10). This lowest income group of Americans represented on Figure 1.10 has an average annual income of $12,222 and would unquestionably be impacted by the doubling of food prices suggested by Secretary Perdue. However, this group is also eligible for federal food assistance programs that would mitigate the risk of food insecurity. Most Americans can afford to pay higher prices for foods.

Despite these facts, the reasoning to keep food production high, to make retail food prices low, continues to justify the current food production system. But how sensitive are food prices to agricultural productivity? The USDA reported that between 2015 and 2019, food prices rose 4.5%, roughly 1% per year, which is a smaller inflation rate than other basic needs such as housing and medical care, which each rose roughly 3% per year during the same period.[94] The average farm price for the top three U.S. field crops (corn, soybeans, and wheat), which encompass the majority of commodity crops that enter into the U.S. food supply, rises or falls by over 10% annually. However, these cost fluctuations of foods produced have relatively no impact on food prices (Figure 1.11).

Food, unlike other basic needs such as water, has become a monetized commodity. The food industry markets the industrialization of these products to Americans with the promise of inexpensive food. However, the environmental, animal, and human costs hidden in the system are not reflected in retail prices. Because of the resources necessary to support the current industrialized agriculture system, it is argued by some that the current system is unsustainable.[2,95] Solutions for reconstructing the current system are proposed in the FSRA legislation, including providing a means for small farms to remain profitable and compete in the market as well as regaining a younger population of farmers. For those opposed to these reforms, an argument continues to support agribusiness with the promise of low food prices, as Secretary Purdue has stated. However, it is also true that people who spend a

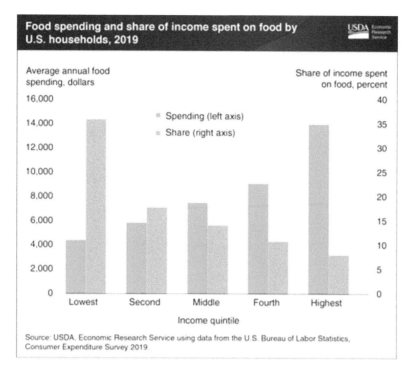

FIGURE 1.10 Food Spending by Income Level in the United States

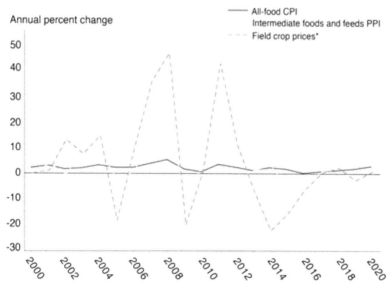

FIGURE 1.11 Trend in Consumer Price Index Stability

larger proportion of their income on food are more likely to shift their demands for food products more frequently. This creates price volatility for farmers and ranchers.[96,97] With a food system such as the United States that already overproduces, price volatility causes instability in the market, which may result in falling profits for producers.

CRITICAL THINKING QUESTIONS AND EXERCISES

1. Choose a commodity crop and describe how that crop is grown and made profitable for the small or larger farmers.
2. Choose a livestock and describe how the animals are grown on large and small farms, what happens once they are grown, and how they get to the retail market.
3. Describe farm labor specific to a commodity crop or raising a specific livestock. What does the work look like? Who is hired to do the work? What are the occupation hazards for the work? What are other work conditions to be concerned about?
4. How has the Agriculture Act helped and hindered farmers and ranchers today?
5. In what ways does the industrialization of agriculture impact what is sold at grocery stores in the United States?
6. Watch the Norman Borlaug video and describe how his work is similar and in contrasts to industrial agriculture practices.
7. Watch the *King Corn* video and explain what you learned about corn production.
8. Watch the Wing Ted Talk video and discuss CAFOs and alternatives for production of livestock.

REFERENCES

1. Institute of Medicine and National Research Council. A Framework of Assessing Effects of the Food System. 2015; https://doi.org/10.17226/18846.
2. Neff R. *Introduction to the U.S. Food System: Public Health, Environment and Equity.* San Francisco: Jossey-Bass; 2015.
3. Community Wealth Organization. Overview: Local Food Systems. 2018; https://community-wealth.org/strategies/panel/urban-ag/index.html.
4. Blount-Dorn K, Scalera L. Modeling an Equitable Michigan Food System. September 14, 2018; www.canr.msu.edu/news/modeling-an-equitable-michigan-food-system.
5. National Park Service. Rise of the Colonial Plantation System. 2017; www.nps.gov/articles/plantationsystem.htm. Accessed November 19, 2020.
6. A & E History Channel. The 13 Colonies. 2010; www.history.com/topics/colonial-america/thirteen-colonies. Accessed November 18, 2020.
7. UShistory.org. The growth of the tobacco trade. *U.S. History Online Textbook.* 2020; www.ushistory.org/us/2d.asp. Accessed November 19, 2020.
8. Public Broadcasting System. Indentured Servants in the U.S. 2014; www.pbs.org/opb/historydetectives/feature/indentured-servants-in-the-us/. Accessed November 19, 2020.
9. A & E History Channel. Slavery in America. 2020; www.history.com/topics/black-history/slavery. Accessed November 19, 2020.
10. LDHI. The Trans-Atlantic Slave Trade. 2020; http://ldhi.library.cofc.edu/exhibits/show/africanpassageslowcountryadapt/introductionatlanticworld/trans_atlantic_slave_trade. Accessed November 19, 2020.
11. Public Broadcasting System. Virginia's Slave Codes, 1705. 2020; www.pbs.org/wgbh/aia/part1/1p268.html. Accessed November 19, 2020.
12. Salmon EJ, Salmon J. Tobacco in Colonial Virginia. January 19, 2013; www.encyclopediavirginia.org/tobacco_in_colonial_virginia. Accessed November 19, 2020.
13. UShistory.com. Economic growth and the early industrial revolution. *U.S. History Online Textbook.* 2020; www.ushistory.org/us/22a.asp. Accessed November 19, 2020.
14. Waterloo. Boulton & Watt Engine. *Age of Revolution and Making the World Over.* 2020; https://ageofrevolution.org/200-object/boulton-watt-engine/. Accessed November 19, 2020.
15. Schur JB. Eli Whitney's Patent for the Cotton Gin. 2020; www.archives.gov/education/lessons/cotton-gin-patent. Accessed November 19, 2020.

16. Dattel ER. Cotton in a Global Economy: Mississippi (1800–1866). 2006; http://mshistorynow.mdah. state.ms.us/articles/161/cotton-in-a-global-economy-mississippi-1800-1860. Accessed November 19, 2020.

17. Congress US. 13th Amendment to the United States Constitution: Abolition of Slavery. In: Washington, DC: National Archives; 1865.

18. BlackPast B. 1724 Louisiana's Code Noir. 2007; www.blackpast.org/african-american-history/louisi- anas-code-noir-1724/. Accessed November 29, 2020.

19. A & E History Channel. Great Depression History. www.history.com/topics/great-depression/great- depression-history. Accessed November 18, 2020.

20. Congress US. Agricultural Adjustment Act of 1933. In: Agriculture US Do, ed. *58-8201-4-197*. Washington, DC; 1933:31–54.

21. Johnson R, Monke J. What Is the Farm Bill? In: Washington, DC: Congressional Research Services; 2019:1–13.

22. Johnson R, Monke J. 2018 Farm Bill Primer: What Is the Farm Bill? In: Washington, DC: Congressional Research Services; 2019:1–3.

23. SNAP to Health. The History of SNAP. 2020; www.snaptohealth.org/snap/the-history-of-snap/. Accessed January 23, 2021.

24. Congressional Research Services. Domestic Food Assistance: Summary of Programs. In: USDA, ed. 2019.

25. Russer J, Anthan G. Why they Love Earl Butz. *New York Times*. June 13, 1976.

26. Goldstein R. Earl L. Butz, secretary felled by racial remarks had died at 98. *New York Times*. February 4, 2008.

27. Welte P. Considering the lessons of Earl Butz. *Ag Weekly*. April 1, 2018.

28. Ozgediz S. *The CGIAR at Institutional Evolution of the World's Premier Agriculture Research Network*. CGIAR; August, 2012.

29. Encyclopedia Britannica. Norman Earnest Borlaug. 2020; www.britannica.com/bibliography/ Norman-Borlaug. Accessed November 11, 2020.

30. Anderson J, Hespeler F, Zwirwn S. *Monocultures in America: A System That Need More Diversity*. College of Natural Sciences, University of Massachusetts Amherst; 2017.

31. Lauck J. After deregulation: Constructing agriculture policy in the age of "freedom to farm". *Drake Journal if Agriculture Law*. 2000;119:2657–2654.

32. Schmitt D. Senate bill aims to eliminate all CAFOs in 20 years. *AG Daily*. November 11, 2020.

33. Mancus P. Nitrogen fertilizer dependency and its contradictions: A theoretical exploration of social-ecological metabolism. *Rural Sociology*. 2007;72:269–288.

34. Economic Research Services. Farming and Farm Income. In: U.S. Department of Agriculture, ed. December 2, 2020.

35. Economic Research Services. Cash Receipts by Commodity, State Ranking. 2019; https://data.ers. usda.gov/reports.aspx?ID=17844. Accessed December 7, 2020.

36. Commission P. Putting meat on the table: Industrial farm animal production in America. 2009; www.pewtrusts.org/en/research-and-analysis/reports/0001/01/01/putting-meat-on-the-table. Accessed November 20, 2020.

37. Kimbrell A. Monsanto vs U.S. farmers. 2005; www.centerforfoodsafety.org/files/cfsmonsantovsfarmer report11305.pdf. Accessed November 23, 2020.

38. Charles D. Farmers' fight with Monsanto reaches the Supreme Court. *National Public Radio*. February 18, 2013.

39. Edwards B, Ladd A. Environmental justice, swine production and farm loss in North Carolina. *Sociological Spectrum*. 2000;20:263–290.

40. Economic Research Services. Farm Labor. In: United States Department of Agriculture, ed. 2020.

41. U.S. Department of Labor. Fact Sheet #12: Agriculture Employers under the Fair Labor Standards Act (FLSA). In: Wage and Hour Division, ed. 2020.

42. Lehmann Y. Interview with Jeremy Peaches, Small Farmer in Texas. In: November 21, 2020.

43. Villarejo D. The health of U.S. hired farm workers. *Annu Rev Public Health*. 2003;24:175–193.

44. Lipscomb HJ, Argue R, McDonald MA, et al. Exploration of work and health disparities among black women employed in poultry processing in the rural south. *Environ Health Perspect*. 2005;113(12):1833–1840.

45. Lipscomb HJ, Loomis D, McDonald MA, Argue RA, Wing S. A conceptual model of work and health disparities in the United States. *Int J Health Serv*. 2006;36(1):25–50.

46. Lipscomb HJ, Dement JM, Epling CA, Gaynes BN, McDonald MA, Schoenfisch AL. Depressive symptoms among working women in rural North Carolina: A comparison of women in poultry processing and other low-wage jobs. *Int J Law Psychiatry*. 2007;30(4–5):284–298.

47. Lipscomb H, Kucera K, Epling C, Dement J. Upper extremity musculoskeletal symptoms and disorders among a cohort of women employed in poultry processing. *Am J Ind Med*. 2008;51(1):24–36.

48. Donham K. Respiratory disease hazards to workers in livestock and poultry confinement structures. *Semiannual Respiratory Medicine*. 1993;14:49–59.

49. Price LB, Graham JP, Lackey LG, Roess A, Vailes R, Silbergeld E. Elevated risk of carrying gentamicin-resistant Escherichia coli among U.S. poultry workers. *Environ Health Perspect*. 2007;115(12):1738–1742.

50. Gray GC, McCarthy T, Capuano AW, Setterquist SF, Olsen CW, Alavanja MC. Swine workers and swine influenza virus infections. *Emerg Infect Dis*. 2007;13(12):1871–1878.

51. Pesticide Action Network. Farmworkers. 2020; www.panna.org/frontline-communities/farmworkers. Accessed November 25, 2020.

52. Network PA. Pesticide Drift: In the Air & in Our Communities. 2020; www.pana.org. Accessed November 25, 2020.

53. Miller C. Disabilities in the U.S. Farm Population. In: U.S. Department of Agriculture, ed. 2019.

54. Graham J, Leibler JH, Price LB, et al. The animal-human interface and infectious disease in industrial food animal production: Rethinking biosecurity and biocontainment. *Public Health Reports*. 2008;123:282–299.

55. Frana TS, Beaham AR, Hanson BM, et al. Isolation and characterization of methicillin-resistant Staphylococcus aureus from pork farms and visiting veterinary students. *PloS One*. 2013;8:e53738.

56. Graham JP, Price LB, Evans SL, Graczyk TK, Silbergeld EK. Antibiotic resistant enterococci and staphylococci isolated from flies collected near confined poultry feeding operations. *Science and the Total Environment*. 2009;407:2701–2710.

57. Cole D, Drum DJ, Stalknecht DE, et al. Free-living Canada geese and antimicrobial resistance. *Emerging Infectious Diseases*. 2005;11:935–938.

58. Rule AM, Evans SL, Silbergeld E. Food animal transport: A potential source of community exposure to health hazards from industrial farming (CAFOs). *Journal of Infectious Disease and Public Health*. 2008;1:33–39.

59. Kindy K. More than 200 meat plan workers in the U.S. have died of covid-19: Federal regulators just issued two modest fines. *Washington Post*. September 13, 2020.

60. Trump D. Executive Order on Delegating Authority under the DPA with Respect to Food Supply Chain Resources during the National Emergency Caused by the Outbreak of COVID-19. In: U.S. Department of Agriculture, ed. The White House; April 28, 2020.

61. Furuseth OJ. Restructuring of hog farming in North Carolina: Explosion and implosion. *Professional Geographer*. 2004;49:391–403.

62. Wing S, Cole D, Grant G. Environmental injustice in North Carolina's hog industry. *Environmental Health Perspectives*. 2000;108:233–238.

63. Tijik M, Mauhammad N, Lowman A, Thu K, Wing S, Grant G. Impact of odor from industrial hog operations on daily living activities. *New Solutions*. 2008;18:193–205.

64. U.S. Environmental Protection Agency. Regulatory Definition of Large CAFOs, Medium CAFO and Small CAFO. 2020; www3.epa.gov/npdes/pubs/sector_table.pdf. Accessed November 20, 2020.

65. Yeoman B. "Suffocating closeness": U.S. judges condemns "appalling conditions" on industrial farms. *Guardian*. November 20, 2020.

66. Shorman J, Hardy K. While Missouri farmers fight plan for 10,000 hogs as neighbors, state sides with big ag. *The Kansas City Star*. December 13, 2020; Government & Politics.

67. Silbergeld E, Graham J, Price L. Industrial food animal production, antimicrobial resistance, and human health. *Annual Review of Public Health*. 2008;29:151–169.

68. Smith TC, Pearson N. The emergence of Staphylococcus aureus st398. *Vector Borne Zoonotic Disease*. 2011;11:327–339.

69. Feingold BJ, Silbergeld E, Curriero FC, van Cleef BA, Heck ME, Kluytmans JA. Livestock density as risk factor for livestock-associated methicillin-resistant Staphylococcus aureus, the Netherlands. *Emerging Infectious Diseases*. 2012;18:1841–1849.

70. Peng H, Hu B, Liu Q, et al. Methylated phenylarsenical metabolites discovered in chicken liver. *Angewandte Chemie International Edition*. 2017:1–10.

71. Stingone JA, Wing S. Poultry litter incineration as a source of energy: Reviewing the potential for impacts on environmental health and justice. *New Solutions*. 2011;21:27–42.
72. Fernandez-Cornejo J, Nehring R, Osteen C, Wechsler S, Martin A, Vialou A. Pesticide Use in U.S. Agriculture: 21 Selected Crops, 1960–2080. In: U.S.D.A., ed. May 2014.
73. Alavanja MC. Pesticide use and exposure extensive worldwide. *Review of Environmental Health*. 2009;24:303–309.
74. Nicolopoulou-Stamati P, Maipas S, Kotampasi C, Stamatis P, Hens L. Chemical pesticides and human health: The urgent need for a new concept in agriculture. *Front Public Health*. 2016;4:e148.
75. Karsten HD, Patterson PH, Stout R, Crewa G. Vitamins A, E and fatty acid composition of eggs of caged hens and pastured hens. *Cambridge University Press*. 2010;12:1–10.
76. Turner KE, McClure KE, Weiss WP, Birton RJ, Foster JG. Alpha-tocopherol (vitamin E) concentrations and case life of lamb muscles as influenced by concentrate or pasture finishing. *Journal of Animal Science*. 2002;80:2513–2521.
77. Dewhyrst RJ, Shingfield KJ, Lee MRF, Scollan ND. Increasing the concentrations of beneficial polyunsaturated fatty acids in milk produced by dairy cows in high forage systems. *Animal Feed Science and Technology*. 2006;131:168–206.
78. Noziere P, Graulet B, Lucas A, Martin B, Grolier P, Doreau M. Carotenoids for ruminants: From forages to dairy products. *Animal Feed Science and Technology*. 2006;131:418–445.
79. Hricko A. Global trade comes home: Community impacts of goods movement. *Environ Health Perspect*. 2008;116(2):A78–81.
80. Hricko AM. Ships, trucks, and trains: Effects of goods movement on environmental health. *Environ Health Perspect*. 2006;114(4):A204–205.
81. Burkholder J, Libra B, Weyer P, et al. Impact of waste from concentrated animal feeding operations on water quality. *Environmental Health Perspectives*. 2007;115:308–312.
82. Allen B. Cradle of a revolution? The industrial transformation of Louisiana's lower Mississippi River. *Technology and Culture*. 2006;47:112–119.
83. Press Briefing with Secretary Sonny Perdue, U.S. Department of Agriculture [press release]. U.S. Department of State's Brussels Media Hub; October 7, 2020.
84. Brown JL. Nutrition. In: Levy BS, Sidel VW, eds. *Social Justice and Public Health*. New York: Oxford University Press; 2006.
85. U.S. Senate. Hunger 1973. In: Select Committee on Hunger and Human Needs, ed. Washington, DC: Government Printing Office; 1973:1–74.
86. Physician Task Force on Hunger in America. *Hunger in American: The Growing Epidemic*. Middletown, CT: Wesleyan University Press; 1985.
87. Brown JL, Allen D. Hunger in America. *Annual Review of Public Health*. 1988;9:503–526.
88. Coleman-Jensen A, Nord M, Andrews M, Carlson S. *Household Food Security in the United States in 2010*. Washington, DC: USDA, ERS; 2011.
89. Economic Research Services. Food Security and Nutritional Assistance. In: U.S. Department of Agriculture, ed. October 16, 2020.
90. Townsend MS, Peerson J, Love B, Achterberg C, Murphy SP. Food insecurity is positively related to overweight in women. *Journal of Nutrition*. 2001;131:1738–1745.
91. Darmon N, Ferguson EL, Briend L. A cost constraint alone has adverse effects on food selection and nutrient density. *Journal of Nutrition*. 2002;132:3764–3771.
92. Karpyn A. Interview with Former Secretary of Agriculture of Delaware, Walter Kee. In: November 18, 2020.
93. Waterhouse B. A sustainable future? In: de Sam Lazaro F, ed. *Death of a Dream*. PBS; 2020; https://www.pbs.org/ktca/farmhouses/sustainable_future.html. Accessed November 19, 2021.
94. Economic Research Services. Food Price and Spending. In: U.S. Department of Agriculture, ed. 2020.
95. Shannon KL, Kim BF, McKenzie SE, Lawrence RS. Food system policy, public health, and human rights in the United States. *Annual Review of Public Health*. 2015;36:151–173.
96. Nelson M. U.S. Food Expenditures at Home and Abroad. November 13, 2019; www.fb.org/market-intel/u.s.-food-expenditures-at-home-and-abroad. Accessed November 21, 2020.
97. Redman R. Grocery shoppers shift to less-expensive brands amid pandemic. *Supermarket News*. 2020; www.supermarketnews.com/consumer-trends/grocery-shoppers-shift-less-expensive-brands-amid-pandemic. Accessed December 9, 2020.

2 The Food Retail Industry

CONTENTS

INTRODUCTION

This chapter aims to take the reader from understanding food production to grasping the driving forces that influence the other end of the U.S. food system, food retail. The purpose of this chapter is to describe the industry of food retailing, with a concentration of selling foods at supermarkets. The history of how foods have been sold in the United States and economic factors such as mass merchandizing and economies of scale that have supported the rise of supermarkets are discussed. Similarities in the food production system, such as the consolidation of farms and ranches are also seen in the food retail market as well as how 'get big' has supported profitability in the food retail sector. Specific factors involved in supermarket profitability are detailed in an interview with former Vice President of Operations at the Kroger Company. This information is provided to support program planners by gaining an understanding of the food retail industry and need for public-private partnerships to strengthen projects aimed to bring these types of retailers to underserved areas.

Equally important to program planners is the documentation of disparities in access to food stores, particularly supermarkets, which is presented along with a landmark report to the U.S. Congress in 2009 describing these disparities and potential impact on residents' health. The chapter also provides an overview of the Food Access Research Atlas, an online interactive tool made available by the United States Department of Agriculture that determines areas that have low access to food stores. However, this chapter begins with reporting from a journalist, Tracie McMillan, on the impact of a new supermarket in an underserved area of Detroit.

In the summer of 2013, Spencertorry Brown, a 49-year-old African American – a woman from Hamtramck, a tiny city within the boundaries of Detroit, did what she often did when her Supplemental Nutrition Assistance Program (SNAP) benefits came in and prompted her monthly grocery-shopping trip. She put on sweats and an Ecko T-shirt, did what she could to remove the patina of pet hair from both, and persuaded her niece to drive her to the grocery store. Today, they aimed for the newest one in town: Whole Foods.

Once there, Spencertorry, who is pretty certain she weighs more than 300 pounds, took her cane and walk-limped to the entryway. Her niece stayed in the car, with her two daughters. Her two sons – Spencertorry's grandnephews – went along with Spencertorry, who procured a green

DOI: 10.1201/9781003029151-3

shopping cart, tossed her cane into the basket, and headed in. While she was contemplating the refrigerated bins stacked with trays of wild-caught salmon, farm-raised tilapia, and step-1-animal-welfare-rated chicken breasts, one of her grandnephews found the make-your-own peanut butter machine amid the bulk bins of quinoa and barley, pressed a button, and churned a smooth dollop of ground peanuts onto the counter before anyone thought to stop him. 'No, no, honey', called out a nutritionist, hired by the store, to educate customers about healthy eating. She ran over and turned off the machine. 'Don't do that'. He scurried wordlessly over to Spencertorry and gripped the side of the cart. Spencertorry looked up and seeing the friendly face of the nutritionist, began to ask for some advice. As it turned out, Spencertorry was looking to turn her diet around.

In Spencertorry, I saw a familiar figure. In my ten years as an investigative food reporter, I've gone undercover in farm fields and Walmart produce aisles; I've hung out on bodega corners in Brooklyn; I've helped keep the kitchen moving at an Applebee's. And nearly everywhere I've worked, undercover or as an open journalist, I've seen the same thing. There are always a handful of people who declare allegiance to burgers and fries and who decry salads as rabbit food. But it's been more common for me to meet people like Spencertorry, people who care about their health but are overwhelmed by the logistics of trading the diet they know for the health of another. For folks like this, diet choices are not solely determined by the stores closest to them. And the food in their cabinets reflects more than a hedonistic desire for fat and sugar and salt. What most people eat, I've become convinced, reflects a complicated set of pressures and structures and priorities. And it's not just the personal priorities we set at home that matter; the priorities we set as a nation matter quite a bit, too.

I ended up spending many hours with Spencertorry, who was earnestly trying to improve her diet. She spent more than $60 on that first visit to Whole Foods, a trip she cut short when her niece came into the store, trailing her daughters and asking when they could go. It was an expensive trip for Spencertorry, who put not just chicken breasts into her cart but marinated kebabs and turkey, spinach patties, barbecue tofu salad, and a rotisserie chicken, ignoring the suggestion of the nutritionist to include a can of steel-cut oatmeal. She justified the spending, in part, by using her $16 in SNAP benefits.

But more notable than my meeting Spencertorry were the circumstances that led to it. I was working on a journalistic assignment that would have been unheard of a decade ago. I was in Detroit not to cover the declaration of the biggest municipal bankruptcy in history, but the opening of that Whole Foods. In 2013, a national news magazine deemed the opening of a grocery store in a broke, and in some ways broken, city to be worthy of in-depth coverage.[1]

OVERVIEW OF FOOD RETAILING AND THE RISE OF SUPERMARKETS

The need for grocery stores in low-income neighborhoods, whether in Detroit or other areas of the United States, has been expressed by community members, like Spencertorry, from areas across the nation.[2-5] The displacement of supermarkets from these regions has been documented for several decades;[6] therefore, a business decision from a chain supermarket like Whole Foods, to break from the norm and locate in a city like Detroit, is of course worth media coverage.[7] The norm of where chain supermarkets locate has been influenced by the same force that have given rise to industrial food production in the United States: profitability.

FOOD SUPPLY CHAIN

Prior to the development of large supermarkets at the beginning of the twentieth century, Americans shopped for food from smaller specialty food stores such as meat markets and produce stands. Large markets that drew multiple vendors, including farmers themselves, into a single public space, such as La Marqueta, in the neighborhood of East Harlem in New York City, were not uncommon.[8] These marketplaces sold both food and nonfood items. Farmers benefitted from a greater share of profit margins by selling directly to consumers even though the volume of sales was relatively small compared to traditional supermarkets. Several factors have contributed to the move away from direct consumer purchases from farmers and ranchers over the past decades. Most notably has been the processing and manufacturing of foods. Figure 2.1 is a diagram that depicts the supply chain from farm and ranch products to retail stores. The figure shows that most foods produced by farmers and ranchers is managed by other parts of the food system before reaching the retail market.[9] Farmers and ranchers sell most of their product to what are known as first-line handlers/processors who provide the initial management and processing of food products. For crops, the yields from many farmers are aggregated, then shipped to wholesalers or manufacturers. These first-line handlers may be for-profit commodity trading companies (used primarily by the larger farms) or farmer cooperatives that aggregate the yield of individual farms to gain economies of scale (used primarily by smaller farms). Economies of scale refers to cost savings gained with a greater volume of production. These first-line handlers also include companies that process foods. For example, farmers may sell products to companies that prepare fresh fruits and vegetables for direct retail sales by washing, wrapping, and packing produce. Other crops may require further processing, such as milling, and therefore farmers may use first-line companies to prepare raw food materials for the manufacturing of finished food products. Some products, such as field corn, are produced and processed specifically to feed livestock. However, by-products from milling of other crops are used to feed livestock or used in other parts of the food system (e.g., ethanol) which are managed by first-line handlers. For livestock and poultry growers, live animals are typically sent off-site to first-line handlers to be slaughtered and processed into raw products fit for human consumption. Finally, there are also companies that convert raw food into higher value packaged and processed food products. This is a large part of the food system. For example, in 2019, 20,062 new foods or beverages came into the U.S. retail market, with the majority being processed and shelf-stable.[10] Regardless of the type of first-line handler/manufacture, food products are then sold to wholesalers who store and distribute these foods

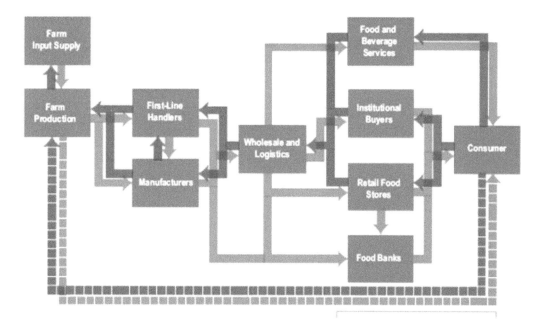

FIGURE 2.1   Conceptual Model of the U.S. Food Supply Chain

(Published with permission from the National Academy of Sciences, courtesy of the National Academies Press, Washington, DC – Institute of Medicine and National Research Council, 2015, A Framework for Assessing the Effects of the Food System (https://doi.org/1-.17226/18846.)

to consumer markets. This wholesale portion of the food systems consists of companies that either own the food products and manage the storage and distribution of foods or are contractors who store and distribute the food products owned by a larger company. As shown in Figure 2.1, these food products then reach Americans through several ways. The most routine way in which Americans obtain food is at food stores and restaurants.[9] This is the retail market, which consists of both the *retail food stores* where foods are purchased primarily for home preparation and consumption (e.g., supermarkets, grocery stores, convenience stores) and the *food and beverage service places*, where foods are purchased for away from home consumption (e.g., restaurants, fast-food outlets, bakeries). Although the retail market is the most routine way for Americans to procure food, foods produced also reach Americans through public schools, hospitals, and other institutional buyers. These programs are often supported by legislation in the Farm Bill discussed in Chapter 1 and may include commodity foods. In addition to institutional buyers, foods are also transported to food banks and other government agencies to prevent hunger.

SHELF-STABLE FOODS

The development of processed nonperishable foods, which came into the U.S. food system after World War II, has been a large contributor to our current food system.[11] Unlike fresh foods that can be sold directly from farmers to consumers, this class of food products are processed after being produced and packaged to become 'shelf-stable'. Shelf-stable means that, unlike fresh foods (e.g., milk, eggs, fresh produce) that will spoil and become harmful to eat after a week or two, shelf-stable foods have longer shelf lives and often do not expire for a year or longer. Since perishable foods result in a business loss if not sold, stocking nonperishable foods has allowed food store retailers to open larger food stores that carry a greater number of products. Michael Cullen opened one the largest supermarkets of its time in the 1930s.[12] At the time, Mr. Cullen managed a number of small Kroger Grocery & Baking stores in Illinois. He visualized and proposed to Kroger's management that grocery stores should expand to be

> monstrous stores, size of some to be about forty feet wide and a hundred and thirty to a hundred and sixty feet deep, and they ought to be located one to three blocks off the high rent district with plenty of parking space, should be operated as a semi-self-service store – twenty percent service and eighty percent self-service.[12]

His vision was not grasped by Kroger (at that time) and therefore he resigned, moved to Long Island and opened the first King Kullen supermarket. His business plan allowed him to accept a low profit margin for foods sold if he was selling a high volume of foods. This is called *mass merchandizing* and is central to the success of Mr. Cullen supermarkets and every supermarket open for business today. By selling nonperishables, it allowed Mr. Cullen to increase the volume of goods sold and provide lower food prices for customers than were available at competitor's smaller grocery stores. The lower prices gain brand loyalty and a greater volume of items purchased by each customer, which in turn, increases the turnover of his products. A typical supermarket sells roughly 38,000 items, which allows for greater product turnover and flexibility of profit margins between products sold.

TYPES OF FOOD RETAILERS

The food retail market consists of places where Americans routinely purchase food, and there are thousands of these stores across the United States.[13] The market consists of a number of types of businesses which are categorized by the North American Industry Classification System (NAICS) which is used by the Economic Census, part of the U.S. Census Bureau.[14]

Food retailers are composed of food stores and food service places. Food stores are defined as places where people typically purchase foods for home preparation and include supermarkets and other grocery stores, convenience stores, gasoline stations with convenience stores, and specialty food stores. Food service places include places where people typically purchase and consume food away from home. These places include full-service restaurants; limited-service restaurants (e.g., fast food restaurants); cafeterias, snack places; alcoholic drinking places; mobile food service; and catering.

Although the NAICS definition provides a categorical system for monitoring industries across the United States, the NAICS index does not clearly delineate small grocery stores from supermarkets and large supercenters. These distinctions are important for understanding disparities in access to food because low-income areas often contain small food stores, if any food stores at all, and these smaller stores have limited inventory that hamper the profits gained with mass merchandizing. Hence to remain profitable, these stores may stock a greater volume of nonperishable food items, snack foods, or require higher prices for products sold. Distinguishing between the stores available for food shopping has been an important part of developing public policies and programs aimed to attract grocers to low-income areas.

Within the NAICS subsectors of 452 (General Merchandizing) and 445 (Food and Beverage Stores), places that sell food are cataloged by the United States Census Bureau. The subsectors include supermarkets and grocery stores as well as smaller specialty stores such as meat markets or donut shops. Here we focus on store distinctions within the category of 445110. Other retailers under the NAICS 445 subsector such as 445210, 445220, 445230, 445291, 445299 are not described because of the limited volume and variety of healthy foods stocked within these types of stores. As stated earlier, because the NAICS does not distinguish between large supermarkets and small grocery stores, and the importance of this distinction in relation to mass merchandizing, others have made distinctions between these food retailers within the 445100 category based on three characteristics: (1) volume of sales; (2) floor space; and (3) the items sold and are described on Table 2.1.[15–17]

Mass merchandizing, the practice of stocking many food items, allows grocers to maintain a profit while offering a wide selection of products to their customers at affordable prices. For example, a full size Whole Foods Market carries 55,000 items[18] and would be considered a supermarket because of the size of the store and the large number of items carried, thus allowing the stores to benefit from mass merchandizing. Whole Foods is similar to the Kroger stores that carry over 69,000 items.[19] A supercenter, like Walmart, is distinguished because this type of food retailer carries nearly twice the number of products as a typical supermarket (approximately 120,000 items).[20] Supercenters typically sell perishable and nonperishable foods intended for home cooking like supermarkets; however they are distinct from supermarkets because foods and beverages are not the primary products for sale in these stores. Smaller stores such as Trader Joe's carry approximately 4,000 perishable and nonperishable food and beverage items, and Trader Joe's characterizes itself as a neighborhood grocery store. Prices at Trader Joe's are kept affordable because the company carries almost exclusively private label brands (another method for controlling profits) and hence falls into the category of limited assortment grocery stores on Table 2.1 along with food stores like Whole Foods 365 and Aldi.[21] Finally, there is a heterogenous group of food stores called *grocery stores* that range in size and nomenclature such as grocery store, corner stores, and bodegas.[22] These businesses primarily sell food, but the stores are smaller with limited inventory compared to supermarkets and supercenters. Some of these stores may be family-owned businesses that sell a full line of groceries such as D'Agostino's in New York, while others may resemble a convenience stores, which contain more snack and nonperishable foods. Because fewer items are sold in these stores compared to supermarkets, grocers must rely on increased prices, stocking more nonfood items, and/or carrying products that will turn over quickly (such as sodas, beer, chips, candy, and other foods that are typically not intended for home cooking) to remain profitable.

TABLE 2.1
Definitions of Places That Sell Food for Home Preparation and Consumption in the United States

General Industry Definition	Type of Retailers	Examples	Retailer Type Definition
Industries in the *General Merchandise Stores subsector (NAICS 452)* retail new general merchandise from fixed point-of-sale locations. Establishments in this subsector are unique in that they have the equipment and staff to be capable of retailing a large variety of goods from a single location. This U.S. industry comprises establishments that are engaged in retailing and merchandise (e.g., apparel, furniture, toys) and contains one subcategory (452311) that includes the sale of foods and beverages with general merchandise.	Superstores and Warehouse Clubs *(NAICS 452311)*	Walmart Target Costco Sam's Club	These general merchandizing stores sell some groceries with a large selection of nonfood products, such as clothes, electronics or toys which make up at least 25% of total floor space. These stores are large (average of 50,000 square feet) and the superstores sell between 30,000 and 120,000 items. The warehouse clubs require a membership fee and sell food and other merchandise packaged for industrial not personal consumption. These warehouses contain fewer products than the superstores (4,000–7,000 food and nonfood items).
Industries in the *Food and Beverage Stores subsector (NAICS 445)* retail food and nonfood items such as dry grocery, canned goods, perishable items and paper products from fixed point-of-sale locations. Establishments in this subsector have special equipment for displaying foods and beverages as well as staff trained in the processing and proper storage of food products. Descriptions of store distinctions within the NAICS 445110 category are described here. Other retailers under the NAICS 445 subsector (445120, 445210, 445220, 445230, 445291, 445292, and 445299) are not described because of the limited volume and variety of healthy foods stocked within these types of stores.	Supermarkets *(NAICS 445110)*	Food Lion Kroger Publix Safeway Whole Foods	These food stores are between 20,000 and 50,000 square feet and offer a full line of groceries including perishables such as meat and produce. These stores also sell nonfood items such as home goods and medicines, but most of the products sold are consumable. Stores average 10,000–40,000 items with sales volume over $2 million annually. These are corporate owned national and regional chains with 100–1,500 store located across state lines.
	Grocery Stores *(NAICS 445110)*	D'Agostino Hollywood Super Mart Weaver Street Market	These food stores are smaller than supermarkets and range in size up to 20,000 square feet. Like supermarkets, these food stores sell a general line of groceries and nonfood items however fewer items (5,000–10,000 items) are sold. Sales volume is typically up to $2 million annually. These food stores may be corporate chains, or family-owned businesses with single or multiple locations. However, there are typically fewer than 100 stores within a chain or family-owned operations nationwide.
	Limited Assortment Grocery Stores *(NAICS 445110)*	Trader Joe's Whole Foods-365 Aldi	These food stores are like grocery stores but restricted further in size and offer even fewer consumable and nonconsumable products, usually between 2,000 and 5,000 items. These stores may have a limited selection of perishables compared to supermarkets and are dominated by private label products.

These designations are intended to aid program planners in identifying the type of food retailer that best fits the underserved community.

THE CONSOLIDATION OF FOOD STORES

Mr. Cullen's business model has since been adopted by other food retailers resulting in other supermarkets (e.g., Kroger, Ralphs, Albertsons) and supercenters (e.g., Walmart, Target) who retail food today. Mass merchandizing has led to increased profitability in the food retail industry. Like the consolidation of farms and ranches, profitability has played a role in the consolidation of food retailing. In 2018, there were 38,307 supermarkets in the United States providing employment for 4.8 million people. The supermarket industry during that year produced over $700 billion in sales.[23] Grocery store mergers and bankruptcies have changed the types of food retailers over time. For example, one of the first supermarkets in the United States opened in 1912, called A&P, went bankrupt in 2015.[24] Alpha Beta was purchased by Ralphs. Dominick's, a well-known supermarket chain in the Chicago area that was founded in 1918 and grew to 72 stores merged with Safeway then finally closed in 2014.[25] These bankruptcies and mergers have been common over the past two decades and have resulted in the emergence of fewer corporations owning a larger proportion of the food retail market. Currently, the four largest food retailers control 72% of sales in the largest metropolitan areas.[26] The share of sales going to traditional food retailers fell from 82% in 1998 to 69% in 2003. Over 500 food industry mergers and acquisitions were recorded in 2016 alone. The top five food retailers in 2019 were: Walmart Stores, Inc., Kroger, Walgreens, CVS, and Costco.[26] The average annual sales for a supermarket is $17.39 million. There are currently (2020) 40,544 supermarkets and grocery stores in the United States.[27] The dominance of supermarkets and supercenters in the proportion of food sales is depicted in Figure 2.2. U.S. supermarkets sales are more than five times greater than other types of food retailers. It is the success of Mr. Cullen's idea of mass merchandising that has now brought nonfood retailers and wholesalers into this marketplace. Retailers such as Walmart have replaced supermarkets such as Kroger as the leader in the field.[28,29] Food retailers have also boosted margins with practices promoting economies of scale with mergers, private label sales, and stronger control over producers.

For the American food shopper, these business practices have translated into greater availability of inexpensive food items. In fact, over the years, Americans are spending less of their

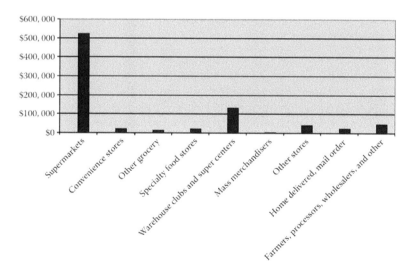

FIGURE 2.2 Food Sales (in millions) in the United States by Type of Food Retailer: 2011

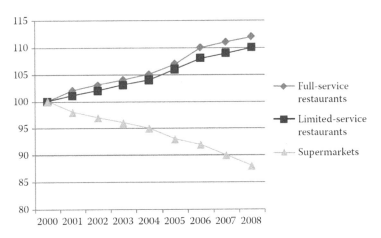

FIGURE 2.3   Number of Supermarkets and Restaurants per Capita, 2002–2008

income on food, even with an increase in the expenditures from foods eaten away from home. It is estimated by the USDA that, in 2009, American families spent an average of $6,389 a year on food, roughly $500 per month. This estimate includes purchases of foods prepared at home as well as those purchased away from home (at limited- and full-service restaurants). This annual food expenditure is 40% higher than in 1984 ($4,552, annual household expenditure).[30] The food service industry has also grown with an increase in the number of full- and limited-service restaurants in the last decade, with a decreasing trend in the availability of supermarkets (Figure 2.3). It is estimated that over 75% of Americans eat outside of their homes at least once a week, and the proportion of caloric intake from foods purchased away from home has nearly doubled since the 1970s.[31] This trend has led to some concern about changes in the nutritional quality of Americans' diets with the understanding that, in general, meals eaten away from home have higher caloric content and are nutritionally poorer than foods prepared at home.[32] Restaurant owners have business goals similar to those of food store owners, which is to make a profit, and prioritize healthy food menu options only to the extent they will achieve that goal.[33,34]

OPERATION OF SUPERMARKETS

Although the food service industry is growing, supermarkets and supercenters remain the main retail food stores for Americans to routinely purchase food for home consumption. Major chain supermarkets and supercenters have replicated successful business models to open and operate profitable chain food stores across the United States. Much of the profitability of these supermarkets involve careful management of three business domains: (a) site location; (b) products sold and cost management; and (c) the staffing of stores. Mr. Bill Green, who has recently retired from his position as Vice President of Operations of Kroger Supermarkets describes this in the following interview.[35]

Interviewer: **Can you briefly explain the approach to opening a supermarket in any location?**
Mr. Green: Well, I get that question quite a bit, and I would say there's a difference between what my experience was and what a first-time grocery store or supermarket opening experience would be like. And the reason I draw that distinction is that when we opened a new store, we had 2,400 stores. So, it was something that we did, it was just boilerplate, we already knew what the store configuration would look like, we

already knew what the market analysis would look like, we pretty much knew what the item assortment would look like. I mean so a lot of the work was already done, because we had opened so many stores. That process would be a little bit different if I were opening-up Bill's Grocery Store for the first time. Because there would not be the same level of certainty about: (a) the market, (b) the product offerings, and (c) how it would work for different customer segments. You know, determining [what] the pricing strategy should be, [the] staffing levels. . . . What are the appropriate staffing levels? So, there is a lot that you'd have to figure out. So, in my experience, we would start a meeting, say, a year and a half out? So, there was a real estate team that would find the best locations. And that real estate team would look at demographics, would look at income levels, who's currently in the market, what stores we currently had in the market, and what the impact would be on those stores and how much in sales we think we can generate. So, let's just say that we think the store could generate $750,000 in sales a week. Then that kind of generates what we think we should build. And so, one of the other things that we would look at is what segmentation should the store comprise? So, we had basically three different main segments. There was like a value segment [for] when we were opening a store in a community that [has] very price conscious customers. There was a segmentation of more affluent customers for whom price is not so much an issue, where customer service and variety were more of an issue for them. There was that middle section, and just like any measurement you take, the middle is going to be the largest portion. So. we would analyze the market on who we thought the potential customers were. . . . You know, going back to that segmentation piece that I shared earlier, if it is a very, very value-based customer, then it doesn't matter much what you build. If your model is more high-end, where it's going to cost more, you may have a whole bunch of rooftops [potential customers] there but they're not going to shop with you.

Interviewer: How do you determine what to sell?

Mr. Green: Again, when you have a long-standing grocery store, those kinds of decisions have already been mapped out. Maybe there's some peculiarities based on a particular store like if it's right across the street from a high school. Maybe there's some other things, elements like maybe there's some school supplies, or you know, grab and go food that you wouldn't have in that standard package. But for the most part we had an idea already. . . . I suspect there was some consultant work that we would engage. But then there were certain processes that were so boilerplate that we just did them every time. And by that, I mean, a lot of real estate data. What's the median home value? What are the real estate taxes in that area? What's the population in the schools? There's a lot of data that you can glean just from, do people own or rent? I mean there's a lot of information in that, that gives you a lot of basic information about them. . . . If it's a food desert, there's somebody who's already serving that community. What are they selling? What are they selling well? What's not selling at all? What's the volume there? . . . In a grocery store, you have to monetize the customer experience. By that I mean, the check-out experience generates no revenue. So, you got check lane candy, gift cards, and maybe some magazines. You got some one-of-a-kind of stuff up there but for the most part it's a cost center. It's not generating any real money for you, so you have to make that a vital part of the store.

Interviewer: How do grocers determine the cost of specific items?

Mr. Green: There's a product mix that is calculated for the grocery store to reach maximum profitability. The product mix will contain some low-margin, high-volume items like canned vegetables, gallons of milk, chips, things that have very low margins, but you expect customers to buy in bulk. But those items will generate top line revenue but not necessarily bottom line. But they are important for a number of reasons. Customers are looking for them. You have to have them, but customers are also not willing to pay an arm and a leg for them. Another part of the product mix is higher margin items that go more to the bottom line as well as the top line. That's why in grocery stores you will see a deli/bakery. Bakery items have extremely high markups. Now they have high shrink and one of the reasons they have high markups is there's also high loss. But it's one of those departments that you have to have. Shrink is anything that does not go through the register. Whether it's any kind of theft, whether it's through spoilage, whether it's through accounting errors, that you thought you received a pallet of product, but you never received it. On paper you received it, but you didn't. So, it didn't go through the registers and it's a loss. Deli is high loss, high shrink. So is produce. Produce is the highest loss department in the store, by far. If you've seen the back of a produce department, back in the prep room, there's garbage cans and garbage cans of product that went bad. Especially a store that prides itself on quality, as soon as that banana gets one brown spot on it, you have to mark it down or you gotta take it off the sales floor. Because if not, it starts to impact your reputation. Theft is a big area of loss as well but produce departments lose a lot of products. It's one of those areas that there's a lot of loss. . . . For everything in the store, there's a price and there's a cost. And so there has to be enough items in the store that have a high margin to pay the bills. And so sometimes those [food] items on the front page are sold at a loss because [of] the calculation that we can lose on all that Coke that you put on the front page because we're gonna make it up in ribs and chicken and hot dog buns and cans of beans and everything else that we sell at the store [e.g., loss leading]. So, this question about price, oftentimes, that is based on supply and demand. But there are other factors as well. So, if a buyer gambled that he or she would be able to sell a certain number of T-bone steaks then went to the distributors and loaded up on T bone steaks. Now the warehouse is loaded up with T-bone steaks. That's when you pull the lever of changing the price. So, then you get the discount on T bone steaks. And now the folks that are selling the beef to the grocery stores can't get a fair price because the grocery store says we're full and we can't buy it unless you bring down the price. So, there are these dynamics that go on at all times, which is the basics of our capitalistic system.

Interviewer: Can you explain a little bit about the supply chain for fresh and processed food items that come into the food store?

Mr. Green: You have to understand that grocery stores now are not just one store, there's several different stores in one. The produce department is a produce business. It has its own suppliers, its own economics, a way of doing business which is completely separate from the meat department. Which is also separate from how the delis and bakeries work. Which is separate from your dry grocery department, which to a certain extent is separate from frozen which is separate from your dairy department. And so, there are all these different kinds of businesses. Which is also separate from your pharmacy. A lot of grocery stores have pharmacies. At one time, they were all stand-alone businesses. And you got some grocery stores, you don't see this as much anymore, but they would have a dry-cleaners or they would have a video store, a bank. So, there are all these different businesses. So, the question of who are the distributors is going to vary by business. It's going to vary by the individual segment of the store.

Interviewer: **Any last thoughts?**

Mr. Green: I've managed stores that are in really tough areas. I've managed stores that struggle to stay clean. . . . There has to be a commitment to staffing [the store]. Therein lies the rub. In order to keep the place clean and running well, you have to put more labor into it, then that decreases the profitability of the store. And [stores in tough areas] have higher liability claims because of incidents that happen at those stores. It just takes the overall profitability of the store down. It's tough. I tell people, running a grocery store is one of the toughest businesses you can have because it's truly low margins. If you can get four cents to the bottom line out of a dollar at a grocery store, you're doing pretty good. It does not leave a lot of room for error, and there's a lot of error in a grocery store.

As stated by Mr. Green in the interview, the placement of a new grocery store involves a careful analysis of real estate to ensure the four cents out of each dollar spent is earned by the grocer. For example, the average home value for areas where Trader Joe's are located is $644,558.[36] Supermarket owners opt for wealthy areas for the placement of their stores, and this sets the stage for low-income neighborhoods to be less likely to be selected by Kroger (or another large chain supermarket) as a location for opening a store. Using Mr. Green's suggested $750,000 of sales per week, the low margins of four cents out of every dollar translates to $30,000 of profit per week, or $1,560,000 of profit per store per year, which is more readily achievable in a higher income area. To many low-income customers, the weekly profit is more than their annual household income. But there is no incentive for large chain supermarkets to lose potential revenue. Like producers, food retailers are in the business of profitability; and they just happen to sell goods that satisfy a basic human need. But perhaps it is the boiler plate business model based on profitability that makes businesses like Kroger less flexible in modifying approaches to serve a wide range of communities. Yael M. Lehmann as Executive Director of The Food Trust says that during twenty years of overseeing the Fresh Food Financing Initiative that, 'Even with all of the business incentives provided by the state and federal governments, I was not able to get a major chain supermarket, like Kroger, to locate in a low-income neighborhood'.

Low-income Americans purchase food just like everyone else and food retailers sell one of the only products that is guaranteed to be purchased by all people, repeatedly. It was estimated by the USDA that the lowest income quintile of Americans each spent an annual average of $4,400 on food in 2019[37] amounting to over $561 million of revenue for food retailers. Owners of supermarkets and supercenters may not be concerned about this lost revenue, or perhaps it is not enough of an incentive for chain supermarkets like Kroger to locate in low-income areas. Some smaller chain supermarkets have aimed to fill the void in underserved areas in the United States. For instance, Jeff Brown, owner of Brown's Grocery Stores, which is part of the ShopRite franchise, has opened and successfully operated chain supermarkets in underserved areas of Pennsylvania[38,39] which is described in a PBS New Hour interview, (https://www.pbs.org/news hour/show/building-oasis-philadelphia-food-desert). To ensure the supermarkets' profitability, Mr. Brown's business plan involves market research, but not with realtors. He works with community leaders to learn about the religions, backgrounds, and the foods desired by local residents. He uses this information to structure store sections and adjust stocking in each store. For instance, one of his stores offers Halal meat in a neighborhood with a greater Muslim population. Another store serves African Americans originally from the South. In this store, Mr. Brown has become famous for their sweet potato pie and other traditional foods that are difficult to obtain in Philadelphia. In addition to stocking specific foods, Mr. Brown also values foot traffic, acknowledging it to be fundamental for large volume of sales that are needed to offset the industries' low profit margins. Therefore, he has added sections to his stores so customers can purchase groceries and conduct other activities of daily living. His stores contain credit unions, nutritionists, social workers, and health clinics. He partners with local nonprofit agencies to provide these services for free or nominal charges and views this part of his business plan to be a 'win-win', stating, 'From our standpoint, each broken social thing hurts business'.[38] Mr. Brown's investment into the communities he serves with his supermarket extends to in-store efforts to attract customers to healthier food options. For example, he takes cues from Whole Foods to hand-stack produce to be visually pleasing to customers and to fire-grill chicken in the store to provide aromas that attract a substitution from fried chicken. Mr. Brown also understands that many of the customers in his community will be traveling to the supermarket using public transportation and therefore makes it a point to lobby the transportation authority to ensure there are bus stations near his stores.[38]

DISPARITIES IN THE LOCATION OF SUPERMARKETS IN THE UNITED STATES

The impact of the business practices of supermarkets has resulted in disparities in the location of supermarkets, with low-income and communities of color having low access compared to wealthier and predominately White areas in the United States. Although the measurement of local food environments and their impact on health began in the late 1990s, consumer advocate groups such as a Consumers Union in the Bay Area of California had conducted studies to measure disparities in retail environments between neighborhoods prior to this time. Others have also documented the influence of economic decline and the decrease of low-cost retailers within American inner cities during the 1960s and 1970s.[40] The urban grocery gap during the late 1980s and early 1990s was captured with the Food Marketing Policy Center of the Department of Agriculture and Resources Economics of the University of Connecticut, where a report on twenty-one American cities and the associations between low-income areas and the presence of supermarkets is presented.[41] The authors report that there were serious distribution problems in some U.S. cities in terms of food delivery and stated that:

> Given the recent cuts at the Federal level in food programs and the clear-cut need to improve the efficiency of distribution of federal food program dollars, the focus on the ability of the supermarket food distribution system to deliver food in an efficient (i.e., reasonably priced fashion) to low-income urban neighborhoods is extremely timely.

These findings were supported by the work conducted by the U.S. House of Representatives Select Committee on Hunger, where it was determined that the migration of supermarkets to the suburbs and lack of transportation contributed to malnutrition among low-income Americans.[6,42] Other economic experts have investigated issues related to attracting supermarkets to inner cities, noting that citywide grocery initiatives are rare within the thirty-two U.S. cities investigated.[43] This earlier work guided the development of new investigations within the public health and medical community to find out how these population and retail shifts, which continue to this day, have impacted Americans' health. The following summarizes twenty-five studies, published between 1997 and 2013, that document U.S. disparities in access to healthy foods.

Most of the public health studies included here have been conducted within urban areas ($n = 23$), particularly New York ($n = 9$) and Los Angeles ($n = 4$). Fewer studies have investigated disparities in access to healthy affordable foods for rural consumers ($n = 4$). Among these studies, most investigators aimed to measure the differences in the placement of food stores (or food items) by economic measures, as had been done in the earlier studies, but also by racial composition of areas. Most of the studies measured food availability based on the presence of types of food stores, such as supermarkets ($n = 16$), although several studies have measured the availability of specific types of foods ($n = 9$) and related costs for those purchases ($n = 7$). Fewer studies have focused on the quality of foods ($n = 1$), eating away from home specifically ($n = 2$), or perceptions and utilization patterns ($n = 1$).

Overall, investigators have consistently documented disparities in the placement of super-markets by either the wealth of areas investigated or the racial composition of area residents.[2,5,44–50] Food options are also associated with inequality in the presence of supermarkets within urban centers.[4,45,48,51,52] Others have documented disparities in the availability of selected healthy food options independent of supermarket presence[53–57] and those differences have been associated with demographic and urbanization factors. Only one study documented lower prices of foods within supermarkets,[3] although other studies that have measured price differences[4,52,58,59] report price not being a significant factor between local food environments.

Fewer studies have measured the changes in local food environments over time. This is an important component of understanding disparities between local food environments and how residents' exposure may be constant over time. One study measured the fluctuation of supermarket presence in Brooklyn from 2007 to 2011 and found that there was an increase in the number of supermarkets during that period; in fact, the greatest proportion of new super-market locations was found in the lowest income areas. The higher wealth areas had the greatest supermarket stability, meaning the greatest proportion of stores remained open during the five-year period of investigation.[50] A better understanding of the types of fluctuations within local food environments may aid in understanding chronic exposure and how motivations for behavior change are influenced by the stability of local food environments. For instance, within an environmental justice project to address poor access to healthy foods, residents opened a new community owned-and-operated food store in East New York. Comments from store patrons as to why they were not using the new food store with any regularity reflected their familiarity with a volatile retail environment, stating they were hesitant to rely on a new food store because they expected it would shut down within a year or two. These comments were despite the recognition by the community that the store was needed and contained foods that were desired and served the community.[60]

REPORT TO THE UNITED STATES CONGRESS: 2009

The preponderance of research showing a lack of access to full-service grocery stores and easier access to fast and convenience foods for low-income and non-White Americans led Congress to include a study to the 2008 Farm Bill. In the Food, Conservation, and Energy Act of 2008, (aka the 2008 Farm Bill) the U.S. Department of Agriculture (USDA) was directed to conduct a study to quantify the limited access to affordable and nutritious food in America. Specifically, the USDA aimed to: (a) assess the extent of the problem of limited access; (b) identify characteristics and causes of limited access; (c) determine the effects limited access has on local populations; and (d) outline recommendations for addressing the causes of limited access in particular areas. The USDA study defined a food desert as an 'area in the United States with limited access to affordable and nutritious food, particularly such an area composed of pre-dominantly lower income neighborhoods and communities' (Title VI, Sec. 7527 of the 2008 Farm Bill).[61]

This study concluded that access to a supermarket or large grocery store is a problem for only a small percentage of American households. For people who did not have access to a vehicle, 2.2% (2.3 million households) lived more than a mile from a supermarket, and an additional 3.4 million households (3.2% of all households) lived more than one-half mile from a supermarket, for a total of 7.7 million households. Area-based measures documented that 23.5 million people who lived in low-income areas (defined for this study as areas with more than 40% of the population having incomes at or below the 200% federal poverty line) are more than one mile from a supermarket or large grocery store. That is more people than currently live in the states of Pennsylvania, New Jersey, and Delaware combined. The study also concluded that urban areas with limited food access have higher levels of racial segregation and greater income inequality, whereas for rural areas with limited food access lack transportation infrastructure. Regarding cost of foods, it was described that those purchases made at convenience stores cost more than similar foods at supermarkets. The study fell short of distinguishing causes for these disparities. The authors discuss both consumer demand and the high development costs for retailers as potential reasons for low access within low-income communities. The higher costs for retailers are supported by statements from Bill Greene earlier in this chapter. Regarding consumer demand, Tracie McMillan, explains it in the following way:[1]

> It hasn't always been like this. A decade ago, the fact that low-income neighborhoods frequently had poorly run grocery stores – when they had grocery stores at all – was considered a fact of life. Grimy supermarkets were considered intractable signs of a lower income, the same as well-worn clothes lacking designer labels, cars that have visibly endured dents and repairs, and tall boys of Budweiser. But while most Americans have understood the omnipresence of battered cars as an indication of limited means rather than a preference for unreliable transportation, the traditional explanation for the lack of supermarkets had been, simply, that there was no market for what they were trying to sell. There was, in other words, no consumer demand for their product. And it is only in the last decade or so that the inherent flaw in this logic has been clearly articulated and set forth: a lack of demand for supermarkets can only exist where people do not, in fact, eat.

THE *FOOD ACCESS RESEARCH ATLAS* (FARA): 2010–2015

Findings from the report to Congress led to the surveillance of supermarket access by the USDA. Beginning in 2010, the USDA launched what is called the *Food Access Research Atlas* (FARA), which is a web-based mapping tool that counts access to food stores at the census-tract level, then rates census tracts with low access to supermarkets. A census tract is a geographic boundary defined by the U.S. Census Bureau, which aims to enumerate the American populations every decade. Census tracts are contained within counties and contain roughly 3,000–5,000 people. The FARA map is interactive and can be accessed at: www.ers.usda.gov/data-products/food-access-research-atlas. The assessment of low access considers: (a) residential proximity to the closest supermarket; (b) available transportation, and (c) income. Census tracts within any geographic area of the United States are rated as a combination of low access and low income. A recent report from the USDA provides estimates of supermarket access using more recent low-income status of Americans (defined as poverty rates at least 20% within census tract or median family income within census tract at or below 80% of the metropolitan area or State median income). The number of census tracts that are characterized as low income and low access in 2010 and 2015 are depicted in Figure 2.4 documenting a decrease in the availability of supermarkets in urban areas between 2010 and 2015.

Low access of a census tract is measured in one of four ways. The first three measures are based on the proximity to the nearest food store only and vary by distance levels for urban and rural areas of the United States (0.5 and 1 mile in urban areas; 10 and 20 miles in rural areas). The fourth measure considers the need for access to private transportation to purchase groceries with a measure of households without vehicles. The USDA reported the following by using the FARA maps regarding access to food stores between 2010 and 2015:[62]

- The number of census tracts classified as low income *increased* from 29,285 in 2010 to 30,870 in 2015, or 5.41%.

- The number of tracts that are classified as *low access (LA) based solely on proximity decreased* across all three measures from 2010 to 2015. These estimates show improvements in the proximity of supermarkets for the total population (regardless of income).

- In contrast, the fourth measure of *low-access tracts increased between 2010 and 2015*. This increase reflects an increase in the number of households without vehicles that are more than 0.5 mile from the nearest store.

The number of low-income, low-supermarket-access census tracts in urban areas rose 5 percent and decreased 5 percent in rural areas from 2010 to 2015

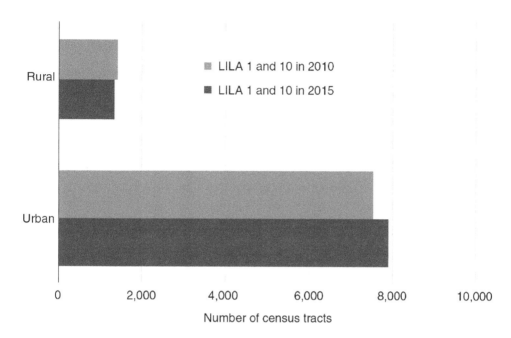

LILA 1 and 10 = A low-income census tract where at least 500 people, or at least 33 percent of the population, live farther than 1 mile from a supermarket in urban tracts or 10 miles from a supermarket in rural tracts.
Urban census tracts have more than 2,500 people, and rural census tracts have fewer than 2,500 people. A census tract is a small statistical subdivision of a county that usually contains between 1,200 and 8,000 people.
Source: USDA, Economic Research Service Food Access Research Atlas.

FIGURE 2.4 Prevalence of Urban and Rural Low-Income and Low-Access Census Tracts: 2010 and 2015

In 2015, there were 34.7 million people living in urban low-income and low-access (LILA) tracts and an additional 4.6 million people living in rural LILA tracts. U.S. population in 2015 was 321 million, therefore 12.2% of Americans were living in LILA areas.

CONCLUSION

Many people in the United States are living in areas without convenient access to supermarkets. There is a disparity in supermarket access that has been documented by the USDA to be associated with low-income areas, and others have documented racial disparities.[2,62] These disparities leave community residents relying on smaller neighborhood food stores or having to travel out of their neighborhood to obtain food for their families. Owners of smaller stores do not have the volume of products to implement mass merchandising in the same way that supermarkets and supercenters do. To maintain profit margins, smaller stores must increase the prices of items sold and/or stock shelves with nonperishable foods. It becomes impractical for a small food store to carry perishable items such as tomatoes, mangos, or lettuce due to the increased risk of shrink for these items. For the residents living in one of those low-income neighborhoods, food choices become limited or difficult to obtain without transportation.

Conversely for a resident living in a neighborhood with a supermarket, these stores provide an average of 36,000 products including an abundance of perishable and nonperishable items available to customers at affordable prices. Often in these neighborhoods, multiple grocery stores will be in the same area offering residents plenty of food choices at competitive prices. It has been argued that food needs to be affordable to prevent food insecurity for low-income Americans. Supermarkets and supercenters provide foods at lower prices compared to all other types of food retailers because of mass merchandising. Therefore, it is important for all Americans, and low-income Americans in particular, to have access to these types of food retailer. Without the large inventory, mass merchandising does not work.

Some low-income Americans are eligible for benefits from government programs intended to stretch food dollars, such as the Supplemental Nutrition Assistance Program (SNAP). In fact, some professionals have reasoned that SNAP food vouchers can offset the high prices at smaller grocery stores and therefore a comparable healthy diet can be obtained with foods purchased from either small food stores or supermarkets. Besides the issue of cost, smaller stores simply lack the variety of healthy perishable foods that are available at supermarkets. The stocking requirements necessary for a store to participate in the SNAP program only call for thirty-six staple food units, of which only six need to be perishable varieties.[63] Staple foods include: fruits and vegetables; meat, poultry, or fish; dairy products; and breads or cereals. So, for instance, an acceptable variety of fruits and vegetables may include a whole orange, but also mushrooms from a can of cream of mushroom soup would meet the criteria, and the nutritional density of those food items vary significantly. The minimum stocking requirement of only six perishable foods allows most small grocers to qualify for the SNAP program, but that qualification does not equate to providing customers with the same selection of perishable healthy foods found in supermarkets.

This issue of the variety of healthy food items available to low-income customers can also be viewed by where SNAP benefits are being used. Most SNAP benefits (82%) are redeemed at supermarkets and superstores, even though these retailers make up only 15% of SNAP authorized stores.[64] Small grocery stores make up only 3.5% of all authorized SNAP retailers, indicating that most small stores do not meet the minimum stocking requirement. These stores redeem less than 1% of SNAP benefits. SNAP participants rely on supermarkets and super-stores to purchase their allowable staples possibly because (1) supermarkets and supercenters have a larger selection of products redeemable with SNAP vouchers or (2) prices are lower at supermarkets and supercenters, and therefore food dollars are stretched even further with SNAP vouchers at these stores.

The bottom line is supermarkets such as Kroger and ShopRite are important components of the current U.S. food system and are needed in all neighborhoods. The consolidation of the supermarket industry places a strain on the variety of large-scale stores that can meet the demand for all Americans. Comparable to food production, a few large corporate food retailers control prices, selection, quality, and, equally important, the locations of where food can be purchased in the United States. The value of supermarkets to all communities is described by Reco Owens, Executive Director of the Neighborhood Progress fund, a Community Development Financing Institution (CDFI) that is involved in funding a supermarket in a low-income neighborhood in Philadelphia:

> Food access is so basic, and it's something that I think most of us take for granted. When we need food, we go get it. For a lot of people, it's something you have to think about and plan. . . . There's a subset of people in our communities that food is a huge focus – you focus on where food is coming from and how am I going to get it. It should be a basic human right and not something we have to worry about. The people who don't understand that don't worry about where their next meal is coming from. It can be hard to fathom the opposite. It's so automatic and part of human existence, it's hard to understand what it might feel like not to have that.[65]

CRITICAL THINKING QUESTIONS AND EXERCISES

1. Watch the Brown's ShopRite video (www.pbs.org/newshour/show/building-oasis-philadelphia-food-desert). Then answer the following question within a class discussion or individually: (a) describe the nutritional and economic impacts the supermarket has on the local community; (b) name three things Mr. Brown has done to ensure his supermarket is profitable in this underserved neighborhood comparing issues raised by Mr. Green; (c) discuss the discrepancy mentioned in the video regarding researchers not finding that a new supermarket improves fruit and vegetable consumption among community members, while Mr. Brown documents his sales for fresh produce is comparable to his suburban markets; and (d) consider how a store like Mr. Brown's Shop Rite would work in an underserved area near you.

2. Use FARA to determine the low-access and low-income status of the student's residential census tract. Count the presence of supermarkets within the tract. Repeat the exercise in a nearby census tract that has the low access and neither low access nor low income.

3. Gain application information for Supplemental Nutrition Assistance Program and determine eligibility for your family's status and amount of benefit. Find out the foods available to purchase and model a low-income American by purchasing foods for one week using this program. Keep a food log of items purchase, consumed, and shared as well as where foods were purchased and amounts spent on food. Be sure you use SNAP retailers.

4. Visit a grocery store or supermarket located in a low-income low-access census tract and conduct a market basket survey of twenty items that are recommended for healthy eating. Record the availability, prices, and quality of the foods.

5. Explain the historical trends that have shaped the current food retail industry in the United States.

6. Describe how food processing and shelf-stable foods have impacted the modern food retail system.

7. Define redlining and the factors that influence the disparities in access to supermarkets and grocery stores for low-income and minority neighborhoods in the United States.

8. Distinguish between food assistance programs and the routine procurement of foods and beverages for low-income community members.

REFERENCES

1. McMillan T. Foreword. In: Morland KB, ed. *Local Food Environments: Food Access in America*. Boca Raton, FL: CRC Press; 2015.
2. Morland K, Wing S, Diez Roux A, Poole C. Neighborhood characteristics associated with the location of food stores and food service places. *Am J Prev Med*. 2002;22(1):23–29.
3. Chung C, Myers SL. Do the poor pay more for food? An analysis of grocery store availability and food price disparities. *Journal of Consumer Affairs*. 1999;33:276–296.
4. Block D, Kouba J. A comparison of the availability and affordability of a market basket in two communities in the Chicago area. *Public Health Nutr*. 2006;9(7):837–845.
5. Sharkey JR, Horel S. Neighborhood socioeconomic deprivation and minority composition are associated with better potential spatial access to the ground-truthed food environment in a large rural area. *J Nutr*. 2008;138(3):620–627.
6. U.S. House of Representatives Select Committee on Hunger. Obtaining Food: Shopping Constraints of the Poor. In: Washington, DC: Government Printing Office; 1987.
7. McMillan T. Can Whole Foods change the way poor people eat? *Slate*. November 19, 2014.
8. NYCEDC. La Marqueta. 2020; https://edc.nyc/la-marqueta. Accessed December 15, 2020.

9. The National Academies of Science Engineering and Medicine. Overview of the U.S. food system. In: Nesheim MC, Oria M, Yih PT, eds. *A Framework for Assessing the Effect of the Food System.* Washington, DC: The National Academies Press; June 17, 2015:31–79.

10. Economic Research Services. New Products. 2020; www.ers.usda.gov/topics/food-markets-prices/processing-marketing/new-products/. Accessed December 22, 2020.

11. Watts L. Processed Food History: 1910–1950. 2021; https://modernpioneermom.com/2012/07/05/processed-foods-history-1910s-to-1950s/. Accessed March 19, 2021.

12. Cullen MJ. About King Kullen. www.kingkullen.com/about-us/. Accessed December 15, 2020.

13. SupermarketPage.com. Supermarkets in the United States. 2021; https://supermarketpage.com. Accessed March 19, 2021.

14. U.S. Census Bureau. NIACS Codes. 2020; www.census.gov/programs-surveys/economic-census/guidance/understanding-naics.html. Accessed December 17, 2020.

15. Food Retail World. Food Retail Definitions and Terminology. www.foodretailworld.com/Definitions.htm. Accessed March 19, 2021.

16. U.S. Census Bureau. The North America Industry Classification System (NAICS). 2021; www.census.gov/naics/. Accessed March 19, 2021.

17. The Food Industry Association. Food Industry Glossary. 2021; www.fmi.org/our-research/food-industry-glossary. Accessed March 19, 2021.

18. Haddon H, Nassauer S. Getting your product on the shelves at Whole Foods just got harder. *The Wall Street Journal.* February 8, 2018.

19. Scrape Hero a Data Company. How Many Products Does Kroger.com Sell. 2020; www.scrapehero.com. Accessed January 5, 2021.

20. Wikipedia.org. Walmart. 2021; https://en.m.wikipedia.org/wiki/Walmart#Walmart_Supercenter. Accessed January 5, 2021.

21. Wikipedia.com. Trader Joe's. 2021; https://en.m.wikipedia.org/wiki/Trader_Joe%27s. Accessed January 5, 2021.

22. Siedenburg K, Sandoval BA, Wooten H, Laurison HB, Johnson-Piett J. *Healthy Corner Stores.* February 2010.

23. FMI. Supermarket Facts. 2020; www.fmi.org/our-research/supermarket-facts. Accessed December 15, 2020.

24. Taylor M. These Beloved Grocery Stores Are Gone Forever. 2020; https://blog.cheapism.com/grocery-stores-we-still-miss/. Accessed December 23, 2020.

25. Lazare L. How Dominick's lost its way in Chicago. *Chicago Business Journal.* October 11, 2013.

26. Statista. Leading Food and Grocery Retailers in 2019. www.statista.com/topics/1660/food retail. Accessed April 8, 2020.

27. IBIS World. Supermarkets & Grocery Stores. 2020; www.ibisworld.com/industry-statistis/number-of-businesses/supermarkets-grocery-stores-united-states/. Accessed December 24, 2020.

28. Food Marketing Institute. *Competition and Profits.* 2008.

29. Watch FW. Consolidation and Buying Power in the Grocery Industry. 2010; www.foodandwaterwatch.org/insight/consolidation-and-buyer-power-grocery-industry. Accessed December 22, 2020.

30. Okrent AM, Alston JM. *The Demand for Disaggregated Food-Away-From-Home and Food-at-Home Products in the United States.* Washington, DC: U.S. Department of Agriculture; 2012.

31. Stewart H, Blisard N, Joliffe D. *Let's Eat Out: Americans Weigh Taste, Convenience and Nutrition.* Washington, DC: U.S. Department of Agriculture; 2006.

32. Lin BH, Frazao E, Guthrie J. *Away from Home Foods Increasingly Important to Quality of American Diet.* Washington, DC: U.S. Department of Agriculture; 1999.

33. Technomics. *Trends in Healthier Eating and Fruit and Vegetable Use in Chain Restaurants.* Wilmington, DE: Produce for Better Health Foundation; 2006.

34. Economic Research Services. *A Revised and Expanded Food Dollar Series: A Better Understanding of Our Food Costs.* Washington, DC: U.S. Department of Agriculture; 2011.

35. Lehmann Y. Bill Green Interview. October 30, 2020.

36. Redman R. Trader Joe's Tops Whole Foods in Nearby Home Values. 2020; www.supermarketnews.com/retail-financial/trader-joe-s-tops-whole-foods-nearby-home-values. Accessed December 24, 2020.

37. Economic Research Services. *Food Price and Spending*. Washington, DC: U.S. Department of Agriculture; 2020.
38. Singh M. Why a Philadelphia Grocery Chain Is Thriving in Food Deserts. 2015; www.npr.org/sections/thesalt/2015/05/14/406476968/why-one-grocery-chain-is-thriving-in-philadelphias-food-deserts. Accessed December 17, 2020.
39. PBS News Hour. Building an Oasis in a Philadelphia Food Desert. August 7, 2015; www.pbs.org/newshour/show/building-oasis-philadelphia-food-desert. Accessed April 20, 2021.
40. Anderson AR. The ghetto marketing life cycle: A case of the underachievement. *Journal of Market Research*. 1978;15:20–28.
41. Cotterill RW, Franklin AW. *The Urban Grocery Store Gap*. Mansfield, CT: University of Connecticut Food Marketing Policy Center; 1995.
42. U.S. House of Representatives Select Committee on Hunger. Urban Grocery Gap. In: Washington, DC: Government Printing Office; 1992.
43. Pothukuchi K. Attracting supermarkets to inner city neighborhoods: Economic development outside of the box. *Economic Development Quarterly*. 2005;19:232–244.
44. Zenk SN, Schulz AJ, Israel BA, James SA, Bao S, Wilson ML. Neighborhood racial composition, neighborhood poverty, and the spatial accessibility of supermarkets in metropolitan Detroit. *Am J Public Health*. 2005;95(4):660–667.
45. Baker EA, Schootman M, Barnidge E, Kelly C. The role of race and poverty in access to foods that enable individuals to adhere to dietary guidelines. *Prev Chronic Dis*. 2006;3(3):A76.
46. Block JP, Scribner RA, DeSalvo KB. Fast food, race/ethnicity, and income: A geographic analysis. *Am J Prev Med*. 2004;27(3):211–217.
47. Moore LV, Diez Roux AV. Associations of neighborhood characteristics with the location and type of food stores. *Am J Public Health*. 2006;96(2):325–331.
48. Morland K, Filomena S. Disparities in the availability of fruits and vegetables between racially segregated urban neighborhoods. *Public Health Nutr*. 2007;10(12):1481–1489.
49. Powell LM, Slater S, Mirtcheva D, Bao Y, Chaloupka FJ. Food store availability and neighborhood characteristics in the United States. *Prev Med*. 2007;44(3):189–195.
50. Filomena S, Scanlin K, Morland KB. Brooklyn, New York foodscape 2007–2011: A five-year analysis of stability in food retail environments. *Int J Behav Nutr Phys Act*. 2013;10:46.
51. Sloane DC, Diamant AL, Lewis LB, et al. Improving the nutritional resource environment for healthy living through community-based participatory research. *J Gen Intern Med*. 2003;18(7):568–575.
52. Jetter KM, Cassady DL. The availability and cost of healthier food alternatives. *Am J Prev Med*. 2006;30(1):38–44.
53. Lewis LB, Sloane DC, Nascimento LM, et al. African Americans' access to healthy food options in South Los Angeles restaurants. *Am J Public Health*. 2005;95(4):668–673.
54. Horowitz CR, Colson KA, Hebert PL, Lancaster K. Barriers to buying healthy foods for people with diabetes: Evidence of environmental disparities. *Am J Public Health*. 2004;94(9):1549–1554.
55. Algert SJ, Agrawal A, Lewis DS. Disparities in access to fresh produce in low-income neighborhoods in Los Angeles. *Am J Prev Med*. 2006;30(5):365–370.
56. Hosler AS, Varadarajulu D, Ronsani AE, Fredrick BL, Fisher BD. Low-fat milk and high-fiber bread availability in food stores in urban and rural communities. *J Public Health Manag Pract*. 2006;12(6):556–562.
57. Fisher BD, Strogatz DS. Community measures of low-fat milk consumption: Comparing store shelves with households. *American Journal of Public Health*. 1999;89:235–237.
58. Cole S, Filomena S, Morland K. Analysis of fruit and vegetable cost and quality among racially segregated neighborhoods in Brooklyn, New York. *Journal of Hunger and Environmental Nutrition*. 2010;5:202–215.
59. Hayes RA. Are prices higher for the poor in New York City? *Journal of Consumer Policy*. 2000;23:127–152.
60. Munoz-Plaza CE, Filomena S, Morland K. Disparities in food access: Inner city residents describe their local food environment. *Journal of Hunger and Environmental Nutrition*. 2008;2:51–64.
61. Economic Research Services. Access to Affordable and Nutritious Foods: Measuring and Understanding Food Deserts and Their Consequences. U.S. Department of Agriculture; June, 2009.

62. Rhone A, Ver Ploeg M, Dicken C, Williams R, Breneman V. Low-Income and Low-Supermarket-Access Census Tracts, 2010–2015. U.S. Department of Agriculture; January 2017.
63. United States Department of Agriculture. Retailer Eligibility-Clarification of Criterion A and Criterion B. In: Washington, DC: Food and Nutrition Service; 2017.
64. United States Department of Agriculture. *SNAP Retailers: Fiscal Year 2020 Year End Summary*. Washington, DC: Food and Nutrition Service; 2021.

3 Federal Food Retail Policies and Programs

CONTENTS

INTRODUCTION

The purpose of this chapter is to describe the U.S. federal public policies and programs that have aimed to invest in low-income communities, both currently and historically, and how lawmakers aimed to connect the Healthy Food Financing Initiative to these existing programs. Lawmakers have acknowledged that redlining bank practices have resulted in a disinvestment of many low-income neighborhoods, preventing these communities from benefiting from resources and services provided in other neighborhoods. Advocacy groups such as the West Coast Regional Office of Consumers Union in San Francisco compared the presence of basic goods and services between three Los Angeles neighborhoods and four neighborhoods of Oakland, California, in the 1990s.[1] The report compared neighborhoods in terms of affordable housing, quality foods, health care, as well as banking and credit needs and documented disparities between low- and middle-income neighborhoods. The authors conclude that the 'Redline of economic discrimination extends throughout the low-income consumer infrastructure, with dramatic effects on low-income consumers and their neighborhoods'. It was argued that, because low-income consumers spend their money for goods and services outside their immediate neighborhood, termed retail leakage, these local areas also miss opportunities for economic growth, which then perpetuates a cycle of redlining and poor credit for businesses within these neighborhoods.

Beginning in the 1990s, the federal government has developed programs aimed to address disparities in access to basic resources among underserved areas across the United States, such as those described by the West Coast Regional Consumer Union office of San Francisco. These programs aim to provide the necessary incentives for corporations and small businesses to locate and operate in low-income areas. Among the goods and services not received in redlined areas are grocery stores. The disparities in the locations of grocery stores are discussed in Chapter 2; however federal assessment of supermarket disparities began nearly two decades after these revitalization programs were funded. It was during the Obama administration that policymakers aimed to connect food retailing to the existing revitalization programs.

DOI: 10.1201/9781003029151-4

The Healthy Food Financing Initiative (HFFI) is a federal program initiated during the Obama administration with leadership from senior nutrition policy advisor Sam Kass and First Lady Michelle Obama.

In the end, as First Lady, this isn't just a policy issue for me. This is a passion. This is my mission. I am determined to work with folks across this country to change the way a generation of kids thinks about food and nutrition.

– First Lady Michelle Obama[2]

After launching her Let's Move! campaign to prevent childhood obesity in 2010, she hired White House assistant chef, Sam Kass, to be its executive director. In this new role, Kass, looking for local, innovative programs that improved access to healthy food and could be scaled to the federal level, saw potential in the Pennsylvania Fresh Food Financing Initiative.

A year earlier, in July 2009, Sam Kass attended a White House event hosted in Philadelphia, the first stop of a 'National Conversation on Urban and Metropolitan America' organized by the Obama administration. The Philadelphia event, led by Adolfo Carrion, Director of the White House Office of Urban Affairs included Cabinet Secretaries Tom Vilsack, Department of Agriculture and Gary Locke, Department of Commerce; and Ron Sims, Deputy Secretary of the Department of Housing and Urban Development. The focus of the event was to learn more about the development of Pennsylvania's Fresh Food Financing Initiative (FFFI) and efforts to encourage supermarket development in urban areas. Kass and others were impressed with FFFI and saw the program as a prime example of the type of collaborative partnership and innovative thinking needed in urban and metropolitan communities across the nation.[3]

Kass soon decided that Philadelphia would be the perfect location for the official launch of Let's Move! along with the announcement of the creation of the Healthy Food Financing Initiative, a new federal program modeled after Pennsylvania's FFFI. On February 22, 2010, Mrs. Obama paid a visit to The Fresh Grocer at Progress Plaza, one of the first FFFI projects – to the great surprise of food shoppers that day. Later, at a local public school, she was accompanied by the U.S. Treasury Secretary Tim Geithner and USDA Secretary Tom Vilsack in announcing that the Obama administration had approved $400 million to create a program (HFFI) to bring grocery stores and other healthy food retailers to underserved urban and rural communities. 'What Pennsylvania has shown us is, if we provide the right incentives, people will invest in these neighborhoods', said Mrs. Obama. 'We want to replicate your success in Pennsylvania all over America'.

This HFFI program was structured to gain resources not only from the USDA Farm Bill, but also from the existing revitalization programs funded through the United States Treasury Department and the United States Department of Health and Human Services. This chapter will describe the programs and infrastructure within these three departments that supports the revitalization of underserved areas and how Community Development Financial Institutions (CDFIs) play a central role in providing capital for local food environment projects.

U.S. PUBLIC POLICIES AIMED TO REVITALIZE LOW-INCOME AREAS

REVITALIZATION ZONES

Several programs have been supported by Congress since the 1990s with an aim to support underserved areas. These programs have changed names, eligibility criteria, and incentives for business owners over time, but the purpose of all the programs have been to draw private corporation to underserved areas. The five different programs are described as follows:

Empowerment Zones (EZs) were introduced in 1993 by the Congress to provide incentives for corporations and government entities to conduct business in distressed communities. The aim of this program was to improve neighborhood economic vitality and provide employment to residents of these communities. Funding for EZs was distributed through local, tribal, and state governments who first needed to apply to be designated as an EZ. Once federally recognized, businesses located in designated EZ areas were then eligible to receive federal grants and tax incentives. Congress authorized the first round of funding to EZs in the Omnibus Budget Reconciliation Act of 1993 and has been funded since with the Taxpayer Relief Act of 1997 and the Consolidated Appropriations Act of 2001. Businesses that operated in EZs qualify for a variety of tax incentives including (a) a tax credit of up to $3,000 per year for each of its employees who resides in the EZ; (b) a Work Opportunity Tax Credit for hiring 18–39-year-old residents of the EZ; (c) a deduction of $35,000 for the cost of eligible equipment purchases under section 179 of the Internal Revenue Code of 1986; and (d) tax exempt private purpose 'EZ Facility bonds' for commercial development. The 111th Congress extended Empowerment Zone tax incentives through December 31, 2011, after which this program no longer existed. During the program implementation however, evaluators found that within EZs, job growth accelerated, there were more EZ resident-owned and minority owned businesses, and approximately 16,000 jobs were created.[4] However, there were concerns about the causal relationships drawn between the program implementation and impact on the targeted communities due to an economic upswing during the time of the evaluation and choice of comparison groups.[5] Nevertheless, reports from the IRS indicate that the programs were well utilized. For example, during 1995–2001, corporations and individuals claimed approximately $251 million in EZ employment credits, and an additional $351 million were dispersed in tax-exempt bonds to businesses located in EZs.[6]

Enterprise Communities (ECs) and Renewal Communities (RCs) which had similar goals of revitalizing area by attracting businesses but offered different incentives.

Promise Zones (PZs) were selected in areas with high levels of poverty by the Obama administration. From 2014 to 2016, 22 PZs were selected to receive federal support for revitalization projects.[7] Unlike EZs, ECs, and RCs, there were no fiscal incentives legislated by Congress for PZs; rather, businesses located in PZs could receive technical assistance from the federal government.

Opportunity Zones (OZs) were initiated by the Trump administration and also aimed to bring investment into economically distressed, predominately urban areas.[8] This program aims to entice Americans to invest their capital gains into low-income areas. Capital gains are profits made by the sale of an investment, such as property, stocks, or other assets. Areas are deemed OZs by state governors and are low-income areas or adjacent to low-income areas in predominately urban cities like Birmingham, AL or Baltimore, MD. These areas have historically lacked capital and therefore private venture capital appeals to investors.[9] Investors in OZ are provided tax incentives to defer up to seven years of capital gains taxes, and if the investment is sold after ten years, taxes on profits are forgiven.[10] Eligible businesses must conduct most of their business in OZs, but there are no other restrictions to the program. This program was initially legislated through modifications to the 2017 U.S. tax code, which was then finalized in late 2019,[9] documenting that the amount of capital gains a stakeholder can invest is limitless.

There are currently more than 8,700 OZs, which are designated census tracts where at least a third of the population is living in poverty. Census tracts are geographic boundaries that are smaller than zip codes and contain approximately 3,000–5,000 people. The current OZs are estimated to contain over thirty million poor Americans. Thus far, the program has attracted predominately real estate investors with more projects for hotels than low-income housing or supermarkets. The program has been criticized that OZs do not appear to be in low-income census tracts. OZ advocates argue that projects may not target the lowest-income areas, but rationalize that these capital investments in the nearby regions will allow more public resources to be available for adjacent needy areas, and hence the program benefits low-income residents indirectly.[9] A second criticism of the program is the lack of transparency of the types of projects funded and no formal evaluation of the program. There is concern the program may not be providing low-income residents with additional jobs or the commerce (such as supermarkets) that are needed to support the local community. Instead, critics claim, the program is simply accelerating gentrification in low-income and minority neighborhoods.[10]

COMMUNITY DEVELOPMENT FINANCIAL INSTITUTIONS (CDFI) FUND

In addition to developing empowerment zones, the Clinton administration developed another fund that has supported underserved areas for the past thirty years. The 103rd Congress passed the Riegle Community Development and Regulatory Improvement Act of 1994, which supports the Community Development Financial Institutions (CDFI) fund. The purpose of the CDFI Fund is to promote economic development in low-income communities through access to basic financial services, affordable credit, and investment in capital. This legislation was in response to an earlier act (the Community Reinvestment Act (CRA) of 1977), which was intended to require commercial banks to serve their entire service area and was not being enforced.

President Clinton was familiar with the redlining practices of banks as well as the lack of enforcement of the CRA in the southern U.S. when he was governor of Arkansas.[11] At that time, President Clinton borrowed practices used by the South Shore Bank of Chicago to model the Southern Development Bancorporation, which was established in 2003, with a mission to revitalize rural economies of the Delta communities. Southern Development Bancorporation is the second largest CDFI, funding more than $520 million worth of development loans and is the largest rural CDFI in the United States. CDFIs are lending institutions, like traditional banks, but have been developed to lend money to economically disadvantaged communities for start-up businesses or to commercial borrowers that would not qualify for conventional bank loans.

This lack of affordable credit and capital in low-income communities began far earlier in U.S. history than the Clinton administration. In fact, in the beginning part of the last century, minority-owned banks opened in low-income areas to provide needed financial services in segregated neighborhoods discriminated against by traditional banks. More recently, credit unions formed, followed by community development corporations that began in the 1960s and 1970s and then nonprofit loan funds in the 1980s. The CDFI Fund is the federal response to promoting economic development in low-income communities through access to basic financial services, affordable credit, and investment in capital; it is a direct response to commercial banks not responding to the credit needs of their entire service area. The CDFI Fund is housed in the U.S. Treasury Department, where it continues to provide funding to CDFIs through its programs that offer grants, loans, and equity investment for projects intended to support the economic growth of disenfranchised neighborhoods served by the specific bank, credit union, or other financial institution. There are currently 1,137 certified CDFIs in all fifty states as well as the District of Columbia, Puerto Rico, and Guam. A list of all the CDFI certified financial institutions by city and state can be found at www.cdfifund.gov.

Reco Owens, the executive director of a CDFI, called *Neighborhood Progress Fund*, commented about the lack of financial resources:

> [I]t all comes down to poverty. Poverty is something [where] . . . you're not just financially constrained, you're isolated in society, and everything is connected. Schools are funded by tax dollars. The value of property is lower, available tax dollars are lower, and schools are worse. And this is a direct line to redlining.[12]

The CDFI Fund aims to promote local economic growth to distressed American neighbor-hoods through assistance with the following programs:[13]

- *New Markets Tax Credit (NMTC) Program*, which allows tax credits to Community Development Entities that provide funding to the private sector investing in low-income communities.

- *Bank Enterprise Award Program* by providing an incentive to banks to invest in their communities and in other CDFIs.

- *CDFI Bond Guarantee Program* by issuing bonds to support CDFIs that make invest-ments for eligible community or economic development purposes.

- *Capital Magnet Fund*, which offers competitively awarded grants to finance affordable housing solutions for low-income people and low-income communities nationwide.

Since its creation, the CDFI Fund has awarded over $3.9 billion to community development organizations and financial institutions; it has awarded allocations of NMTCs to attract private-sector investments totaling $61 billion, including $1 billion of special allocation authority used for the recovery and redevelopment of the Gulf Opportunity Zone, and has guaranteed more than $1.7 billion in bonds through the CDFI Bond Guarantee Program. The economic impact of the CDFI Fund program has been seen through the reinvestment of infrastructure, the cre-ation of jobs, and financial literacy. For example, in 2017, $5 billion in financing was provided to homeowners, businesses, and commercial and residential real estate developments through this program. This financing contributed to more than 4,000 jobs; more than 300 affordable housing units; 8.3 million square feet of commercial real estate, and nearly 500 businesses receiving financial counseling or other services. As of 2013, the CDFI Fund has also focused on improvements to food environments. For example, in 2015 the CDFI Fund awarded $22 million in HFFI financial assistance to CDFIs, which used the funding to finance businesses providing healthy foods.

New Markets Tax Credit (NMTC) Program

One of the CDFI programs that has been used extensively to fund HFFI projects is the NMTC program and is therefore described in more detail here. The U.S. government authorized the NMTC Program to incentivize businesses to locate in low-income underserved areas.[14] The NMTC Program is one of the programs offered with the CDFI Fund that has been central to the success of the HFFI. The way the program works is that Congress authorizes an amount of credit annually. Then U.S. Department of Treasury allocates the funds through a competitive application process with participating Community Development Entities (CDEs).[15] Most CDEs participating in this program are CDFIs or mainstream financial institutions (73%), although gov-ernment, nonprofit, and for-profit institutions have also become certified to receive awards from the CDFI Fund. Like CDFIs, CDEs provide allocations to businesses investing in low-income areas. Then investors are eligible for tax credits against their federal tax obligation. Typically, CDEs must invest at least 85% of their qualified equity investments in qualified low-income com-munity investments to be eligible for the program. Approved projects must be in highly distressed areas of the United States, of which 43% of the United States qualify. These qualified businesses, called *Qualified Active Low-Income Community Businesses* (QALICBs), benefit from the NMTC through the CDEs. QALICBs can be any type of business. However most businesses participating in this program are for-profit (69%) and range from start-up companies to businesses with annual gross revenue up to $7 billion. Although fourteen different industries have participated in the program, most of the businesses supported have been retail, manufacturing, and food process-ing. The NMTC program is flexible, allowing for funding to be used for a variety of expenditures, including but not limited to the following: equipment, operations, and real estate.

The NMTCs investors are given the incentive of a seven-year tax benefit on the cash value of the investment and on average, the NMTC decreases the amount of equity the owner must contribute to the project by 20%–25%, making this program a powerful financing tool for supermarket owners wanting to locate in a new underserved market. In addition to program requirements regarding location in underserved areas and length of time in business (seven years, after which time a balloon payment is due), there are other complexities to the NMTC program. For example, because NMTC federal documentation may not be familiar to investors with commercial loans, added costs for attorneys and CPA time are likely to be needed. Hence, NMTC may work best for large projects (e.g., $5 million or more) because these additional costs become a smaller proportion of the larger projects.

The NMTC program is a utilized federal program. For example, the Reinvestment Fund (a CDFI) allocated $8 million in NMTC to supermarket projects alone during the first round of awards from the United States Treasury Department. Since the enactment of the Community Renewal and Tax Relief Act (P.L. 106–551) in 2001, where $15 billion was allocated by Congress, the NMTC has been reauthorized seven times, demonstrating the bipartisan support of the program and its use by investors.[16] The NMTC program costs roughly $1.4 billion per year and has supported over 5,000 projects across the United States with roughly $27 billion of tax credits since its inception. The program was reauthorized by Congress on December 22, 2020 as part of the FY21 government funding bill and will extend for 5 years, until December 2025.

U.S. PUBLIC POLICIES AIMED TO ATTRACT SUPERMARKETS TO UNDERSERVED AREAS

HEALTHY FOOD FINANCING INITIATIVE (HFFI)

In February of 2010, First Lady Michelle Obama arrived in Philadelphia to kick off her Let's Move! campaign and announce the Obama administration's commitment to reducing the disparities in access to food retailers across the nation. The Healthy Food Financing Initiative (HFFI) is the first federal program to address food retail specifically, and it is modeled on the Pennsylvania Fresh Food Financing Initiative (FFFI), which is described in Chapter 4. Briefly, the PA FFFI was seeded with a $30 million investment by the state of Pennsylvania to attract supermarket owners to locate stores in low-income, underserved neighborhoods. In total, the PA FFFI has funded food retail projects which have resulted in the placement of eighty-eight food markets in underserved communities across the state.

The Obama administration created an intradepartmental funding platform to support the first federal program that addressed limited food retailers in low-income neighborhoods. The Healthy Food Financing Initiative (HFFI) initially was funded through existing programs within three federal departments: Treasury, Health and Human Services, Agriculture. On September 14, 2011, the Department of the Treasury announced that twelve CDFIs were awarded a total of $25 million, which is to be made available to food retail businesses through the HFFI.[11] Later in 2013, additional formal federal legislation was passed in order to solidify the earlier commitment.

Department of the Treasury

The Department of Treasury will support projects using discretionary funds that aim to strengthen, expand, and innovate within the food retail supply chain. Grant and tax benefits are available to assist many types of organizations that require capital for ventures with the goal to process, distribute, aggregate, market, and/or sell healthy, fresh, and affordable foods to underserved communities and markets. Tax credits and grant funds are available for corporations and other organizations by working with regional CDFIs.[17] These programs are discussed in the earlier section of this chapter, including the reinvestment zones and program within the CDFI Fund. As stated in the CDFI fund HFFI fact sheet:

> The businesses supported by CDFIs with these funds may take many forms, including grocery stores, farmers markets, bodegas, food co-ops, and urban farms. They may work on the production, distribution, or retail aspects of the business cycle. Most importantly, however, they are often the single source of fresh produce or organic products for an entire neighborhood, a vital resource to which the CDFI Fund is committed.[24]

Department of Health and Human Services

The Department of Health and Human Services supported the HFFI legislation through the Community Economic Development Program within the Office of Community Services. Federal grants through this program supported employment and commercial development projects designed to provide economic self-sufficiency to low-income individuals and their communities. Projects included the development of grocery stores, farmers markets, and other sources of fresh nutritious food for underserved communities. These funds were provided to organizations that are considered Community Development Corporations (CDCs). CDCs are organizations that have a third-party board of directors that includes residents of the community served, local business, and civic leaders whose purpose is planning, developing, or managing low-income housing or community development projects.[18] The HHS component of the FFFI was an initial carve out (i.e., program dollars were carved out from other established programs for this purpose) used in 2011 and again in 2016 as a mechanism to bolster program resources, but since that time has largely been replaced by the USDA's permanently authorized program as well as the resources provided by the Department of the Treasury.

The program was funded by the Office of Community Services at the HHS Administration for Children and Families and in 2016 announced plans to award $7.4 million to eleven community-based organization to address the lack of healthy affordable foods in low-income neighborhoods.[19] This grant program allowed local, nonprofit and community development corporations to apply for as much as $800,000 to improve access to healthy foods in low-income areas. Allowable costs include the development of businesses that increase access to healthy foods for these communities, for example, grocery stores, farmers markets, and food distribution businesses. While exact outcomes are not yet published, funds were used to create thirty-eight food retail business and 347 full-time jobs whereby 271 of those jobs were to be filled by low-income community members. The grant program aimed to leverage an additional $121.3 million in public and private funds. Since 2011, the CED-HFFI has awarded $51.89 million in grant funding; however funds were not added to this aspect of the program between 2016 and 2021.

Department of Agriculture

The United States Department of Agriculture (USDA) supports the HFFI through discretionary funds legislated through Title XI of the Farm Bill of 2018. These discretionary funds (e.g., $5 million in 2020) are dispersed to one CDFI called the *Reinvestment Fund*. The Reinvestment Fund also dispersed state funds for the Fresh Food Financing Initiative (FFFI) in Pennsylvania. To gain access to these funds, food retailers may gain a Request for Applications (RFA), which are available annually through the Reinvestment Fund's website by using the following link: www.investinginfood.com. Information regarding the most current RFA, called *America's Healthy Food Financing Initiative Targeted Small Grants Program (HFFI TSG Program)*, has allocated $3 million for the 2021 fiscal year.[20] The Reinvestment Fund is looking to support projects aiming to strengthen, expand, and innovate the food retail supply chain. The funds from the USDA support a wide range of projects that may impact underserved communities, including those that require capital to process, distribute, or sell healthy, fresh, and affordable foods. Projects need to demonstrate they are targeting underserved areas, which is defined as a geographic area where residents have limited access to affordable healthy foods, a high rate of hunger or food insecurity, and/or a high poverty rate. For the purposes of the TSG program, the full definition is detailed in the RFA and related to the low-income/low-access definitions provided in the U.S. Department of Agriculture Food Access Research Atlas. Grant awards between $20,000 and $200,000 are made available to for-profit business enterprises, tax-exempt non-profit corporations, higher education institutions, and other organizations. The process for applying for funds requires a letter of intent from the organization, which is reviewed by program staff at the Reinvestment Fund and if approved, the organization will be asked to submit a full application.

The Agricultural Adjustment Act (the Farm Bill)

The Agricultural Adjustment Act from Franklin D. Roosevelt (discussed in Chapter 1) continues to govern the U.S. food system and is known more commonly as the Farm Bill. This legislation is passed by Congress approximately every five years, and costs are budgeted for mandatory programs (such as the SNAP program). Other programs are authorized to receive discretionary funds (also called appropriated funds) through this legislation. Unlike mandatory funds that are set aside by the USDA to ensure that specific Farm Bill programs can be executed, appropriated funds are made available by Congress through the federal budget.

The Farm Bill of 2014

The USDA required that the allocation of department funds to the HFFI must be incorporated into the Farm Bill. The HFFI was brought to the 113th Congress by Senator Kristen Gillibrand on April 25, 2013. This bill aimed to attract investment in underserved communities by providing grant and loan financing. This was designed to help businesses involved in retailing food to make investments in healthy foods availability for low-income communities with limited access to supermarkets. The legislation was supported by seven other senators. The purpose was:[21]

> to establish a program to improve access to healthy foods in underserved areas, to create and preserve quality jobs, and to revitalize low-income communities by providing loans and grants to eligible healthy food retailers to overcome the higher costs and initial barriers to entry in underserved, urban, suburban, and rural areas.

The legislation was justified by Congress (S.821, section 2):

> Developing high-quality fresh food retail outlets creates jobs, expands markets for agricultural producers in the United States, advances health, and supports economic vitality in underserved communities. Model programs in several States and cities (including the States of California, Illinois, New York, and Pennsylvania and the city of New Orleans) have shown success in creating public/private-partnerships that leverage millions in private capital and grant funds to establish successful retail outlets in low-income underserved communities. As a result of those programs, thousands of jobs have been developed, hundreds of thousands of people are gaining access to healthy food, and sustainable businesses have been developed. Despite those successes, more than 25,000,000 people in the United States live in low-income communities with very limited access to supermarkets, grocery stores, and healthy food. With an increasing demand for fresh local foods, regional food hubs are rapidly expanding, with well over 200 food hubs operating in the United States as of the date of enactment of this Act. Regional food hubs are part of a growing local food system that strengthens rural economies by lowering entry barriers and improving infrastructure to establish, as well as expand, regional food markets. Many food hubs are designed to move locally produced food into underserved communities. Supermarkets and

grocery stores often face barriers to opening stores in communities with very limited access to healthy food, also known as food deserts. The supermarket industry operates on a historically thin profit margin. According to the 2011 National Grocers Association Independent Grocers Survey, the average net profit margin before taxes for independent grocers in 2010 was 1.08%. Urban operators face barriers, including (i) increased real estate costs or limited availability of suitable commercial real estate in the community; (ii) increased employee training needs and costs; (iii) elevated security expenses; and (iv) often zoning restrictions. Supermarkets and grocery stores in rural food deserts also face barriers, including increased food delivery costs due to distance from distributers, dispersed customer base, and low volume. The United States faces an obesity epidemic in which 30.5 percent of children ages 10 through 17 are overweight or obese. The obesity epidemic contributes to increasing rates of chronic illness, including diabetes, heart disease, and cancer. The obesity epidemic cost the United States $147,000,000 in medical expenses in 2008, and this cost is expected to rise in the future. More than 170 studies show that access to healthy food is particularly a problem in hundreds of low-income, rural, and urban communities, as well as communities of color in the United States. The opportunity to access healthy food is linked to lower levels of obesity, diabetes, and other food-related chronic illnesses, leading to better health outcomes. Children from low-income families are twice as likely to be overweight as children from higher income families. African American and Hispanic children are more likely than Caucasian children to be obese. Studies show that when healthy foods are available, people will increase consumption of fruits and vegetables. Leading public health experts, including the Centers for Disease Control and Prevention, the American Heart Association, the Institute of Medicine, and the American Public Health Association agree that providing improved access to supermarkets and grocery stores is needed to improve public health and prevent obesity. Access to affordable capital is a significant problem for rural and urban supermarkets, grocery stores, regional food hubs, farmers markets, and healthy food retail business enterprises. By providing seed capital and technical assistance, the Federal Government, through time-limited investments, can attract private sector investment to create and retain much-needed jobs; and provide long-term, sustainable solutions to the decades-old problem of limited access to healthy food in underserved, low-income urban and rural communities. With legislation establishing a national fund modeled on successful programs in Pennsylvania and other States and localities will help create much needed jobs and economic revitalization, address an important part of the obesity epidemic, and solve the healthy food access problem in hundreds of communities across the United States.[21]

The 2014 Farm Bill authorized the HFFI at the USDA at up to $125 million, but the program did not receive any mandatory funding, and the first appropriated dollars for HFFI were distributed beginning in 2017 in the amount of $1 million.

Farm Bill of 2018

Congress has since passed the Farm Bill of 2018 reauthorizing and expanding the national HFFI within the current Farm Bill. The new bill expands on HFFI investment beyond retail food enterprises to also support job growth in communities with access to food stores. The HFFI Act of 2018 aims to have a direct nutritional benefit to residents of underserved areas, but the expanded HFFI views healthy food retail to have an even greater reach on the economic health and well-being of communities. By revitalizing struggling business districts, healthy food businesses help to create jobs across the food system, increase or stabilize home values in nearby neighborhoods, generate local tax revenues, provide workforce training and development, and promote additional spending in the local economy. Creating supermarkets is seen as a central part of revitalization of underserved communities and therefore this legislation has sought to impact multiple levels that may reduce disenfranchisement of a low-income community.

The HFFI Reauthorization Act of 2018 (H.R.5017, 115th Congress 2017–2018) was sponsored by Marcia L. Fudge (D-Ohio), Dwight Evans (D-PA), and Barbara Lee (D-CA) who introduced it to the House of Representatives on February 14, 2018 and then was referred to the subcommittee on Nutrition and the House Committee on Agriculture.[22] The bill is an amendment of the Department of Agriculture's Reorganization Act of 1994, which has reauthorized and modified the HFFI. The initiative authorizes the Department of Agriculture to provide financial and technical assistance to food retailers, including supermarkets, farmers markets, food hubs, and others to improve access to healthy food in underserved U.S. communities. As stated earlier, this legislation has a further reach than simply attracting supermarket owners to low-income communities. The legislation aims to build the economic vitality of distress economies by bringing food stores and other businesses that supply healthy foods to these areas of the United States. The legislation intends to not only improve access to healthy foods in underserved communities, but also create quality jobs for residents and improve the economic status of low-income areas with successful commerce. Specifically, the H.R. 5107 of the 115th Congress states the purposes of the initiative includes:

> improving access to, and expanding the supply of, healthy food in low-income, underserved communities; creating and preserving quality jobs and businesses; revitalizing distressed rural, urban, and small town economies; supporting the development of local and regional food systems; increasing the distribution of locally produced agricultural products; and strengthening farm-to-consumer relationships.[22]

HFFI discretionary funds were distributed the following total amounts per year: 2018 ($1 million); 2019 ($2 million) and 2020 ($5 million).

Other USDA Programs. There are additional programs unrelated to the HFFI that support healthy foods for communities in need. Those programs are listed as follows.

- *Community Facilities Program* provides low-interest direct loans and grants for land acquisition, professional fees, and purchase of equipment in the development or support of local food systems such as community gardens, food pantries, community kitchens, food banks, food hubs, or greenhouses. These funds are intended to support rural areas including cities, villages, townships, and towns as well as federally recognized tribal lands with no more than 20,000 residents. This program prioritizes small communities of 5,500 residents or less.[23]

- *Farmers Market Promotion Program* provides federal grants to support the development, promotion, and expansion of direct, producer-to-consumer marketing and consumption of local and regionally produced agricultural products. The program will support organizations that are domestic agricultural businesses and cooperatives, Community Supported Agriculture (CSA) networks and associations, food councils, economic development corporations, local governments, nonprofit and public benefit corporations, producer networks or associations, regional farmers market authorities, and tribal governments.[24]

- *Community Food Projects Competitive Grants Program* provides grant funds ranging from $35,000 to $400,000 to support community food and planning projects. This program is designed to create community-based food projects with objectives, activities, and outcomes that are in alignment with Community Food Projects Competitive Grants Program (CFPCGP). The purpose of a Planning Project (PP) is to complete a plan toward the improvement of community food security in keeping with the primary goals of the CFPCGP. PPs are to focus on a defined community and describe in detail the activities and outcomes of the planning project. Public food program service providers as well as tribal organizations and private nonprofit businesses are encouraged to apply.[25]

CONCLUSION

Overall, through the three departments, the Healthy Food Financing Initiative has invested $220 million in grants and loans to more than 35 states with the mission to improve access to healthy foods, create and preserve jobs, and revitalize communities. The program's public-private partnership has enabled recipients to receive funds and leverage over $1 billion in additional resources to expand nearly 1,000 healthy food businesses such as supermarkets, grocery stores, farmers markets, co-ops, and other enterprises that increase the supply of healthy foods in under-served rural and urban communities.[26]

The HFFI program is flexible and comprehensive enough to support innovations in healthy food retailing to assist retailers with different aspects of the store development and renovations. Regardless of the origination of department funds, HFFI is administered with fund managers at Community Development Financial Institutions (CDFIs). CDFIs are financial organizations that have received certification to participate in the federal government sponsored CDFI Fund programs and are integral to the HFFI funding. The federal departments support the HFFI by utilizing CDFIs, which then work with local communities to offer grants, loans, and tax credits for projects aimed to reduce disparities in access to healthy foods across America. The purpose of CDFIs is to garner economic growth in disadvantaged communities across the United States and be a resource for flexible financing that may not be available at commercial banks. The CDFIs invest federal dollars along with private capital to support the infrastructure of neighborhoods that lack access to financing.

As stated earlier, the CDFI Fund (at the Department of Treasury) was established by the Riegle Community Development and Regulatory Improvement Act of 1994 with the purpose of promoting economic development in low-income communities through access to basic financial services, affordable credit, and investment in capital. Community Development Financial Institutions have played important roles in working with both federal and state governments to administer funds earmarked for bringing supermarkets to disenfranchised areas of the United States. Mr. Owens, Executive Director of Neighborhood Progress Fund states:

> Those types of subsidies [referring to state funding for Pennsylvania's Fresh Food Financing Initiative – FFFI] help make projects make sense to developers and operators. In north Philadelphia, you have Progress Plaza. Without FFFI, you would not have the Fresh Grocer there. Same with the Parkwest Center and Jeff Brown. That was financed with tax credits, some subsidy dollars. Without that, the community wouldn't have been invested in. There wouldn't have been a ShopRite.[12]

By offering flexible financing and being a financial institution within the local community, CDFIs are in a unique position to solve specific issues that may arise during these ventures. Mr. Owens goes on to comment on the need for subsidies to support the supermarket development in urban areas:

> Without the Center, you don't have a grocery store. In order to build a retail power center you need 30, 40, 50 acres of land. Not only for the buildings, but for the parking. To find that much continuous land in an urban area, a lot [may not be] environmentally safe. You need even more subsidy to develop. Tax credits allow you to build a $50 million center for $40 million. Those subsidies are critical to put a full-service grocery store in the community. And you need operators that have experience, that can do it.[12]

The federal government's continued support for underserved areas was reiterated on June 14, 2020, with the announcement from the Biden administration that $1.2 billion in funds have been allocated to 863 CDFIs for the purpose of improving the infrastructure of underserved communities such as food stores.[27] As these new programs develop from the funds authorized from the Consolidated Appropriated Act, 2021 (Pub. L 116260) and the existing HFFI funds are distributed through the three federal departments, public-private partnerships are called upon to work together to develop program plans. Program plans are mutually beneficial for public-private ventures because these partnerships allow store owners to gain information on the food products that are desired by the community they will be serving, as well as understand barriers residents might have for adopting the store as a primary grocery store. This information will increase sales. For consumers who have been trained to shop for food outside of their neighborhoods, a voice in the planning builds confidence by residents that the food store will address their perceived food access problems, and this will generate customer loyalty.

CRITICAL THINKING QUESTIONS AND EXERCISES

1. Describe and contrast the types of revitalization zones, and discuss the strength and limitations of the types of zones in attracting supermarket retailers to low-income communities.
2. Go to Congress.gov and look for the Healthy Food Financing Initiative legislation. Read the entire legislation and discuss the rational and intended laws as well as outcomes planned from this legislation.
3. Discuss what a Community Development Financial Institution is and how they have been leveraged to bring supermarkets to underserved communities.
4. Discuss other options for public policy initiatives to guarantee that supermarkets are available equitably in all U.S. areas.
5. Explain the rationale for the Healthy Food Financing Initiative (HFFI) of 2013 and what the goals of the legislation are.
6. Describe how the HFFI is integrated into the USDA's Agricultural Act.
7. Distinguish the HFFI from other federal programs aimed to reduce food insecurity.

REFERENCES

1. Troutt D. The Thin Red Line: How the Poor Still Pay More. In: Consumers Union West Coast Regional Office, ed. San Francisco, CA; 1993.
2. U.S. White House. Let's Move: America's Move to Raise a Healthier Generation of Kids. 2014; https://letsmove.obamawhitehouse.archives.gov/about. Accessed July16, 2021.
3. Lucey C. White House urban affairs team coming to Philly. *The Philadelphia Inquirer*. 2009.
4. Gruentein D, Herbert S, James F. Interim Assessment of the Empowerment Zones and Enterprise Communities (EZ/EC) Program: A Progress Report and Appendices. In: U.S. Department of Housing and Urban Development, ed. Washington, DC: U.S. Department of Housing and Urban Development; 2001.
5. U.S. Government Accountability Office. Empowerment Zones and Enterprise Community Programs: Improvements Occurred in Communities, But the Effect of the Program Is Unclear. In: U.S. Government Accountability Office, ed. Washington, DC; 2006.
6. U.S. General Accounting Office. Federal Revitalizations Programs Are Being Implemented, But Data on the Use of Tax Benefits Are Limited. In: U.S. General Accounting Office, ed. Washington, DC; 2004.
7. Stoker RP, Rich MJ. Obama's urban legacy: The limits of braiding and local policy coordination. *Urban Affairs Review*. 2019;56(6):1607–1629.
8. Stoker RP, Rich MJ. Old Policies Ad New Presidents: Promise Zones and the Trump Administration. 2020; https://urbanaffairsreview.com/2020/02/21/old-policies-and-new-presidents-promise-zones-and-the-trump-administration/. Accessed December 28, 2020.
9. Gagiuc A. Reviewing Opportunity Zones with Steve Glickman and Ira Weinstein. January 5, 2021; www.multihousingnews.com/post/amp/reviewing-opportunity-zones-with-steve-glickman-and-ira-weinstein/. Accessed January 5, 2021.
10. Drucker J, Lipton E. How a Trump tax break to help poor communities became a windfall for the rich. *The New York Times*. August 31, 2019.

11. Benjamin LRJS, Zielenbach S. Community development financial institutions: Current issues and future prospects. *Journal of Urban Affairs*. 2004;26:117–195.
12. Lehmann Y. Interview with Reco Owens. August 27, 2020.
13. U.S. Department of the Treasury. Community Development Financial Institutions Fund. 2020; www.cdfifund.gov/about/Pages/default.aspx. Accessed January 4, 2021.
14. The Reinvestment Fund. *New Markets Tax Credit and Urban Supermarkets*. Philadelphia, PA: The Reinvestment Fund CDFI; 2011.
15. Tax Policy Center. Key Elements of the U.S. Tax System. 2020; www.taxpolicycenter.org/briefing-book/what-new-markets-tax-credit-and-how-does-it-work. Accessed January 4, 2021.
16. Ibanez B. What is the likelihood of the NMTC reauthorization beyond 2020? *NMTC Resource Center*. October 12, 2020; www.novoco.com/notes-from-novogradac/what-likelihood-nmtc-reauthorization-beyond-2020. Accessed January 12, 2021.
17. U.S. Department of the Treasury. New Markets Tax Credit Program. 2020; www.cdfifund.gov/programs-training/Programs/new-markets-tax-credit/Pages/default.aspx. Accessed January 7, 2021.
18. U.S. Department of Health and Human Services. Community Economic Development. 2020; www.acf.hhs.gov/ocs/programs/ced. Accessed January 7, 2021.
19. Administration for Children and Families. CED-HFFI Grantee Map FY 2016. 2021; www.acf.hhs.gov/ocs/map/ced-hffi-grantee-map-fy-2016#CA_5208. Accessed January 4, 2021.
20. The Reinvestment Fund. America's Healthy Food Financing Initiative. 2020; www.investinginfood.com/. Accessed January 7, 2021.
21. Gillibrand K. S.821 Healthy Food Financing Initiative. In: 113th Congress (2013–2014), ed. Washington, DC: Congress.gov; 2013.
22. Fudge MHR. 5017 Healthy Food Financing Initiative Reauthorization Act of 2018. 115th Congress (2017–2018); 2018.
23. U.S. Department of Agriculture. Communities Facilities Direct Loan and Grants. 2020; www.rd.usda.gov/sites/default/files/fact-sheet/508_RD_FS_RHS_CFDirect.pdf. Accessed January 7, 2021.
24. U.S. Department of Agriculture. USDA Agriculture Marketing Services: Farmers Market Promotion Program. 2020; www.ams.usda.gov/services/grants/fmpp. Accessed January 7, 2021.
25. U.S. Department of Agriculture. Community Food Projects (CFP) Competitive Grants Program. 2020; https://nifa.usda.gov/funding-opportunity/community-food-projects-cfp-competitive-grants-program. Accessed January 7, 2021.
26. The Reinvestment Fund. *HFFI bill would expand healthy food access, revitalize communities*. Philadelphia, PA: The Reinvestment Fund; 2018.
27. U.S. Department of the Treasury. *U.S. Treasury Awards $1.25 Billion to Support Economic Relief in Communities Affected by COVID-19*. June 15, 2021.

Section II

State Food Environment Initiatives

For many years, food advocates in cities and states across America have recognized the disparities in access to healthy food among low-income and Black, Indigenous, and People of Color. Beginning in 2002, advocates in cities such as Philadelphia organized and led a charter through city and state governments to promote funding for food retailers to locate in underserved areas. Most states have now initiated policies that provide funding to this effort. In this section, five of those states' initiatives are described: Pennsylvania, Louisiana, New York, Colorado, and Michigan. The chapters are titled with cities that were key in pioneering the work. In each chapter, the unique circumstances by which task forces are developed, programs and funding are garnered, and funds are administered are described. In addition, the role of United States policies, beginning with emancipation and migration of African American slaves away from southern states to the systematic racism within the banking industry are also discussed, with regard to their part in the development and preservation of underserved areas in the United States. Food retailers supported by these state initiatives are depicted, and their success is the foundation for the federal Healthy Food Financing Initiative described in Chapter 3.

DOI: 10.1201/9781003029151-5

4 Philadelphia, Pennsylvania

CONTENTS

INTRODUCTION

Chapter 4 is the first of five chapters in Section II. These five chapters aim to highlight state-led initiatives that have addressed disparities in local food environments across the United States. The five states selected have been used as examples of success to justify the federal Healthy Food Financing Initiative legislation.[1] The section begins with Chapter 4 regarding Pennsylvania's Fresh Food Financing Initiative (FFFI) because Pennsylvania was the first state to provide state funds to address disparities in local food environments for underserved areas of the state. The purpose of this chapter is for readers to understand the historical circumstances that have created disparities in access to supermarkets in Philadelphia (and other areas of Pennsylvania) and how the Fresh Food Financing Initiative (FFFI) encouraged grocery stores to locate in low-income neighborhoods, thereby providing both economic growth and food to underserved communities.

The chapter reviews several notable examples of the impact of the financing work, including the opening of new stores such as Progress Plaza, which is an early national example of Black American owned-and-operated retail spaces that include a grocery store. The process by which The Food Trust began the supermarket campaign in Philadelphia by working with community groups, advocating for supermarkets, and establishing a task force is reviewed. In addition, the chapter describes the program process of selecting underserved areas for FFFI funding and how the Pennsylvania FFFI became the model of other State Health Food Financing Initiatives as well as the federal program. The chapter concludes with a reflection on the ways in which redlining impacted the city, and how community members effectively worked to self-invest in their own neighborhoods.

DOI: 10.1201/9781003029151-6

PHILADELPHIA, PENNSYLVANIA

Philadelphia, with 1.5 million residents, is Pennsylvania's largest city. It is an incredibly significant city in American history as it was the nation's first capital. Independence Hall is where the Declaration of Independence was signed and where the first and second presidents (George Washington and John Adams) served their terms. Philadelphia is also a centerpiece of the northern civil rights movement; a place where beginning in 1910, Black southerners began to relocate to the City of Brotherly Love as part of the Great Migration. As a result, the city's Black population increased more than twofold with residents seeking to work in factories in need of labor. While racial segregation was not as prominent as in the South, it was visible in the city in hotels, restaurants, theaters, neighborhoods, and workplaces. The NAACP formed its Philadelphia Chapter in 1912, and by 1935 the organization led the passage of legislation that banned racial discrimination in public accommodations across Pennsylvania. Despite progress, discrimination remained visible, for example, in the employment sector where Black residents struggled to gain access to professional occupations and in access to housing where Black Philadelphians were largely restricted to living only in the city's worst neighborhoods. While the 1950s is known as a time of housing boom, with federally subsidized mortgages enabling home ownership for many working-class families, these opportunities were largely closed to Black families. By 1955 only three subdivisions in suburban Philadelphia were not marketed according to race, leaving Black residents to remain in the inner-city, high-density neighborhoods and its stock of aging homes. During this time, areas of the city such as North and West Philadelphia became home to most Black residents.

REDLINING IN PHILADELPHIA

The New Deal was responsible for the first Farm Bill in the 1940s (Chapter 1), but it also represents a key piece of legislation that developed and funded programs aimed to help Americans prevent foreclosures, purchase new homes, and provide low-cost shelter after the Great Depression. While private banks were still a bit tentative to make larger, or riskier, investments, the government sought to stimulate the economy with its own plan to support development. As part of this effort, the Home Owners' Loan Corporation (HOLC) was created, and the Federal Housing Administration (FHA) began loan programs for new homes, which also provided employment opportunities in construction. New public housing was also prioritized with the New Deal.[2] As early as 1920, racial homogeneity of neighborhoods was fostered with the institution of restrictive covenants by real estate boards and homeowner associations, targeting Black Americans in particular. Under these covenants, property owners would sign agreements to not allow Black Americans to own, occupy, or lease their properties. These types of contracts were used in the United States until 1948 when the U.S. Supreme Court finally declared they were unenforceable.[3] However, up until this time, these restrictive covenants were commonplace and supported by the official policies of the National Association of Real Estate Brokers in their code of ethics in 1924 which stated; 'a Realtor should never be instrumental in introducing into a neighborhood . . . members of any race or nationality . . . whose presence will clearly be detrimental to property values in that neighborhood'.[4] These policies were also supported by bankers who would not grant loans to Black applicants; hence, for these financial and institutional reasons, Black Americans have been systematically relegated to specific regions of the United States.[5]

The HOLC's mission was to work with commercial lenders to provide the loans. To provide creditworthiness of areas to bankers, the HOLC created 'Residential Security Maps', that graded and colored on maps residential neighborhoods on four tiers of risk (A = Best – green; B = Still Desirable – blue; C = Definitely Declining – orange; and D = Hazardous – red). The determinants of risk or 'creditworthiness' operated under the assumption that older neighborhoods could not be restored. In addition to the age of the neighborhoods, the HOLC hired local real estate agents (who had developed the restricted covenants) to appraise areas and often employed discriminatory judgments against Black American neighborhoods because areas populated by

Black Americans were considered high-risk and therefore colored red on the maps. These practices led to a disinvestment in inner-city neighborhoods and Black neighborhoods as well as an
over-investment in suburban residential areas.

The policies of the FHA followed those of the HOLC and perpetuated the segregation of
American neighborhoods with an underwriting manual that stated: *'If a neighborhood is to
retain stability, it is necessary that properties shall continue to be occupied by the same social
and racial classes'.*[6] Additionally, FHA loans favored single-family homes and therefore put
residents of attached dwelling and row housing (common in inner cities) at a disadvantage for
benefiting from this federal program. The trend to support the growth of the suburbs continued
through the 1970s to such an extent that private and government lending to inner-city residents
led to the depreciation of homes in predominantly Black and low-wealth areas. Although these
federal initiatives focus on housing, the disinvestment of these areas by the federal government
was also supported by a disinvestment by commercial entities.

More than a half century after the implementation of the New Deal, Philadelphia, like many
other U.S. cities, continues to feel the impact of that legislation. Maps of Philadelphia, developed by real estate agents to appraise properties, positioned Black American neighborhoods in
the worst category (D-Rated) while placing White neighborhoods most favorably. New Italian
and Jewish immigrant neighborhoods were also seen as higher risk.[7] The maps, while striking
visuals of discrimination, may have been as much a reflection of pre-existing discrimination as
they were the cause; those areas labeled as hazardous were already experiencing disinvestment.

Today, the former D-rated, or redlined, neighborhoods continue to struggle for investment
and face environmental disparities, from higher densities of toxic brownfield sites to limited
access to healthy affordable food. As David Bartelt, an established and deeply respected geography and urban studies scholar in Philadelphia has described, the political economy of a
neighborhood defined largely by the stream of capital that flows through it, is a primary force
which shapes that community.[8] The redlined map of Philadelphia is shown in Figure 4.1. Reco
Owens, Executive Director of Philadelphia's Neighborhood Progress Fund, an organization

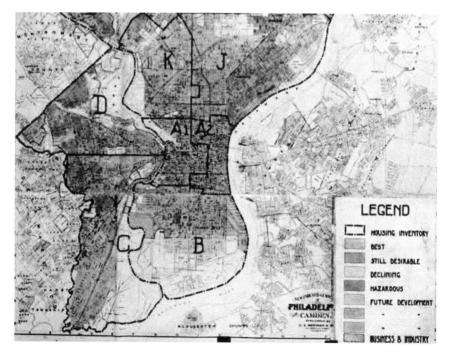

FIGURE 4.1   Redline Map of Philadelphia, PA

responsible for redeveloping disinvested urban areas, explained the impact of redlining as a cause and effect of poverty, with its impact still rippling today:

> [As] a direct line to redlining, people were unable to get a mortgage. Oftentimes the owners of these properties left the community, they rented, and they had no incentive to improve the properties. In North Philadelphia, the vast number of owners do not live in that community so it's not about the value of the community. So, it [poverty and lack of opportunity] just continues from generation to generation. This is the result of redlining and segregation.

PROGRESS PLAZA: FOOD RETAIL IN AN ERA OF REDLINING

Despite banking policies of the day, there are examples of areas of Philadelphia that were able to develop needed retail corridors despite disinvestment. Located in the Yorktown neighborhood, on Broad Street in North Philadelphia, is the site of Progress Plaza, an area designated as hazardous on HOLC maps in 1936. On a crisp October day in 1968, 10,000 people gathered to mark the opening of the large new shopping plaza, which would become the country's first Black American–owned shopping center. Despite the challenges associated with its poor rating, the crowd was celebrating the new shopping center, anchored by a big, beautiful A&P Supermarket, owned and operated by sixteen surrounding Black American businesses, which brought much-needed services and jobs to the community.

The story of the community succeeding to establish supermarket retail despite the political economy of the time, can be traced to 1962, when Zion Investment Associates was formed by a visionary Black American leader, Rev. Dr. Leon H Sullivan, who himself had served in prominent roles in corporate America, including as the first Black board member of General Motors. Seeking to expand opportunity for Black American residents, the investment company served as a backbone for Black American enterprise development. Opening its doors in 1968, Progress Plaza became home to a much-needed supermarket and other shopping amenities. The project was financed not through a typical bank loan, but was the result of cash deposits, accruing over years. In total, 650 members of the nearby Zion Baptist Church financed the project with $10 monthly contributions every month, for three years. The effort not only demonstrated the collective capacity of the Black American community in Philadelphia, but through its example, stimulated future federal investments, including some controversial Black American investment philosophies of the Nixon administration, such as work to promote 'Black Capitalism'.[9]

Political in nature, the term *Black Capitalism* is reflected in the history books in both positive and negative light. It is evoked as a testament to Nixon's commitment to civil rights or, conversely, as a misguided attempt to ignore long-standing injustices and suppress Black protests. The approach, which has been adopted widely since, and is credited with stimulating concepts like Opportunity Zones, is also criticized for its lack of focus on government jobs, housing, and welfare support. The emphasis is instead on the importance of the free market and the opportunity that tax credit policies can have in opening investment markets and in promoting equity among those who historically lacked access to such mechanisms. These policies are controversial, however, and for some, Black Capitalism is an example of the ways in which America's roots in White privilege are ignored in an embrace of a good ole' pick yourself up by the bootstraps mentality forced upon Black Americans. As noted in a 2019 opinion article in the *New York Times*, 'The Real Roots of "Black Capitalism", Mr. Nixon Pointed Blacks to the Free Market and Wished Them Luck'.[10]

THE COMMUNITY REINVESTMENT ACT

The federal government became increasingly aware of the need to address discriminatory lending and repayment practices, in part due to the U.S. Commission on Civil Rights, which documented consistent refusal to invest in specific areas. In an effort to address redlining and reduce discrimination in lending, Congress passed the Community Reinvestment Act (CRA), situated as Title VIII of the Housing and Community Development Act of 1977 (see Chapter 3).[11] The Act sought to require banks backed by the FDIC to extend credit across communities, regardless of its relative wealth or poverty. Specifically, it requires that any bank that receives deposits must offer equal access to lending, investment, and services to all those located within a 3- to 5-mile radius of the location. If the bank had many locations, it could require equal lending to an entire county or state. Between 1977 and 1991 $8.8 billion was invested through the CRA in communities.

As banks reopened their doors to communities that before were not able to obtain mortgages, investments in housing increased, which in turn stimulated food retailers to relocate to the suburbs. As noted, the 1960s and 1970s were marked by a suburban 'flight', a reaction to both the push of urban decline and the pull of large new construction with green lawns in communities funded with government-backed mortgages. Supermarkets followed White residents to the suburbs where there was ample land to build larger stores, with sizable parking lots; Safeway alone closed 600 urban stores between 1968 and 1984 in one large city.[12,13] Between 1970 and 1990, 34 of 50 chain supermarket locations in Boston closed, while in Los Angeles County, the number of supermarkets plummeted from 1068 to 694.[14]

EVOLUTION OF FOOD RETAIL, SUPERMARKETS, AND LOCAL FOOD SALES

As described in Chapter 2, after World War II the supermarket industry started to become less of a patchwork of mom-and-pop specialty stores and instead was dominated by larger supermarket chains to increase profitability. In this larger market format, revenue was driven by a higher volume of sales rather than relying on the markup of the price of goods alone.[15] The consolidation of the industry was born with the arrival of this new philosophy, and in the 1950s supermarkets became the dominant outlet for grocery purchasing. Such a shift in food retail industry left many smaller stores and farmer owned-and-operated stands with declining profitability. For example, in Philadelphia, there is the history of the Reading Terminal Market, a central market for local food dating back to the late 1800s. In the early 1900s the market was a vibrant cornerstone of food commerce in Philadelphia, boasting 250 food dealers and more than 100 farmers together in a central location with modern refrigeration in the heart of Philadelphia. The market succeeded well into the 1940s and was able to provide the city with food during the Great Depression because of its deep local network and regional food supply chains.[16] Later, during World War II, when rationing limited the food supply for residents, the market persisted in providing a needed outlet for a variety of locally grown food and sales from local farmers.

However, the 1960s marked a shift in the vitality of the Reading Terminal Market. Disinvestment and the emergence of the supermarket industry led to the once-modern facility falling into disrepair; the railroad which runs over the market (and once an important mechanism for aggregating and selling products) ceased to operate as it once had, declaring bankruptcy in 1971. The railroad was the backbone of the market's vibrancy, and by 1976, its bankruptcy caused the Reading Terminal Market to dwindle, with only the most committed operators willing to endure the increasing rents and declining operational conditions (Figure 4.2). By this time, this market, located in a low-income and predominately Black residential area of Philadelphia was the most proximal retailer of food for the community.

During the 1980s however, the Reading Terminal Market began to make a comeback with strong community support and an improved management structure that better supported vendors and provided a more realistic fee structure and, hence, a renewed sense of purpose. At the same time the city was planning the construction of the nearby Philadelphia Convention Center. The project afforded an opportunity for the Reading Terminal Market operators to capitalize on this investment into the area, and, by partnering with the Convention Center project, they were able to garner $30 million in public funding to upgrade the infrastructure of Reading

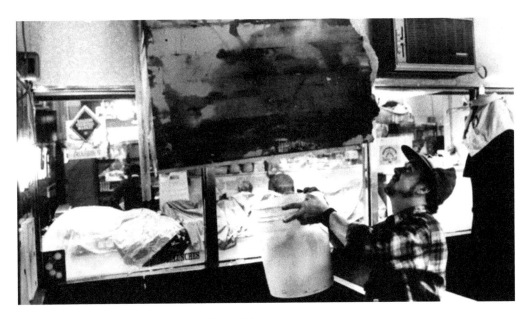

FIGURE 4.2   Reading Terminal: Down Home Diner

Terminal Markets and reorganize the business structure, allowing a nonprofit corporation to manage the market.

The new management recognized that while the Reading Terminal Market remained a place of commerce for residents, it did not provide the local communities with the affordable foods offered by supermarkets. Therefore, Philadelphia city planner Duane Perry, then the executive director of the Merchant Association for the Reading Terminal Market, was one of the first people to raise the issue of disparities in food access in Philadelphia in 1990. He observed residents from many neighborhoods in Philadelphia shopping at the Reading Terminal Market to purchase fresh produce because it was not available in their communities.

Mr. Perry proposed the expansion of Reading Terminal Market to bring affordable and nutritious foods to more residents of the underserved neighborhoods. This would also benefit local farmers by providing an additional outlet for the region's farmers to sell their products. Mr. Perry initiated his idea with the development of the nonprofit corporation called the *Farmers Market Trust*, whereby nutrition education and outreach services were made available to low-income residents and provided at farmers markets located in multiple locations throughout the city. The nonprofit organization initially operated farmers markets in communities where supermarkets no longer were located, helping residents to obtain seasonal access to affordable nutritious foods. The Farmers Market Trust later became known as The Food Trust.

One of the first agency efforts was a farmers market in the lower-income community of Tasker Homes, a public housing development in South Philadelphia. Each week The Food Trust, with the help of the Tasker Homes tenant council, set up one long table with an array of fresh vegetables and fruits for residents to purchase. 'People hadn't seen that kind of quality produce in their neighborhood before', Perry recalled. Residents told the market staff about traveling long distances to buy healthy food for families and often complained of the prices and lack of quality or variety in small neighborhood corner stores. The market was a tremendous success, confirming Perry's hypothesis that there was demand for healthy foods in neighborhoods underserved by supermarkets and other fresh food retailers. The Tasker Homes market and the profitability of each new farmers market opened by The Food Trust demonstrated that lower-income families, just like middle- and upper-income families, desired fresh produce for their families.

As the success of the farmers markets grew, The Food Trust recognized that products available through a farmers market are only available for part of the year, leaving these targeted community residents with few local options for purchasing fresh produce before June and after November when the growing season ended. Further limitations of the program were acknowledged, such as the fact that farmers markets are only open once or twice a week for a few hours a day, limiting the availability of these food products. Customers also recognized this limitation and informed The Food Trust that fresh produce and other healthy foods had previously been available in their neighborhood at supermarkets, and that they were frustrated that those stores had closed with no plans for replacing them.

As Mr. Perry surveyed other low-income areas in Philadelphia, these comments from community members seemed more than isolated observations. In fact, a study conducted in 1995 found that the Greater Philadelphia region had a low ratio of supermarkets to population [17] and needed approximately seventy supermarkets to meet national standards in other areas of the United States. And like other supermarkets that were closing in low-income areas across the city, after three decades of operation, the Progress Plaza supermarket also closed in 1998 leaving the Yorktown community, a predominantly Black area of Philadelphia, without access to healthy affordable food in their neighborhood. With the closure of this supermarket, the once-proud Progress Plaza fell into decline, and Yorktown residents then needed to travel nineteen blocks, via two buses, to the nearest supermarket to obtain fresh fruits and vegetables and other healthy foods for their dinner tables. It would take another decade and another innovative community effort before a supermarket came back to this neighborhood.

PHILADELPHIA'S SUPERMARKET CAMPAIGN

ADVOCATING FOR SUPERMARKETS

The profitability of the farmers markets made it clear there was customer demand for the products sold within the city's lower-income communities. So where were all the supermarkets that could provide perishable goods such as fresh produce to residents year-round? And why were supermarkets in many low-income areas of Philadelphia no longer operational? The Food Trust set out to answer those questions. With the help of Dr. Amy Hillier of the University of Pennsylvania, then a student, The Food Trust used geographic information system software to map the locations of supermarkets in Philadelphia and discover the extent of the city's food access problem (Figure 4.3). The maps layered income data from the 1990 U.S. Census supermarket sales and diet-related mortality data (including deaths due to neoplasms or tumors; endocrine, nutritional, and immunity disorders such as diabetes; and diseases of the circulatory system) provided by the commercial data firm Trade Dimensions and the Philadelphia Department of Public Health, respectively to sales and health statistics.

This diet-related element offered a new perspective on the issue of food access. Early conversations with city officials about Philadelphia's lack of supermarkets had not been encouraging. The social justice aspects of food access were a tough sell in a city mired in a bad economy. And talk of supermarkets as an economic development strategy was not initially popular in a city that saw its future, as it had its past, in manufacturing. But these maps showed something more compelling to city officials: the city's lower-income communities also had some of the lowest supermarket access and these lower-income, low-access communities had the highest rates of diet-related deaths. The maps, published in the 2001 report called 'Food For Every Child: The Need for More Supermarkets in Philadelphia', showed that food access was not simply a social justice issue, nor simply an economic development issue; it was an urgent and expensive public health concern for Philadelphia.[18] This data collection and dissemination was the first step in The Food Trust's fledgling supermarket campaign. The process, which would later be named The Food Trust Framework, and would

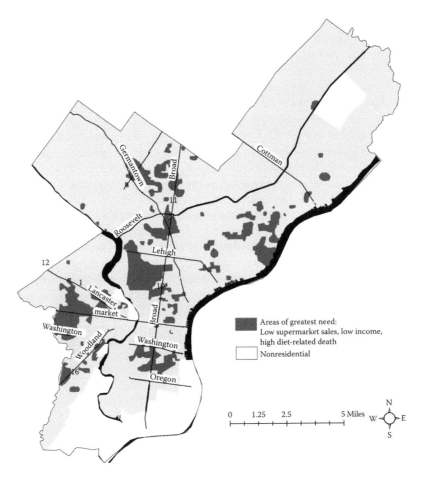

FIGURE 4.3   Areas of Greatest Need for Supermarkets

be replicated across the country, grew out of the on-the-ground education and coalition building work the organization had been conducting in Philadelphia for a decade.

In 2002, the Philadelphia City Council, spurred by The Food Trust's report, called for hearings on the issue of supermarket access in Philadelphia. The hearings, which included testimony from dozens of concerned community members and leaders, generated wider awareness of the issue. One leader became increasingly engaged. State Representative Dwight Evans grew up in a northern section of Philadelphia, in the Germantown and West Oak Lane neighborhoods, a part of the community he represented at the time. He knew what it was like growing up without convenient access to a supermarket; the Oak Lane neighborhoods were among the lowest-income, lowest-access communities identified by The Food Trust's maps. Now Evans saw that the problem was not unique to Oak Lane and nearby Olney; it affected communities throughout the city, including large portions of North Philadelphia, the near Northeast, South Philadelphia west of Broad Street, and West Philadelphia. 'I already knew that there was a problem', Evans said. 'The map just made it real. It put a face on it. It was like an exhibit in a courtroom'. As he continued to research the issue of food access, it became clear that the problem was not unique to Philadelphia either. It plagued other Pennsylvanian cities such as Pittsburgh (a five-hour drive from Philadelphia in the western section of the state) and rural, agricultural towns such as Apollo and Gettysburg, traditionally agricultural towns about a three-hour drive west of Philadelphia.

The Food Trust and key city and state leaders now knew the extent of the problem, but it was not clear how to solve the issue. What would it take to bring supermarkets back to these underserved communities?

ESTABLISHMENT OF THE FOOD MARKETING TASK FORCE

In 2003, at the request of the Philadelphia City Council, The Food Trust organized the Food Marketing Task Force. This task force included high-level representatives from many disciplines including public health, government economic development, and businessmen from the grocery retailing industry. These groups that did not typically work together but gathered as members of the Food Marketing Task Force for the sole purpose of addressing the disparities in access to food in Pennsylvania.

The co-chairs were Walt Rubel, an executive of the ACME/Albertsons, Inc. grocery chain, and former President of the Grocer Association, and Christine James-Brown, who was the president and chief executive officer (CEO) of the United Way International, PCCY child health advocate group and Commerce Department. The majority of the thirty-member Task Force, was comprised of grocery store executives, bankers, and community leaders. The Food Trust intentionally did not invite journalists or community residents to be members of the Task Force, in order to enable frank conversation and to allow retailers to explain needs and concerns in a familiar context, absent strong criticism. Task force members were also vetted to ensure that they were high-level decision-makers with strong industry knowledge and respect, who could pave a path to make swift changes to the food retail environment in Philadelphia. The members of the task force and their affiliations are described in Table 4.1.

TABLE 4.1
Thirty-Member Food Market Task Force[20]

Member	Professional Affiliation	Contribution and Development Specialty
Bill Anderson	President, Longview Development LP	Real Estate
Murray Battleman	Owner, Richboro Shop N Bag	Grocery
William Bradley	Senior GIS Analyst, Neighborhood Transformation Initiative	Community Development
Lorraine Brooks-Body	Site Location Analyst, Wakefern Food Corporation	Grocery Retailer-Owned Cooperative
Jeffrey Brown	Owner, ShopRite	Grocery
Duane Bumb	Deputy Director, Commerce Department	Economic Growth and Development
Hannah Burton	Program Coordinator, The Food Trust	Food Access
Cathy Califano	Deputy Secretary, Office of Housing and Neighborhood Preservation	Community Development
Della Clark	President, The Enterprise Center	Economic and Community Development
Beverly Coleman	Program Director, Philadelphia Neighborhood Development Collaborative	Community Development
Larry Collins	Owner, ShopRite	Grocery
Donna Cooper	Director, Governor's Policy Office	Public Policy
James Cuorato	Director and City Representative (former), Commerce Department	Economic Growth and Development
Jacob Fisher	Policy Analyst, Neighborhood Transformation Initiative	Public Policy and Community Development
Kathy Fisher	Welfare and Public Benefits Coordinator, Philadelphia Citizens for Children and Youth	Youth Development

(Continued)

TABLE 4.1 (Continued)
Thirty-Member Food Market Task Force

Member	Professional Affiliation	Contribution and Development Specialty
Eva Gladstein	Executive Director, Philadelphia Empowerment Zone	Economic and Community Development
Lori Glass	Director, Capitalization and Investor Development, The Reinvestment Fund	Economic Development in Underserved Communities
Bob Gorland	Vice President, Matthew P. Casey & Associates	Grocery Development
Rob Graff	Senior Project Manager, The Reinvestment Fund	Economic Development in Underserved Communities
Kevin Hanna	Secretary, Office of Housing and Neighborhood Preservation	Community Development
David Hollinger	Chairman, Four Seasons Produce	Grocery
Christine James-Brown	Past President and CEO, United Way of Southeastern Pennsylvania President and CEO, United Way International	Economic and Community Development
Peter Longstreth	President, Philadelphia Industrial Development Corporation	Economic and Community Development
Joseph Mahoney	Vice President, Public Policy, Greater Philadelphia Chamber of Commerce	Economic Growth and Development
Richard Matwes	Senior Real Estate Representative, Wakefern Food Corporation	Real Estate
David McCorkle	President and CEO, Pennsylvania Food Merchants Association	Food and Grocer Trade Association
Rich McMenamin	Owner, ShopRite	Grocery
Stephen Mullin	Principal, Consult	Urban and Real Estate Economic and Community Development
Jeremy Nowak	President and CEO, The Reinvestment Fund	Economic Development in Underserved Communities
Carlos Peraza	Senior Program Officer, LISC	Community Development
Duane Perry	Executive Director, The Food Trust	Food Access
Bilal Qayyum	Economic Development Coordinator, Department of Commerce	Economic Growth and Development
Samuel Rhoads	Senior Vice President, Philadelphia Industrial Development Corporation	Economic and Community Development
Walter Rubel	Director, Government and Community Relations, Acme/Albertsons, Inc.	Grocery
Rich Savner	Director, Pathmark	Grocery
Mark Schweiker	President and CEO, Greater Philadelphia Chamber of Commerce	Economic Growth and Development
Patricia Smith	Director, Neighborhood Transformation Initiative	Community Health Development
June Spring	Senior Real Estate Manager, Wawa, Inc.	Grocery
Patrick Temple West	Director of Nutritional Services, The Archdiocese of Philadelphia	Church Organization
David Thornburgh	Executive Director, Pennsylvania Economy League	Economic Growth and Development
Shelly Yanoff	Executive Director, Philadelphia Citizens for Children and Youth	Youth Development

The group was initially called together to broadly discuss opportunities for supermarket retail in Philadelphia and specifically share the food retailers' perspectives about the critical needs, issues, and potential solutions that surrounded the lack of food retailers in the city. At the same time, the process worked to establish a common understanding of the current location of stores, population densities, and areas of greatest risk for diet related mortality. These data took the form of a report, 'Food for Every Child'. The convening was not the first of its kind—several had raised the issue of lack of access to supermarkets in prior years. However, prior efforts to promote supermarkets had focused on economic development needs alone and on specific locations where residents thought a market should go. This new approach created momentum to understand the food retail industry needs from both an economic and health perspective and opened the eyes of leadership to the ways in which the grocery gap has a ripple effect in communities. This new health-economic vantage point created important momentum, which helped to generate solutions posed by the highest-level industry leaders, ultimately becoming actionable recommendations that would address these challenges at an industry level.[19]

After four meetings in 2004, The Food Trust published 'Stimulating Supermarket Development: A New Day for Philadelphia', which laid out the Task Force's ten recommendations for encouraging supermarket development in Philadelphia and throughout Pennsylvania (Table 4.2).[20] Key among these recommendations was the development of a business-financing program at the state level to encourage supermarket development in underserved communities. This recommendation aimed to solve the central barrier for grocery retailers interested in opening supermarkets in underserved communities (which often required higher development investment to address issues like land assembly and workforce development), which was lack of access to capital. Jeff Brown, a fourth-generation grocery store owner in Philadelphia, and member of the Food Marketing Task Force said:

> During that first task force meeting in Philadelphia, I was completely convinced that this was an opportunity to grow my business profitably and serve society in a profound way. One of the key elements was the platform to discuss the challenges and how government, nonprofits and businesses were willing to work together to mitigate some of these challenges. If we could find a way to address the financial gap created by the low profit margins typical of the supermarket industry and the higher expenses associated with opening in an underserved community, I knew we could bring supermarkets back to these neighborhoods.

TABLE 4.2
Ten Task Force Recommendations[20]

The city should adopt food retailing as a priority for comprehensive neighborhood development.

The city should employ innovative, data-driven market assessment techniques to highlight unmet market demand in urban neighborhoods.

The city should identify targeted areas for supermarket development and promote them to real estate developers and the supermarket industry.

The city should give priority to assembling land for supermarket development.

The city should reduce regulatory barriers to supermarket investment.

The city should market available public incentives to maximize impact on supermarket site location decisions.

City and state economic development programs should be made available to the supermarket industry.

The Commonwealth of Pennsylvania should develop a business-financing program to support local supermarket development projects.

The appropriate city, regional, and state transportation agencies should develop safe, cheap, and convenient transportation services for shoppers who do not have access to a full-service supermarket.

The city should convene an advisory group of leaders from the supermarket industry and the civic sector to guide the implementation of these recommendations.

IMPLEMENTING PHILADELPHIA'S FRESH FOOD FINANCING INITIATIVE

AVAILABILITY OF FUNDS

With strong support from all sectors represented on the task force and Representative Evans as its champion, the recommendation for a business-financing program was realized in 2004 when the Pennsylvania state legislature established and funded the Fresh Food Financing Initiative (FFFI). The state funds were allocated to address the lack of access to capital for supermarket owners and through flexible grant and loan funding aimed to open new grocery stores or expand healthy food offerings at existing supermarkets in underserved Pennsylvania neighborhoods. The Food Trust; Reinvestment Fund, a Community Development Financial Institution (CDFI); and a Philadelphia based nonprofit, the Urban Affairs Coalition, were charged with implementing FFFI.

The Pennsylvania legislature seeded the FFFI with $30 million in three annual installments of $10 million. This money was leveraged by Reinvestment Fund to create a comprehensive, multifaceted $120 million financing program for grocery stores and supermarkets. Through the FFFI, grocery retailers were eligible for loans of up to $5 million and grants of up to $250,000 per store. On rare occasions, projects that demonstrated both a special need and high potential for impact were eligible for up to $1 million in grant funding.

Recognizing that the barriers to food access are unique in each community, FFFI was designed to be flexible to best meet the needs of grocery retailers responding to the context of their local communities. For example, full-size supermarkets were the primary focus of the funding; however, smaller healthy food retailers, including corner stores and farmers markets were also eligible. The FFFI was also flexible on how the funds could be used, ranging from ground-up construction; renovations to existing grocery store structures; as well as employee training and other justifiable costs that are necessary to achieve the end goal of reducing the disparities in access to food in Pennsylvania.

ADMINISTRATIVE STRUCTURE

The FFFI structure is the key to this pioneering program's success which is a public–private partnership initiated by the partnerships established within the Task Force. The rollout of the FFFI has involved three key stakeholders. First, the state provided funding for FFFI through the Pennsylvania Department of Community and Economic Development (CED). The CED offered program management and tracked the economic impacts of the FFFI. Second, the Reinvestment Fund, a Philadelphia-based community development financing institution (CDFI) functions as the bank, whereby the grocers can access the state funding through grants, loans, and tax-credits. The Reinvestment Fund also leveraged the state's seed funding with additional investments from public and private sources and evaluated the applicants' financial eligibility. The third partner in this public-private partnership is The Food Trust. The Food Trust conducted outreach; marketed the FFFI to food retailers and community leaders in underserved areas; and had the responsibility of determining the potential community impact of the proposed food retail project before recommending it to the Reinvestment Fund for financing. The Food Trust also partnered with the Urban Affairs Coalition to outreach specifically to women- and minority-owned businesses.

IDENTIFYING IMPACTFUL PROJECTS TO BE FUNDED BY THE FFFI

The Food Trust took on the role of marketing the FFFI and identifying qualified grocers from across the state among rural and urban areas. To effectively promote the program, the agency built relationships with the statewide grocery association, wholesalers, and grocery store operators by attending trade shows, presentations at grocer board meetings, one-on-one meetings at their existing stores, connecting with operators via word of mouth, and on the ground in communities. In addition to marketing directly to grocery operators. The Food Trust also reached out to key community and economic development contacts in every county across the state. This outreach proved helpful in identifying regions of need.

PROGRAM ELIGIBILITY

There is a two-step process for applicants – developers or grocery operators – to gain access to FFFI funds. First, The Food Trust evaluated the initial site eligibility application, which was designed to encourage applicants.[21] A short application gaining information about the site location and general store development plans was evaluated by The Food Trust within ten business days. Developing a nuanced understanding of each community and each project was important to the evaluation process. Initially the location was considered using census tract information to determine a region's economic level. Then The Food Trust consulted socioeconomic data at the borough and township level, especially in rural areas with large census tracts, and considered free and reduced-priced school lunch data as another indicator of poverty in an area. The Food Trust judged applications on three main criteria:

- Is the project located in a low- to moderate-income census tract?

- Is this community underserved by food retail, as determined by the food retail density of the area?

- Will the project meet the needs and expectations of the residential community for improved access to healthy and affordable foods?

To determine if a region was underserved, The Food Trust looked at the number of stores in the trade area. Trade areas were developed with industry partners and were based on the size of the store. Stores of less than 10,000 square feet were assigned a half-mile trade area; those of 10,000 to 25,000 square feet, a 1-mile trade area; and those larger than 25,000 square feet, a 2-mile trade area. When evaluating the community fit of a proposed project, The Food Trust considered several qualitative measures such as: (a) community support for the store; (b) quality, affordability of proposed food and beverage products; (c) location within the community; and (d) economic potential impact for the community, such as new jobs. This part of the process involved interviews with local stakeholders, community meetings, and other ground testing of the data used to determine income level and retail density to ensure it reflected the actual experiences of the residents in each community.

If the criteria for site eligibility were met, applications progressed to be evaluated by the Reinvestment Fund for financial evaluation of the grocery store owners and proposed project strength, plans for management, budget integrity, appropriate collateral, as well as the project's competitive advantage in the marketplace. Unlike traditional lenders, the Reinvestment Fund sought to work with applicants to strengthen their applications and design an appropriate FFFI financing package, often including a combination of grants, loans, and New Markets Tax Credits to support the proposed food retail project. Jeremy Nowak, then president and CEO of the Reinvestment Fund said the following about the FFFI.

> We can attract the private capital to match public investment in healthy food choices in our communities. These investments can drive the health and economic vitality of these communities, particularly during difficult economic times.

NEIGHBORHOOD IMPACTS OF THE FFFI

The first iteration of the PA FFFI, which began in 2004 and continued until 2010, funded ninety projects. In 2018 the program was recapitalized, and in partnership with 3 CDFIs across the state of Pennsylvania (TRF, Community First Fund and Bridgeway Capital), funded an additional twenty-five projects, although more are anticipated. In 2020, the Department of Agriculture also made an investment in the state program, creating a separate, time-limited COVID-19 relief fund effort which provided an additional $10 million in support of food retailers who were impacted by the pandemic and as of 2021 has supported 115 projects.

The FFFI program supports stores across the state in more than half of Pennsylvania's counties. The size of the stores supported by the FFFI funding has ranged from 12,000 to 65,000 square feet, with the larger, full-service supermarkets employing 150 to 200 full-time and part-time employees, with weekly sales of $200,000–$300,000.[22] In total, the program has generated more than 5,000 jobs to date and has improved access to food for an estimated half-million Pennsylvania residents. Table 4.3 includes a summary of selected funded projects by the FFFI.

Most notably is Jeffery Brown who opened his first food store in 2004 in a low-income area of Philadelphia. He currently owns twelve grocery stores and half are in underserved neighborhoods. As part of the FFFI Task Force, Mr. Brown has taken advantage of the FFFI funding to open grocery stores that maintain profits in neighborhoods that previously left residents without consistent access to food within their communities. Part of his process for making his supermarkets successful involves meeting the local residents before he opens a new store. During one meet-and-greet, Mr. Brown was asked by a local resident, 'The Great White Hope (referring to a grocery store) has been here before and failed. Why are you different?' To this Mr. Brown responded, 'I want to be here, that's the difference'.[23] The ShopRite grocery store has become a protected resource to the local community, which is expressed clearly by the community's response to the looting of the grocery store during protests of the George Floyd murder in 2020.[24]

> We developed a plan to get 300 men to come to ShopRite to stand guard', Pastor Johnson told Brown. 'But as of this morning, there were 3,700 people . . . to stand in solidarity with you.

In addition to Jeff Brown, there are many other examples of food stores funded by the FFFI that have had important impacts on the foodscapes and residents throughout Pennsylvania. For example, in Blossburg, PA, funding from FFFI provided Melanie and Ryan Shaut, a young, local couple with entrepreneurial goals, with the financing needed to purchase the Bloss Holiday Market from the retiring owners. The Bloss Holiday Market is the only source of fresh produce for nearly 8 miles in this north-central Pennsylvania town.[25] Second, in south-central Adams County, Kennie's Market, a family- and employee-owned supermarket located in the heart of Gettysburg received FFFI funding for the construction of a new 32,000-square-foot store. The expanded store offers residents convenient access to an expanded selection of fresh food and created fifty new jobs for the city.[26] Third, in Apollo, near Pittsburgh, experienced supermarket operators Randy and Brenda Sprankle bought two stores on the verge of closure due to the previous owners' retirements with assistance from FFFI; both stores were the only supermarkets in their respective communities.[27] Finally, and quite significantly, more than a decade after the supermarket has closed and Reverend Sullivan and his congregation built Progress Plaza, FFFI funded Fresh Grocer to open a new 46,000-square-foot supermarket at Progress Plaza, which has anchored the rebuilt plaza. Fresh Grocer has improved food access and economic opportunities for the Yorktown community as well as serving as a hub for nutrition education with tastings and marketing materials about healthy food options.[28] A longtime Yorktown community member, Anita Chappell, recalled as Fresh Grocer prepared to open in Progress Plaza:

> To see it come back to its strength and vibrancy the way he imagined it, it took years, it took money, it took patience, it took tears, a lot of prayers. So, it is just marvelous to see it there. I'm just thrilled that I lived to see it.

TABLE 4.3

Pennsylvania's Fresh Food Financing Initiative Selected Funded Projects

Food Retailer	Description	Location in PA	FFFI Grant/Loan Amount Awarded	Use	Intended Community Impact
ShopRite of Island Ave.[39,40]	Supermarket chain in the Northeast U.S.	Philadelphia	$250,000 in grants	Workforce development and training costs	Provide fresh and affordable food, community connection through new community meeting rooms, and investment in local prepared food vendors. Created 258 jobs, most of which qualify for employee benefits.
Ha Ha's[40]	Specialty Food Store, Korean-owned neighborhood fish market, est. 1989	Philadelphia	$25,000 in grants $30,000 in loans	Renovated refrigeration units, repaired HVAC equipment, purchased a much-needed new ice machine, replaced store windows, expanded the store, increased fresh food options	Increase fresh produce, fish, and spice offerings to the community
Fresh Grocer of Progress Plaza[28]	Supermarket chain with seven stores in the tristate area	Philadelphia	$250,000 in grants $2.3 million in loans	Predevelopment costs as well as renovations, new equipment, security, and staff training	Created 272 jobs, 80% of which are filled by neighborhood residents
Weaver's Way Cooperative[41]	Cooperative food market focused on local sustainable producers	Philadelphia	$126,715 in grants	Developed second location	A source of both fresh and affordable foods and community engagement.
First Oriental Market[42]	Asian specialty supermarket	Philadelphia	$500,000 in loans	Purchased property that had previously been leased, enabling owners to make building improvements including roof repairs, paving the parking lot, and installing new security gates	Employs 32 people and is one of the largest Asian supermarkets in the city. The supermarket has been at its current site in this low-income neighborhood for ten years and has had its present owners since 1999.
Romano's[26]	Convenience Store	Philadelphia	$60,000 in grants	Demolition, predevelopment, and operating expenses of implementing energy-efficient measures	Provide 13 fresh fruits and vegetables, frozen fruits and vegetables, whole grains, 100% juice, low-fat dairy options, and eggs to a community with an above-average obesity rate. A model for energy-efficient and eco-friendly building.
Boyer Family Market[39]	Supermarket chain in Northeastern PA	Orwigsburg	$500,000 in grants	Purchased energy-efficient supermarket equipment, furniture and fixtures, leasehold and tenant improvements, and employee training	The 17-store supermarket chain employs more than 950 people, expanded food offerings to the community of organic and fresh produce, prepared foods to go, fresh seafood and meats

(Continued)

TABLE 4.3 (Continued)
Pennsylvania's Fresh Food Financing Initiative Selected Funded Projects

Food Retailer	Description	Location in PA	FFFI Grant/Loan Amount Awarded	Use	Intended Community Impact
Bloss Holiday Market[25]	Specialty food store, store specializing in meats	Blossburg	No data	Purchased refurbished meat and deli cases, purchased better lighting with energy efficient features, replaced dial-up checkout, added catering services, re-organized store to remove clutter	The only community, family-owned market for 15 miles in an area dominated by Walmart
Cassville Country Store[25]	Full-service restaurant and catering with grocery and deli	Cassville	No data	Purchased two produce coolers and prep table with refrigerated storage to prepare food to order. Partnered with local farmers to provide seasonal produce.	The only grocery store within 15 miles
Hurley's Fresh Market[25]	Grocery store with two locations in PA	North Towanda	No data	Expanded store's bakery, deli, and fish counter, doubling revenue with increased food offerings	Provide offerings of seasonal local produce, perishable foods, meat, and fish to the community
Right By Nature[39]	Grocery store opened in 2008 and closed in 2011	Pittsburgh	$250,000 in grants	Purchased equipment, inventory, and working capital, plus preopening labor costs, and supporting professional services	Provide affordable, fresh, and organic produce to the neighborhood, as well as provides 60 part-time and 20 full-time jobs
Shop 'n Save in Heldman Plaza[26]	Limited Assortment Grocery Store, store closed in 2019	Pittsburgh	$1 million in grants	Development and new construction	First grocery store in nearly 30 years, brought 100 jobs to the area
Kennie's Market[26]	Grocery Store	Gettysburg	$250,000 in grants	Rebuilt and expanded, purchased energy-efficient coolers, and new equipment	The only grocery store in a town of 7,500 people. Created 50 jobs and increased fresh produce offerings to the community
Sprankle's Neighborhood Market[40]	Grocery Store	Vandergrift and Apollo	$248,000 in grants $1 million in loans	Purchased two closing markets from retiring grocery owners, upgraded equipment and inventory to make stores full-service supermarkets with fresh produce, meat, deli, and grocery departments	The only supermarkets in either town, providing walkable access to residents of these moderate-income communities, including many nearby seniors
Mastrorocco's Market[42]	Specialty Food Store, a wholesale meat company	Derry	$25,000 in grants $600,000 in loans	Renovated the store, installed a new HVAC unit, built a new loading dock, and upgraded the store's lighting units	The only full-service supermarket in town
Lancaster Central Market[42]	Historic public market located in Penn Square, and is the oldest farmers market in the U.S.	Lancaster	$100,000 in grant funding	Improved infrastructure to support 60 plus small business vendors selling local fresh produce, meats, and seafood	Allowed the market to remain a crucial food source and economic generator for Lancaster City

FOUNDATION SUPPORT AND IMPACT ON FEDERAL AND STATE PUBLIC POLICIES

With its mission to increase access to healthy 'food for every child', Pennsylvania's Fresh Food Financing Initiative (FFFI) was launched in 2004. Its success in funding supermarket projects across the state in low-income and underserved areas – quickly – was evident within just a few years. In recognition of FFFIs success in increasing accessibility of nutritious foods while also providing job opportunities and fostering neighborhood revitalization, in 2008, Harvard University recognized the Pennsylvania FFFI as one of the 'Top 15 Innovations in American Government'.[29]

Concurrently, rising childhood obesity rates in the United States were causing great alarm among those dedicated to improving child public health. In fact, some policymakers declared childhood obesity 'as one of the most critical public health threats of the twenty-first-century'.[30] Also of significant concern was that while the obesity 'epidemic' was affecting children of all ages, income groups, races and ethnicities across the country, Black Americans, Hispanics, and American Indian children were disproportionately affected.[31]

Government agencies and private foundations dedicated to improving public health started looking for solutions. In 2001, the U.S. Surgeon General issued the Call to Action to Prevent and Decrease Overweight and Obesity to stimulate the development of specific agendas and actions targeting this public health problem. In recognition of the need for greater attention directed to prevent childhood obesity, Congress, through the fiscal year 2002 Labor, Health and Human Services, Education Appropriations Act Conference Report, directed the Centers for Disease Control and Prevention (CDC) to request that the Institute of Medicine (IOM) develop an action plan targeted to the prevention of obesity in children and youth in the United States.[32] In addition to the CDC, the study was supported by the Department of Health and Human Services' Office of Disease Prevention and Health Promotion (ODPHP); National Institute of Diabetes and Digestive and Kidney Diseases (NIDDK); the National Heart, Lung, and Blood Institute (NHLBI); the National Institute of Child Health and Human Development (NICHD); the Division of Nutrition Research Coordination of the National Institutes of Health; and the Robert Wood Johnson Foundation.

The Institute of Medicine Committee on Prevention of Obesity in Children and Youth was charged with developing a prevention-focused action plan to decrease the prevalence of obesity in children and youth in the United States. One suggested solution was to implement strategies that would improve both the access to and affordability of fruits and vegetables. To achieve this, many believed that there needed to be increased focus on improving the physical environments (including neighborhoods, schools, and playgrounds) that children interact with so that healthy behaviors like healthy eating were better supported.

The focus on improving and investing in the environment for low-income children and children of color mattered to many in the racial justice and racial equity movement. For decades, community development efforts, defined as 'the work of building and sustaining neighborhoods',[33] to improve Black neighborhoods and neighborhoods with a high proportion of residents who are people of color or low income, had primarily focused on affordable housing. Angela Glover Blackwell, racial equity leader and founder of PolicyLink,[34] a national research and action institute advancing racial and economic equity explained,

> I remember a community development conference I attended nearly thirty years ago. The people in the room focused on building attractive, affordable housing as the way to revitalize severely distressed neighborhoods and improve the lives of residents, most of them people of color. I questioned the premise. Why concentrate affordable homes in neighborhoods without transportation, good schools, grocery stores, jobs, and all the other resources that people need to thrive? Would nicer apartments in and of themselves strengthen the economic and social fabric of a neighborhood stripped of investment or put its residents on a path to financial security and success? . . .

Rather than revitalize communities, billions of dollars in housing investments fueled concentrated poverty and further constricted opportunity for generations of people of color who needed and deserved better.[35]

As Blackwell points out, racist policies and practices that led to racially segregated neighborhoods throughout the United States also starved these neighborhoods of resources and access to a range of much needed basic public services and businesses, including banks, playgrounds, public transportation, high-quality schools and supermarkets. 'Racial inequity is the result of structural racism that is embedded in our historical, political, cultural, social, and economic systems and institutions'. A critical approach to addressing this was through public policy, as policy 'is the key to reversing the racial, social, and economic exclusion it fostered in the first place'.[35]

The Robert Wood Johnson Foundation (RWJF), the nation's largest health philanthropy, was one of the private foundations that supported the idea that improving the built environment through public policy initiatives was critical – for improved health and to support racial equity. Former RWJF President and CEO Risa Lavizzo-Mourey, MD was quoted as saying, 'We all have a role to play in our homes, schools, and neighborhoods to ensure that all kids have healthy food and safe places to play'. In 2007, RWJF, under Lavizzo-Mourey's leadership, made a commitment of $500 million to end the childhood obesity epidemic (eventually the foundation dedicated more than $1 billion to reversing the childhood obesity epidemic) and was looking to invest in proven public policy solutions that could be replicated across the United States.[36]

The foundation made their rationale for the investment clear, as evidenced by this public statement:

> When we think about what it takes to live healthy, having easy access to nutritious food is critical. For millions of households, a lack of reliable access to healthy food hinders children's growth and development and increases risk for obesity and challenges to health and well-being throughout life. This is especially true in low-income communities in inner-city and rural areas, where convenience stores and fast-food restaurants are widespread but major grocery stores are often scarce.

The Greater Philadelphia Urban Affairs Coalition is another example of a funder which supported the work to help supermarket developers to 'enhance contracting opportunities for minority and women-owned businesses and to ensure that women, minorities, and local residents have access to employment in the new supermarkets'.

The Pennsylvania Fresh Food Financing Initiative was viewed by RWJF (and others in philanthropy and government) as a promising policy that could be replicated in other states and increase access to healthy food in low-income neighborhoods. Some promising aspects included: 'its use of flexible capital, a single point of entrance for gaining funds, the cooperation and utilization of specialty organizations and nonprofits, and its application of industry knowledge to program administration'.[29] A public-private partnership that combined the private capital raised by Community Development Finance Institutions (CDFIs) and public funds, FFFI was widely viewed as a successful program that could promote community development and job creation in low-income and historically racially segregated neighborhoods and potentially narrow the racial disparities in childhood obesity rates by facilitating the opening of grocery stores offering healthy food options. After the establishment of the FFFI, the foundation provided funding to The Food Trust to establish similar programs in other parts of the country – beginning with Illinois and Louisiana.

The Food Trust's role in advocating for the replication of the PA FFFI in other states included[21]: (1) conducting research and publishing reports on the health impacts in neighborhoods with low supermarket access; (2) convening a local task force to review the problem, consider possible solutions, and make policy recommendations; (3) produce and distribute reports highlighting the task force's final recommendations; and (4) advocate for policy changes endorsed by the task force. Typically, a task force would offer up to ten policy recommendations, with one of the recommendations being the creation of a financing initiative based on the Pennsylvania FFFI model.

If advocacy for a healthy food financing program was successful, The Food Trust also, in some states, helped with implementation of the new financing program, in partnership with a CDFI and a local government agency (and an additional private foundation in some cases). Implementation activities might include reviewing applications for funding and determining eligibility, marketing the program to grocers, and hosting community meetings to solicit feedback on what community grocery needs were. For example, as we discuss later in the text in the chapter dedicated to New Orleans, once their Fresh Food Retailer Initiative was established, The Food Trust partnered with a CDFI called *HOPE Enterprise Corporation* and other partners to administer the program and evaluate applications to determine eligibility.[37]

CONCLUSION

While the level of state funding varies from year to year (including no funding at all for several years), the Pennsylvania Fresh Food Financing Program continues to provide grants to food retailers across the state and adapt to the food access needs of underserved Pennsylvania residents. In response to COVID-19, the state channeled additional grant support to the PA FFFI, made available through federal stimulus dollars, also known as the CARES Act.[38] The program continues to have a focus on racial equity. The stimulus funding made available in 2020 gave special prioritization to food retailers, food distributors and other food businesses that 'are owned by and serve low-income BIPOC [Black, Indigenous, and People of Color] communities'. Redlining, the racist practice of identifying areas where high proportions of Black and other minority Americans resided, and then restricting mortgage lending to those areas specifically, resulted in disinvestment in many Philadelphia communities and shifted investment to growing White suburbs. The negative effects of racism, redlining, and segregation continue to this day – and are largely responsible for creating the food access problem in urban (and some rural) areas in America. The lack of investment in racially segregated and redlined areas resulted in inadequate delivery of many basic services (transportation, trash pick-up, even mail delivery) and a lack of thriving businesses, including grocery stores offering healthy foods like fresh produce.

In Philadelphia, the response was to have community members, nonprofit groups, community development banks, grocers, and policymakers come together to bring needed services and critical businesses, such as supermarkets, to underserved neighborhoods throughout the city. Initially, Black American leader, Rev. Dr. Leon H Sullivan organized community members to take matters into their own hands and self-invest in their own neighborhoods. Thanks to monetary support from members of Dr. Sullivan's congregation, Zion Baptist Church, the first Black American owned shopping center, Progress Plaza was opened in 1968 and a much-needed supermarket was brought to north Philadelphia. Later, nonprofit groups such as The Food Trust and the Urban Affairs Coalition, Reinvestment Fund, and policymakers including Congressman Dwight Evans (formerly PA state representative) joined together to create the Pennsylvania Fresh Food Financing Initiative to increase investment in formerly redlined areas and bring high-quality grocery stores back to urban and rural areas throughout the state of Pennsylvania.

The success of this first-of-a-kind program gained national attention from government, academia, and philanthropy. As a result, The Food Trust received funding to replicate the program in other parts of the country. In the words of Congressman Dwight Evans: 'Food is at the center of our daily lives. Food is nourishment. Food is sustenance. But more than this, food is the cement that sets a foundation for strong neighborhoods within our communities'.

CRITICAL THINKING QUESTIONS AND EXERCISES

1. Why is Progress Plaza such a landmark area for access to food for the Yorktown community?
2. Identify an underserved local food environment and discuss the Food Market Task force that might provide insight for changes to that community's food environment.
3. Play the role of the members of the Food Marketing Task Force and develop a list of barriers and solutions to opening a grocery store in an underserved area from the perspective of the role being played.
4. Describe the reasons why food stores were not located in low-income areas of Pennsylvania incorporating lessons learned from Chapters 2 and 3.
5. Explain who initiated state policy changes to address local food environment disparities.
6. Describe the process for developing the FFFI.
7. Document how funds are made available through the FFFI, what the status of the program is today, how funds can be used and types of projects funded with the FFFI.
8. Articulate how the FFFI has impacted underserved areas in Pennsylvania.

REFERENCES

1. Gillibrand K. S.821 Healthy Food Financing Initiative. In: 113th Congress (2013–2014), ed. Washington, DC: Congress.gov; 2013.
2. Blumgart J. *How Redlining Segregated Philadelphia*. Philadelphia, PA: WHYY; 2017.
3. Drake SC, Cayton HR. *Black Metropolis: A Study of Negro Life in a Northern City*. Chicago: University of Chicago Press; 1970.
4. Code of Ethics. National Association of Real Estate Boards; June 6, 1924.
5. Massey DS, Denton NA. *American Apartheid: Segregation and the Making of the Underclass*. Cambridge, MA: Harvard University Press; 1993.
6. Administration FH. Underwriting Manual: Underwriting and Valuation Procedure under Title II of the National Housing Act with Revisions to February, 1938. In: Washington, DC: Federal Housing Administration; 1939.
7. Jackson KT. *Crabgrass Frontier: The Suburbanization of the United States*. Oxford: Oxford University Press; 1987.
8. Bartelt DW. Urban housing in an era of global capital. *The ANNALS of the American Academy of Political and Social Science*. 1997;551(1):121–136.
9. Weems RE, Randolph LA. The national response to Richard M. Nixon's black capitalism initiative: The success of domestic detente. *Journal of Black Studies*. 2001;32(1):66–83.
10. Baradaran M. Opinion: The real roots of "black capitalism". *The New York Times*. 2019; https://www.nytimes.com/2019/03/31/opinion/nixon-capitalism-blacks.html
11. PolicyLink. Community Reinvestment Act: Equitable Development Toolkit. In: 2001.
12. Weinberg Z. *No Place to Shop: The Lack of Supermarkets in Low-Income Neighborhoods*. Washington, DC: Public Voice for Food and Health Policy; May 1995.
13. Kane J. The supermarket shuffle. *Mother Jones*. 1984;7.
14. Blay-Palmer A. *Imagining Sustainable Food Systems: Theory and Practice*. Farnham, Surrey, England; Burlington, VT: Ashgate; 2010.
15. Sarkar P. Scrambling for customers: The supermarket was born 75 years ago: One-stop shopping has come a long way. *San Francisco Chronicle*. 2005.
16. History. *Reading Terminal Market*. 2017, 2020; https://readingterminalmarket.org/about-us/history/.
17. Cotterill RW. The urban grocery store gap. In: Franklin AW, ed. *Food Marketing Policy Center*. Mansfield, CT: University of Connecticut; 1995:82.
18. Perry D. Food for Every Child: The Need for More Supermarkets in Philadelphia. In: Philadelphia, PA: The Food Trust; 2001.

19. Giang T, Hillier A, Karpyn A, Laurison HB, Perry RD. Closing the grocery gap in underserved communities: The creation of the Pennsylvania fresh food financing initiative. *Journal of Public Health Management and Practice*. 2008;14:272+.

20. Burton H, Perry D. Stimulating Supermarket Development: A New Day for Philadelphia. In: Philadelphia, PA: The Food Trust; 2004.

21. Lang B, Harries C, Manon M, et al. The Healthy Food Financing Handbook. 2013; http://thefoodtrustorg/uploads/media_items/hffhandbookfinaloriginalpdf.

22. Treuhaft S, Karpyn A. The Grocery Gap: Who Has Access to Healthy Food and Why It Matters. In: Oakland, CA: PolicyLink and the Food Trust; 2010.

23. Feeding The Soul: Grocer Jeff Brown Tackles Philadelphia's Food Deserts. [Online article]. 2019; www.ypo.org/2019/06/feeding-the-soul-grocer-jeff-brown-tackles-philadelphias-food-deserts/.

24. Panaritis M. ShopRite returns after the looting, but this is not enough: Jeff Brown is not enough. *The Philadelphia Inquirer*. June 18, 2020.

25. The PA Fresh Food Financing Initiative: Case Study of Rural Grocery Store Investments. Philadelphia, PA: The Reinvestment Fund; 2012.

26. *Healthy Food Retail Financing at Work: Pennsylvania Fresh Food Financing Initiative*. 2011.

27. The Reinvestment Fund. *Pennsylvania Fresh Food Financing Initiative*. Philadelphia, PA: The Reinvestment Fund; 2008.

28. Progress Plaza. Philadelphia, PA; 2005, 2020; https://nmtccoalition.org/project/progress-plaza/.

29. *Fresh Food Financing Initiative: 2008 Finalist Commonwealth of Pennsylvania*. Cambridge, MA: Harvard Kennedy School of Government; 2008.

30. Institute of Medicine Committee on Prevention of Obesity in Children and Y: The National Academies Collection: Reports funded by National Institutes of Health. In: Koplan JP, Liverman CT, Kraak VI, eds. *Preventing Childhood Obesity: Health in the Balance*. Washington, DC: National Academies Press (US) National Academy of Sciences; 2005.

31. Ogden CL, Carroll MD, Kit BK, Flegal KM. Prevalence of obesity and trends in body mass index among US children and adolescents, 1999–2010. *JAMA*. 2012;307(5):483–490.

32. Institute of Medicine. *Preventing Childhood Obesity: Health in the Balance*. Washington, DC: Institute of Medicine; 2005.

33. Building the Engine of Community Development in Detroit. What Is Community Development in Detroit? 2016. Accessed March 24, 2021.

34. PolicyLink. Angela Glover Blackwell. 2021. Accessed March 24, 2021.

35. Blackwell A. Why the Equity Movement Needs Its Elders. *Journal of the American Society on Aging*. 2017;41(4):64–68.

36. Robert Wood Johnson Foundation Doubles Its Commitment to Helping All Children Grow Up at a Healthy Weight [press release]. www.rwjf.org/en/library/articles-and-news/2015/02/rwjf_doubles_commitment_to_healthy_weight_for_children.html#:~:text=Princeton%2C%20N.J.%E2%80%95Recognizing%20that%20obesity,they%20are%20or%20where%20they2015.

37. Committee. NOFA. *Building Healthy Communities: Expanding Access to Fresh Food Retail*. New Orleans: Robert Wood Johnson Foundation; 2007.

38. Coronavirus Aid Relief and Economic Security Act. In: 2020.

39. Evans D. Pennsylvania Fresh Food Financing Initiative. In: Committee HA, ed. Budget Briefing, ed. 2010.

40. The Reinvestment Fund. *The Economic Impacts of Supermarkets on Their Surrounding Communities*. Philadelphia, PA: The Reinvestment Fund; 2007.

41. Lenzi M. Healthy food: A key to the future of urban and metropolitan America. *The Shuttle*. September 2009.

42. Weidman J. FFFI Examples. In: 2020.

5 New Orleans, Louisiana

CONTENTS

INTRODUCTION

New Orleans has a deep, complex history with food. From its early roots in the slave trade, driven in part by the sugar cane industry, to supermarket destruction from Katrina, food access often reflects an underlying power struggle and meaning for residents which encapsulates more than food alone. Layered on top of the infrastructure and justice issues is the bureaucracy that guides programs, including disaster response funds. Despite challenges, public-private partnerships can work. This chapter describes a brief history of New Orleans, including the ways in which equity influences place. This chapter also explains the historical differences of food disparities between Black and White neighborhoods in New Orleans. It describes in detail the way in which the New Orleans Fresh Food Retailer Initiative was formed and the parameters by which the program operates. The stories of Circle Food Store and Whole Foods, two supermarkets which were able to open their doors in part because of the financing programs developed, are also shared.

Before Katrina, 14,000 people lived in the Lower 9th Ward, yet in 2014 only 3,000 residents had returned. Since the storms' devastation, the 9th Ward had not had any grocery stores until Burnell Colton opened the Lower 9th Ward Market and said the following about the store:

> It's bigger than me, it's bigger than them [my family] it's about the whole entire community. It's become a second home to some of the kids, I have people drive to the window and just cry and want to take pictures with me. The store has changed people's entire life.[1]

A Brief History of New Orleans

In the words of the first Creole cookbook author (1877) Lafcadio Hearn, New Orleans 'resembles no other city upon the face of the earth, yet it recalls vague memories of 100 cities.' Deeply steeped in French, Spanish, and West African traditions and rooted in a history of immigration and slavery, it is an American food story that like many, depicts the value of food retail in communities where racial injustice and inequity have a long history. New Orleans was officially founded in 1718 by the French, who were eager to develop a city on the continent, in part to keep up with the established British colonies in Philadelphia and Boston that had already been in place for nearly a century. Financing for the city itself came because of an investment scheme attributed to a Scottish economist named John Law. The failed approach was later dubbed the Mississippi Bubble. By 1720, the bubble burst, leaving investors destitute and New Orleans without ongoing capital funds. The result was a French population disillusioned about the potential of a prosperous city once promised. In concert with financial challenges, France had trouble populating its new city, and reports of early efforts indicate that the government went to extreme lengths to relocate French speaking people to the city, including relocating French prisoners recently paired with Parisian prostitutes.[2]

In the late 1790s the expanding United States was granted access to the Mississippi River ports and infrastructure, enabling the nation to prosper from the growing sugar and cotton industries. Wealthy settlers, with privileged access to surveyor's maps, purchased land that occupied the elevated geologic ridges of the often-wet marsh land from a city situated in the Mississippi floodplain. Sugar plantations occupied vast stretches of land between the Mississippi river to Lake Pontchartrain, across what today is the lower 9th Ward. During this time, the city's population dramatically increased, becoming the site of the largest slave market in the Deep South. New Orleans was an economy and city developed by enslaved people, evidenced in part by the slave-built levees, and the more than 100,000 people, many who were children younger than 13, bought or sold between 1804 and 1862.[3]

Redlining in New Orleans

Following the 1929 stock market crash, New Orleans, like much of the United States, benefited from federal efforts to revive the housing market and make home ownership available to many American families. The 1934 Federal Housing Administration policies enabled long-term (30-year) home mortgages, and as a result, provided the economic conditions that stimulated the single-family suburban home boom. In New Orleans, like Philadelphia and many other cities across the United States, maps were drawn to depict which areas of the city would be eligible for the federal mortgage insurance that backed the home loans.[4] The result was that neighborhoods where Black and Brown residents resided were often deemed 'hazardous', while many White neighborhoods were not. Mortgage rules for 'single-family' areas excluded Blacks from 'desirable' neighborhoods to restrict the 'blighting of property values and the congesting of the population, whenever the colored or certain foreign races invade a residential section'. Economically, home ownership became an important mechanism for White families to establish wealth, while Black and Brown families were largely denied mortgage capital, perpetuating segregation (Figure 5.1).

Pontchartrain Park: An Example of a Black Middle-Class Suburban-Style Community

While many of the Black and Brown residents of New Orleans were unable to access the new suburban lifestyle, a relatively rare instance of rebellion against the FHA criteria changed that for 1,000 families. The New Orleans Mayor at the time, DeLesseps Morrison, backed by survey data demonstrating adequate incomes among Black residents as well as a verbal financial commitment by the philanthropic daughter of the founder of Sears, Roebuck & Company, negotiated an exception to the FHA criteria, which enabled the construction in 1954 of a

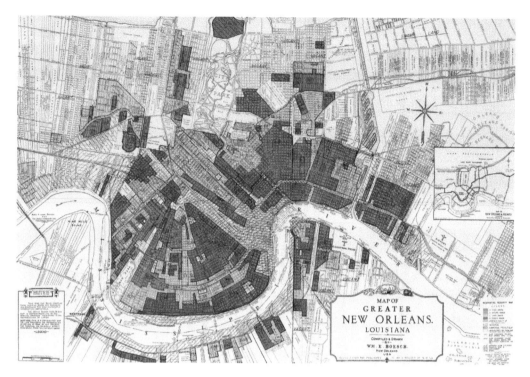

FIGURE 5.1   Map of Redling in Greater New Orleans, Louisiana

suburban-style Black middle-class community called Pontchartrain Park (PP). The community offered new homes with fenced yards, a golf course, new schools, playgrounds, fishing lagoons, and a shopping center complete with a supermarket. 'Everything was perfect [in PP]. It was a perfect place for a kid to be raised'.[5] Research on the impact of the community confirms the neighborhood cohesiveness. Interviews with children who were raised there finds that the neighborhood created conditions that enabled social capital, education, and spiritual development, along with long-lasting communal bonds. Together these resources helped to confront racial hostility and improved potential for health and prosperity, including valuable networks for job opportunities. The example is one of few early policies that effectively promoted equity among those in greatest need.

GROCERY STORES IN NEW ORLEANS

Grocery stores in New Orleans have for more than 200 years served as a mechanism to 'create a thriving residential and commercial neighborhood' as part of mixed use communities.[6] In the city, residents have for generations 'made groceries' with the passion and care that you would expect from a place with such rich and historic food culture. The local neighborhood store was a staple in the community, and although the same trends that many cities felt to shift to larger suburban stores happened in New Orleans as well, local retailers survived, recognized by residents as an important part of the 'fabric of the city'.

TOWARD DEVELOPMENT OF THE NEW ORLEANS FRESH FOOD RETAILER INITIATIVE

In late August 2005 Hurricane Katrina, made landfall near New Orleans with 120-mile-per-hour sustained winds.[7] About a month later, the already damaged city was subjected to a second storm, Hurricane Rita, which, along with a levee failure, collectively had profound effects throughout southeastern Louisiana, including flooding across large areas of the state. In total, the storms led to more than $108 billion in damage to homes and infrastructure and 1,800 lives lost, nearly half due to chronic disease exacerbated by the storms' effects. While the disparities in food access were apparent before the natural disasters, they opened the realities of the inequities at a time when much of the country was watching the media coverage of the stores. The wide scale destruction exposed several deeply entrenched inequities that had been a reality long before Katrina. Victims were disproportionately low income, Black, and suffered from inadequate housing, poor diets, and compromised health. Further, those that had the means to leave the city for shelter did, resulting in more than 400,000 residents displaced by the storm. Staff member Julia Koprak at The Food Trust, a nonprofit organization that helped to support the food access work in the city, recalled the time during an interview.

> New Orleans was a city that had already faced centuries of systemic inequities before Katrina, and those just exacerbated after Katrina. Like we saw in Philadelphia and many other cities, a history of redlining, racism and other issues led to a lack of investment in healthy food retail. In New Orleans, people were already struggling to buy groceries in many neighborhoods, and that became a much bigger struggle.

To rebuild the city and bring back food retail to struggling communities, a series of efforts began to take shape to examine how to stimulate the redevelopment of food retail outlets in the city.

New Orleans, like many areas in the United States, has a history of a preponderance of smaller food stores that serve local communities and are a staple in more disadvantaged areas, as compared to larger supermarkets.[8] Community markets are particularly valuable in the context of a city where many do not have easy access to a vehicle. One New Orleans' study found that more than 60% of residents reported living greater than 3 miles from a supermarket and at the same time, more than 40% of these residents relied on transportation other than a car for their major grocery trips.[9,10] For these residents being able to shop close to home and walk to the store is an important part of food access. Ms. Koprak detailed the city's struggle to food access as such:

> There was a strong history of corner grocery stores and food culture. Many New Orleans residents recall a time not too far back when there was a robust amount of fresh seafood and fresh produce readily available in many neighborhoods.

Local grocery stores however are particularly vulnerable to economic shifts, and after Hurricane Katrina, considerable efforts were needed to reestablish grocery stores across the city.[11] The rebuilding effort included both state and city planning processes.

FOOD POLICY ADVISORY COMMITTEE IN NEW ORLEANS

The Food Policy Advisory Committee (FPAC) grew out of prior efforts, including early work to create a network called *Grow New Orleans*, which was organized by the New Orleans Food and Farm Network. Many community and committee members knew that access to fresh, nutritious food was inadequate in New Orleans prior to hurricane Katrina, but the circumstances had worsened considerably after the storms. By 2007 the group added members and formed a more formal FPAC (Table 5.1). The FPAC convened representatives from both the public and private sectors to initially share and then to create policy-oriented recommendations. (We discuss the process and activities of this group and parallel groups like it later in this section.) The New Orleans FPAC was formally established with a unanimous

TABLE 5.1
New Orleans Food Policy Advisory Committee Members

Committee Member	Title	Organization
Sr. Anthony Barczykowski	Executive Director	Department of Community Services
Eric Baumgartner	Director, Policy and Program Development	Louisiana Public Health Institute
Dwayne Boudreaux	Owner	Circle Food Store
Jay Breaux	Perishables Director	Breaux Mart Supermarkets
David Cody	Office of Recovery and Development Administration.	City of New Orleans
Jessica Elliott	Director, Governor Affairs	Louisiana Retailers Association
Dana Eness	Executive Director	The Urban Conservancy
Randy Fertel	President	The Ruth E. Fertel Foundation
Greta Gladney	Executive Director	The Renaissance Project
Denny Gnesda	Regional Vice President	Supervalu
Ashley Graham	Director	Share Our Strength Louisiana
Sandra M. Gunner	Director, Intergovernmental Affairs	New Orleans Chamber of Commerce
Natalie Jayroe	President and CEO	Second Harvest Food Bank of Greater New Orleans and Acadiana.
Jim LeBlanc	President and CEO	Volunteers of America of Greater New Orleans
Clayton Lester	Vice President	Corporate Marketing and Special Services Associated Grocers
Shaula Lovera	Program Director	Hispanic Apostolate for New Orleans
Veda Manuel	Community Member	Grow New Orleans
Richard McCarthy	Executive Director	Market Umbrella.org
Carl Motsenbocker	Professor of Horticulture	Louisiana State University AgCenter
Loretta Poree	Business Development Specialist	Small Business Administration
Darlene Robert	Secretary and Treasurer	Robert Fresh Market
Sandra Robinson	Deputy Director	New Orleans Health Department
Diego Rose	Nutrition Section Head	Tulane University School of Public Health and Tropical Medicine.
Donald Rouse	President	Rouse's
Bill Rouselle	President and CEO	Bright Moments Public Relations
Gregory St. Etienne	Chief Operating Officer	Ultimate Technical Solutions
Laurie Vignaud	SVP/ Senior Director	Community Development Banking Capital One N.A.
Judy Watts	President and CEO	Agenda for Children
John Weidman	Deputy Executive Director	The Food Trust
Michelle Whetten	Director, Gulf East	Enterprise Community Partners
Gary Wood	Senior Commercial Loan Officer	ECD/Hope Community Credit Union
Roy Zuppardo	Vice President	Zuppardo's Family Supermarket

city council resolution vote to enhance legitimacy in May 2007. The resolution is described as such:

> Whereas it is the belief of the city council of the city of New Orleans that everyone deserves equal access to healthy and nutritious foods, and this could serve as an economic catalyst for recovering neighborhoods; now, therefore be it resolved at the council of the city of New Orleans strongly supports the creation of a food policy advisory panel and . . . [t]hat a final report with recommendations for programs and policies to alleviate the problem be delivered to the special projects and economic development committee by January 31, 2008.

At the time the FPAC was established, New Orleans had been in recovery for nearly two years, struggling to understand how they should rebuild their community and attract residents back to New Orleans. Ms. Koprack describes the rebuilding in the following way:

> After Katrina, the rebuilding process in New Orleans was definitely uneven. Some neighborhoods in more affluent or tourist areas were rebuilt very quickly, though even many of those areas still lacked grocery stores. And then in other parts of the city, grocery store development really lagged, and it made the rebuilding of communities so much harder.

Without supermarkets and other local resources, the City struggled to appeal to the many residents who had fled and had not yet returned. At the state level, a regional plan called the *Louisiana Speaks Regional Plan* considered how reinvestment in specific regional resources could help to rebuild the parishes affected by the storm, ad how the investment could further support sustainable, diverse communities.

The Tulane University Prevention Research Center led the FPAC organizing effort locally, with strategic guidance from The Food Trust, who had staff funded in part by the Robert Wood Johnson Foundation to support national work developing programs that would establish supermarkets in underserved areas of the country. Julia Koprak, quoted throughout this chapter, was one of those staff. Ultimately, seven organizations formed the foundation of the FPAC, including Second Harvest Food Bank of Greater New Orleans and Acadiana, Louisiana Public Health Institute, City Health Department, Renaissance Project, New Orleans Food and Farm Network, TUPRC, and The Food Trust. Building from this framework, leaders from a cross-sector of organizations were added to the committee with the intention of achieving broad representation from the following areas: (1) the grocery sector, (2) farmers markets and local agriculture, (3) nonprofit organizations, (4) public health agencies and local government, (5) academic institutions, and (6) financial institutions. In total, thirty-two leaders participated, and among these included a strategic effort to invite and include food retailers; ultimately retailers or representatives from the food retail industry held nine of the thirty-two committee seats (Table 5.1).

The goal of the work was to identify ways to improve access to fresh food retail outlets. The mission was intentionally broader than grocery and supermarkets and included conversations about needed policies and programs to support small food stores and farmers markets as well. In this way the program sought to expand to include Pennsylvania as part of the Pennsylvania Fresh Food Financing Initiative. With a common goal, the committee worked together as part of a study process to generate a common understanding of the issues and then identify recommendations that would help to address areas of need. In total, the committee work lasted for six months, although the results of their work took several years to see fruition.

The first phase of the work undertaken by the FPAC was to conduct a needs assessment and examine relevant statistics as well as collect data about the extent of the problem. Data on the number of stores before and after the storms hit, the distance residents were traveling to shop for food, disparities in health outcomes, including obesity, as well as documentation of the interest in local residents to have more healthy local food, was presented at the meetings and in a report for wide-scale dissemination.[12]

Many realities were presented as part of the process. Among them was the fact that in 2007, fewer than half of the original full-service supermarkets had reopened in the city, and many smaller stores had been put out of business. Further, while the city's population had shrunk to only about 70% of its pre-storm size, the number of residents per supermarket had ballooned. Pre-Katrina there were about 12,000 residents for each supermarket in the city and afterward, even several years later, the number had risen to 18,000 residents per supermarket; a common standard is 1:10,000 residents.[13,14] This was in comparison to a national average of 8,800 residents per supermarket at the time.[12] In addition, a Tulane University study published in 2008 found that nearly 60% of New Orleans Parish residents who are low income needed to drive more than 3 miles to get to a supermarket. The challenge was further compounded because only about half of those in the study reported having their own car. Despite a lack of access to healthy food, nearly 70% said that they would or might buy fresh produce items if they were available in their neighborhood. Another local study done by Tulane found that as fresh vegetables became more available to residents, consumption increased significantly. Obesity was another concern for the committee and one discussed as part of the process. Data from the Centers for Disease Control for Louisiana indicated high rates of obesity and obesity-related comorbidities such as diabetes and heart disease. In 2008 nearly 28% of adults were obese, a statistic which reflected a dramatic rise over the past fifteen years; in 1991 only 16% of the Louisiana population were obese.

Unified New Orleans Plan and Other Simultaneous Rebuilding Efforts

Another process, called the *Unified New Orleans plan* (the UNOP process), was underway in New Orleans as well. Using participatory methods, including grassroots outreach, local meetings, surveys, and large community congresses, the UNOP process intended to catalyze the intense concern that many residents had for racial equity, including government mistrust and concern for financial equity and oversight in the redevelopment process. As such, the approach to develop a plan focused on hearing the voices of concerned residents in an inclusive and responsive manner. The concern was for a community with strong divisions along race and socioeconomic lines.

Among many issues discussed as part of the plan, access to healthy food was repeatedly raised as a critical factor for the recovery of neighborhoods. In fact, as drawings and urban planning designs were unveiled as part of the strategic recovery and rebuilding plan process, nearly every neighborhood plan included a supermarket or grocery store as part of its community. In tandem with the participatory process to understand an outline of vision for recovery efforts was the reality of the need for strategic financial investments that were equitable and assurances that resources would go where they were needed. Planning processes resulted in community members expressing concern for economic stewardship while calling for the creation of a state community reinvestment trust fund. This resource could provide grants to support plans and projects to reinvigorate existing commercial corridors. The fund could support other efforts to identify financial or tax incentives for developers and workforce development training funds for community members and businesses alike. Ms. Koprak described the effort in the following way:

> With food retail being so key to a community's vitality, it gained the attention of the city, Tulane University (specifically their Prevention Research Center) and Second Harvest Food Bank, along with many other partners. And it was around the same time when The Food Trust had recently launched this concept of 'healthy food financing' for the first time in Pennsylvania with Reinvestment Fund. Many leaders, including then Senator Mary Landrieu, looked to the Pennsylvania Fresh Food Financing program to learn more about this model and explore if these same efforts could be replicated in New Orleans.

In the eyes of many, the storm created an important policy window of opportunity for policy change in New Orleans.

Supermarkets as an Economic Development Strategy

The FPAC saw supermarket access as not just a way to provide food to community members but also as an important economic development strategy. Supermarkets create jobs, on average between 100 and 200 permanent jobs, although larger stores can create more.[15,16]

Furthermore, supermarkets often establish a commercial corridor and serve as an anchor tenant attracting other retail to the area.[17] The reestablishment of commercial corridors and supermarkets was seen as a mechanism to improve the physical landscape of the city and reduce blight. Research has also shown that an issue called retail leakage can be responsible for the loss of keeping retail demand local. Retail leakage occurs when residents want to buy food but cannot find it locally, which leads them to go to areas outside of their community and results in the loss of local dollars in local communities.

Another economic benefit of strong food retail in the city was its potential to create strong local sales tax revenue, which in turn could be used to fund other community needs. By creating more jobs and encouraging more spending locally, supermarkets and other new food retailers were highlighted to restore, and potentially enhance, the viability of New Orleans for all residents.

RETAILER CONCERNS VOICED

While supermarkets hold considerable potential for rebuilding communities, they are expensive to build and maintain, as described in Chapter 2. The industry is competitive and in general profits average about 1% of sales, leaving a small margin for error. Retailers in recent years have faced stiff competition from Walmart as well as dollar stores, particularly in the low- to moderate-income markets. In New Orleans, these challenges were magnified by the Hurricanes. Through the FPAC process, retailers were invited to share their challenges, in part as a mechanism to reach solutions. Retailers in Louisiana shared concerns about many issues, including the considerable challenges they faced in obtaining financing for new stores in the city, the prohibitively expensive costs of required insurance coverage for stores following the storms, their need for current market research data which could provide insight into population demographics, and spending potential so that they could site stores in a sustainable manner. Retailers further expressed concerns about the potential for crime and theft and the cost that such activities could incur in losses for their stores. As a result, additional comments were made related to addressing the concerns with costly added security measures (personnel, cameras, lighting, etc.). Retailers noted too the importance of having a strong qualified employee base and expressed concern over the potential to staff stores given the stark reduction in the population that the city felt following the storm. Regulatory and zoning processes were also raised as an issue. Retailers shared that these administrative processes can be complicated and that it often took considerable time and frustration to get the approvals necessary to rebuild in the city.

FOOD POLICY ADVISORY COMMITTEE RECOMMENDATIONS

After reviewing data and hearing retailer needs and concerns, the FPAC moved to develop policy recommendations as required by the Council of the City of New Orleans resolution. A list of ten recommendations were developed and reported less than one year after the FPACs formal establishment. Recommendations sought to increase access to a variety of retail outlets to benefit those who are most in need of nutritious foods. The committee specifically issued ten recommendations for the city, city and state, and state alone. They called for the city specifically to follow the action steps on Table 5.2. Furthermore, the committee made recommendations that both the city and the state make economic development programs available to fresh food retailers and address the need for transportation to supermarkets, grocery stores, and farmers markets for residents.

Regarding recommendations at the state level, the group requested that Louisiana prioritize the development of a financing program to provide grants and loans to supermarkets, smaller grocery stores, and other fresh food retailers that enhance healthy food access and

TABLE 5.2
Food Policy Advisory Committee's Recommendations and Actions Steps

Recommendation	Action Steps	Level of Recommendation
Adopt fresh food retailing as a priority for comprehensive neighborhood and direct development the Office of Recovery and Development Administration to provide grants and loans to food retail projects located in target areas Reduce regulatory barriers to businesses that sell fresh food Provide tax incentives to encourage the sale of fresh food Prioritize security for supermarkets and grocery stores	• A one-stop shopping approach for businesses making inquiries and submitting applications for licenses and permits • Making explanatory information and forms available via the City's website • A fast-tracked permitting process for fresh food retailers planning to locate in underserved communities	City of New Orleans
Make economic development programs available to fresh food retailers Address the need for transportation to supermarkets, grocery stores, and farmers markets	• The City and State should actively market programs to existing independent and smaller grocers • Establish a temporary grocery shuttle program that link the transit dependent families in underserved neighborhoods to full-service food retailers	City of New Orleans and the State of Louisiana
Develop a financing program that will provide grants and loans to supermarkets, smaller grocery stores, and other fresh food retailers that enhance healthy food access in underserved areas Expand participation in federal nutrition programs that enable more residents – especially seniors and families with children—to purchase locally grown fresh fruits and vegetables at famers' markets Partner with fresh food retailers to create vocational training opportunities in the fresh food retail sector	• Establish of a public-private partnership • Create a public-private partnership to provide EBT terminals, marketing materials, and training to farmers markets' managers at no charge • Partner with the fresh food retail sector to develop an industrywide vocational training program	State of Louisiana
The New Orleans Fresh Food Policy Advisory Committee serve as an ongoing, multistakeholder advisory to the City Council	• Adopting a Community Food Charter that outlines the strategies necessary to move the vision of a healthy New Orleans forward • Improving the nutritional value of food served in our schools • Supporting our local and regional food producers • Promoting environmental, nutritional, cultural, culinary, and horticultural awareness • Developing infrastructure and resources for fresh food growing throughout the city • Launching a full-scale market analysis of the city's untapped economic potential that can be used by a variety of fresh food retail	City Council of New Orleans

underserved areas. Further, they recommended the expanded participation in federal nutri-tion programs, which would enable more residents to purchase fruits and vegetables at farm-ers markets and other locally grown sources. Last, they requested that the state partner with food retailers to create vocational training opportunities within the fresh food retail sector. To manage the process and ensure that the forthcoming strategies would be comprehensive and diverse, the committee's final recommendation was to formally establish the New Orleans Food Policy Advisory committee as an ongoing multistakeholder advisory body for the New Orleans City Council.

After presentation to the FPAC, the group unanimously adopted the list of ten recommenda-tions, which included advising the city to establish a fund that would provide loans and grants for fresh food retail development targeted toward underserved areas of the city. After passing these recommendations FPAC introduced a resolution to create a new task force that would provide advice and recommendations about the parameters of program implementation. The now termed FPAC *Task Force* worked closely with the newly formed City Office of Recovery and Development Administration (ORDA) along with other civic and private sector groups to guide the development of the healthy retail policies. The task force operated for more than a year, working with the city to provide input and ultimately develop a proposal for how the city could use available disaster recovery funds to support the strategies prioritized by the FPAC. In 2008, $7 million was identified by the ORDA to support supermarket financing efforts, and another $3 million was identified to support smaller garden and farmers market efforts. In 2009 the budget was approved; however, it was not until more than two years later (2011) that the program was initiated. Administrative turnover within ORDA and political shifts, including a new mayoral administration, contributed to significant delays in the launch of the program; and the reality was that, only 2% of the recovery dollars for the city were earmarked for fresh food access and in the context of rebuilding. The effort took a back seat to other priorities. Funds for the city needed to come through the state. The process was long, requiring separate state approvals at every step.

THE NEW ORLEANS FRESH FOOD RETAILER INITIATIVE

In 2011, because of the determined FPAC efforts, a city financing program called the *Fresh Food Retailer Initiative* (FFRI) was created to support the development of supermarkets, gro-cery stores, and other fresh food markets across New Orleans' low-income and underserved neighborhoods. The program was based on the initial allocation of $7 million from the city for this purpose. A Community Development Financial Institution called *Hope Enterprise Corporation* (HOPE) and The Food Trust jointly administered the New Orleans program. Hope Enterprise Corporation (HOPE) is a Community Development Financial Institution (CDFI) ded-icated to strengthening communities, building assets, and improving lives in economically distressed areas of the mid-South by providing access to high-quality financial products and related services.

The program was seeded with an initial $7 million in Disaster Community Development Block Grant (D-CDBG) funds, which would be matched 1:1 by HOPE using other available funding sources. Under the FFRI program, HOPE has been responsible for the financing side of the work and provides lending support and grants to qualified retailers in a combination with forgivable and interest-bearing loans for predevelopment, site assembly and improvement, construction and rehabilitation, equipment installation and upgrades, staff training, security, and inventory and working capital for start-up costs. The Food Trust, the Philadelphia-based nonprofit involved in the development of the FFFI, brought their experience in establishing and partnering on the operation of financing programs. They were responsible for recruitment and community-oriented concerns and worked to evaluate applications to determine eligibility for the program as they had done for the FFFI. Of note in this process is the fact that a non–New Orleans organization (The Food Trust, Philadelphia, PA) played a key role in the implementation of the initiative. Ms. Koprak, explains her involvement:

> At the time, The Food Trust began to play a role across the country in helping to implement or train others to implement fresh food financing programs. We were able to use our experiences from other states as the New Orleans Fresh Food Retailer Initiative was getting launched, and formed a three-way partnership between the city, HOPE and The Food Trust.

Funding Parameters

The New Orleans FFRI program is still in existence as of 2021, and an applicant organization may have a for-profit or nonprofit status and can be a national grocery store chain, regional grocery chain, singular grocery retail outlet, and smaller neighborhood or cooperative food store (but not a farmers market). The program is limited to applicants who can demonstrate that they either plan to open a new store or renovate an existing building, and that the store they operate is a self-service supermarket or other grocery retail outlet that primarily sells 'affordable fresh produce, seafood, meat, dairy, and other groceries'.[18] A store may also qualify for funding if it is an existing store that sells less healthy food and is interested in expanding offerings to include a variety of fresh fruits and vegetables. The program is not open to other food businesses that process or manufacture food (e.g., a company that makes salsa) or restaurants.

To provide resources to the communities most in need, the program limits funding to specific community criteria. To be eligible for FFRI funds, the store or prospective store needs to be: (1) in the Orleans Parish; (2) a location where resident incomes are low or moderate (within a census tract OR service area where at least 51% of persons or households are low to moderate income); and (3) in an underserved grocery retail area (defined as an area of below average supermarket density or below average grocery sales). A provision was also made for stores that may be currently operating and serving the community but at risk for closing its doors. In this case, a grocery store or supermarket may also be eligible if it intended to retain permanent jobs, at least 51% of which (computed on a full-time equivalent basis) were available to, or held by, local residents.

Beyond economic parameters, program stakeholders, especially those representing public health, were genuinely concerned about the types of foods offered in the prospective retail stores and wished to include a minimum shelf space dedicated to fruits and vegetables. However well-intentioned, a requirement for shelf-space specific parameters would have led to some challenges in implementation and compliance monitoring. As a result, the program guidelines included a recommendation whereby significant shelf space (suggested minimum of either 15% of the current or future store shelf space or twenty-four linear feet of shelf space, whichever is greater) is dedicated to the sale of fresh fruit and vegetables.[18] As described by Ms. Koprak,

> What we wound up including in the guidelines [see previous paragraph] was that the applicant must demonstrate that there's a meaningful commitment to selling fruits and vegetables, though it wouldn't be realistic for program staff to go into stores with a measuring tape to ensure compliance.

The grants or loans received by the store owners through the program can be used for a variety of types of activities, all of which are determined to support the operational capacity or direct provision of healthy food in the community. For example, funds can be used to cover the cost of professional fees (e.g., architectural, engineering, etc.), market research studies, as well as for land or down payments for space. Funds can be used for demolition, environmental remediation, unstable foundations and soil conditions, and other costs associated with site and infrastructure improvement, for construction, or for equipment in the store. Often, stores have old, inefficient refrigeration that is costly to operate, and funds can be needed to install or upgrade equipment, since fruits and vegetables often need to be stored in cool temperatures. The program further recognizes that the business of selling fresh food requires that staff become specially trained in safe food handling techniques, sanitation, and management of fresh fruits and vegetables. As such, program funds are eligible to be used for these purposes. Further, and in response to the earlier committee recommendations, funds are able to be used to cover costs associated with store security and theft, including security staff, security training, and security related equipment and site design features to create a safe environment in a neighborhood setting. Last, the program made a provision for operators that the initial inventory costs for selling produce and other healthy food items can be covered by the funds in the program. This includes funding for first-time inventory or other working capital expenses necessary to the sale of fresh fruits and vegetables and the initial operations of the business.

The program includes several phases of application review, first to determine suitability of the proposal for the community as part of the eligibility application[18] and second for its economic viability. To examine the suitability of the application from a community perspective, the application is reviewed by the nonprofit organization, The Food Trust, in order according to parameters found in Table 5.3.

In addition to their responsibilities to review applications for adherence to these guidelines, The Food Trust in the early years of the program supported outreach to new potential projects

TABLE 5.3
Business Eligibility Guidelines

Review	Description of Parameter
Degree of Benefit to Underserved Populations	The project has a measurable impact on the level of affordable fresh foods provided to low- and moderate-income residents of the area that the project serves
Promotion of Fresh Foods and Vegetables	The applicant demonstrates a commitment to promoting the sale of fresh fruits and vegetables, e.g., the projects details strategies to promote fresh produce sales beyond simple availability, such as product placement, marketing, providing recipes and demonstrations, and outreach
Organizational Experience and Capacity	The applicant demonstrates the capacity to implement and sustain the project, e.g., through a sound financial/business plan and relevant experience in fresh food retail
Project Need	The project requires an investment of public funding to move forward, to create impact, or to be competitive with similar projects in the region
Community Support	The project demonstrates community support and/or partnerships as evaluated by letters of support from community-based organizations and community groups
Consistency with 'Green Community' Objectives	The project incorporates environmentally responsible practices into the project plan, such as integrated design, site improvements, water conservation, energy efficiency, and use of materials beneficial to the environment
Market and Demographic Evaluation	The applicant will examine the quality and accessibility of any local competition, site geography, and demographic profile of the census tract in which the site is located
Consistency with Plans	The applicant will coordinate with the City of New Orleans Master Plans, local community plans and community development program
Land Use and Urban Design	The project will adhere to sound land use and urban design principles

and retailers to help recruit applications. Ms. Koprak explained the recruitment in the follow-ing way:

> We conducted info sessions with many grocery wholesalers in the area, including Associated Grocers of Baton Rouge and Associated Wholesale Grocers. There's a large presence of independent, family-owned grocery stores in New Orleans, many of whom had served on the Food Policy Advisory Committee and helped advocate for the creation of the FFRI program. Many were either still operating grocery stores or had shuttered grocery stores which they were hoping to bring back.

Once a project is determined to adequately meet the eligibility criteria, the application advances to the financial review of the business loan application to determine whether the potential borrower met the required economic terms for the loan.

Applications for this phase of review are sent to HOPE Enterprise Corporation's Credit Committee so that the business and funding plan are reviewed to determine if the project complies with the requirements for an acceptable loan. Several general criteria apply in this phase of the process, although there are many additional details regarding funding terms that are not fully described here for simplicity. First, applicants cannot request more than $1,000,000 per store from this fund, inclusive of forgivable loans, such as grants, and loans that would be repaid. Second, those borrowing funds must have a minimum of 10% cash equity on hand for the project. Loan applicants must also have a credit score greater than 550, no prior history of bankruptcy, and have a minimum of five years of grocery store management experience with a preference of eight years. After the committee review is complete, and all necessary information gathered and determined eligible, the loan officer then must go through a formal credit approval process at HOPE. Following that approval, all program loans are then required to be reviewed by the City of New Orleans, which has authority to approve, modify, or deny applications. After approval, the financing program recipients are required to maintain and submit audited financial records and tax returns as well as other evidence of compliance with the terms just described. One such review is an environmental assessment to determine if the project follows current environmental regulations.

PROGRAM OUTCOMES

The rigorous and complex process described in the previous section takes time – time to identify viable applicants, time to compile the paperwork necessary to put forward the needed documentation of their viability, and time to work through the administrative lay-ers required by the partners. Before providing a description of the programs that have been funded, it is important to pause here and reflect on these guidelines and what they entail. Essentially this process is one that requires someone with strong credit, cash on hand, and with substantial retail experience plus the resources to assemble an application with the city and the patience to wait for layers of review. It can be tough to find this unique combination of characteristics of an applicant, which hinged not only on the upstanding financial back-ground of the applicant but also on the practical experience in grocery operations and dem-onstrated capacity to keep a grocery outlet in business while offering fresh food to residents.

To date, a handful of stores, including Whole Foods and Circle Food Store, have successfully opened with available funds, while several other projects have entered the pipeline but ulti-mately have not been able to open their doors, often because of project logistics and changes in leadership. Ms. Koprak explains:

> Many applicant projects had strong ideas and commitment but lacked a grocery expert on the ownership team and intended to hire a manager with retail experience. However, if that candidate didn't come through or left the project, then the project lacked the capacity and the expertise needed to see things through.

That said, several have opened and remain in operation today. The next sections explores two examples: Whole Foods and Circle Food Store.

WHOLE FOODS

Whole Foods is not a supermarket typically associated with serving low- to moderate-income communities; however the store on Broad Street in New Orleans sought to do just that.[19] The supermarket was included as part of a larger, multipurposed space ultimately called the *ReFresh Project*, which houses other social programs including a teaching kitchen and non-profit organizations dedicated to community service. Ms. Koprak explained the project:

> There had been an empty vacant grocery store (Schweggmann's) which was eventually pur-chased by a community group, Broad Community Connections, and converted into a multi-purpose site where there's now a smaller format Whole Foods, culinary training program and Tulane-led teaching kitchen.

The total project cost $20 million and of that, the supermarket obtained $1 million in financing from the FFRI. The new Whole Foods is 25,000 square feet of the total 60,000-square-foot space that was developed by a local community development company, Broad Community Connections. The redevelopment effort brings back to life a site which, dating back to 1965 had a supermarket, but after Katrina had been vacant.

Whole Foods is considered the anchor store in the ReFresh Project's development, a project that residents saw as critical to bringing back the health and economic strength of the city. Residents at its grand opening commented,

> This is where the culture resides. . . . These are the neighborhoods where it is the people that make New Orleans New Orleans. And for 50 or 60 years, Broad Street, just like Claiborne Avenue, just like a lot of these other avenues, has been completely disinvested in.[20]

The store's product mix emphasizes the less expensive 365 brand, as well as, featuring over 330 local products from producers including sauces and other value-added products. One producer's items for example featured Creole BBQ sauces named Who Doo and Beer Bee-Q, created by a local company called *NOLA foods*, which is owned and operated by a successful local resident entrepreneur.

CIRCLE FOOD STORE

At almost the same time the Whole Foods opened, so too was Circle Food Store preparing its reopening.[21] Unlike Whole Foods, Circle Food Store is a long-time staple store in the New Orleans community, traditionally owned and operated by local families and a highly valued socially integrated community resource. Many felt that if a supermarket initiative were to support stores that served the community, Circle Food Store would be at the top of the list. Those work-ing on the program felt the importance of rebuilding Circle Food Store. Ms. Koprak explained Circle Food Store like this:

> From when the FPAC convened, I think there was always a thought there should be a program to support grocery stores and I think in the background of all that was Circle Food Store which had been integral to the community. There were pictures of the flooded stores all over national news. Of course, there was interest in food access in many neighborhoods, but people often specifically asked, 'What can we do to bring back Circle?'

Circle Food Store, as it is known today, was originally one of a series of indoor markets and served as a community gathering space which included a grocery store, but also offered residents a bakery, pharmacy, and other retail resources dating back to 1854. Then called the *St. Bernard Market*, this historic location was one of several dozen public markets the city of New Orleans operated until around 1940.

The current Circle Food Store is the result of construction by prominent New Orleans architect Sam Stone Jr. The store opened its doors in 1938, named after the traffic circle that was at the intersection prior to construction. The store continued to serve the community, despite the addition in the 1960s of a large, raised interstate freeway (I-10). The highway changed the local environment for residents and took what was once a neighborhood of beautiful homes and Black-owned businesses along a tree-lined road, into a much different, denser, noisier urban neighborhood. However, the importance of the market to residents remained.

The effects of Katrina devastated the store and caused it to close its doors. An interview with 7th Ward resident Doris Burbank captures the sentiments of the community well.

> My name is Doris Burbank, I've been here over 53 years and I love my neighborhood, and I have some very good memories. This community which was around Claiborne and St. Bernard Ave. was a very vibrant, active, loving area. . . The Circle had been such a big part of this community. It's hard for those of us who have lived here for years to imagine going on without the Circle. That store was like glue, a community center. When you went in there to do your shopping you met people from all over. We deem it our neighborhood store, but this is a city store, people come from all over this city and shop in this store. Everybody loved going in the Circle because you could find everything you needed, even down to school uniforms.

When asked the question, 'What is it going to mean to you when and if the Circle opens?' Ms. Burbank responded:

> Oh, I'll be in 7th heaven when it opens, oh I'll be ecstatic I can go from this house to the Circle with my shopping cart. I don't have to ask anyone to bring me to the store; I can buy everything I want and need. Everything; there was a pharmacy in there. All you had to do was go.

**(Interview reported in the brochure, Circle Food Store:
The rebirth of the one stop shop, Tulane University, n.d.)**

Facing expensive damage, the owner Dwayne Boudreaux, who successfully operated the store from 1991 to 2005, immediately called upon the community and the city to help support and fund the market's reopening. The project required substantial investment however, and to obtain the capital needed, several sources were accessed. Ms. Koprak recalled:

> In terms of the total project cost for Circle, it was roughly a $9 million project. When it got rebuilt, $ 1 million was from the city's FFRI dollars, and the other $8 million came from other public and private sources, including a state loan and a New Markets Tax Credit transaction. The city wasn't the only source of funding in any of the FFRI projects and brought in significant other leveraged investments.

Eventually in 2014, nearly ten years after it closed, the iconic Circle Food Store reopened to residents. However, the impact of the many years of closure, coupled by more damages from flooding in 2018, caused its doors to again close. In 2019, the store was acquired by Rick L Jahari and Sydney Torres IV at a foreclosure auction for $1.7 million. In 2020, the store was reopened with an additional $1.2 million in funds for upgrades and renovations. It continues to operate today and provides fresh food access to 'make groceries' in the Seventh Ward.

CONCLUSION

Efforts to develop a financing initiative in New Orleans came together in part because of the additional resources and undeniable challenges the city faced after Hurricane Katrina. The hurricanes and levee failures caused unprecedented destruction to a city with a history of disparities dating back to its founding, magnifying their impacts. The community was determined to rebuild however, and national resources became an important part of the way forward. From local entrepreneurs and grocers to local organizations and networks, to university leadership, persistence to overcome is a hallmark of the New Orleans Retail story. The work built upon existing local efforts in tandem with strategic approaches advanced in other cities and states (Philadelphia and Pennsylvania). Like the story of Circle Food Store, efforts to rebuild and support grocery retail in the city of New Orleans are marked by progress, challenge, and disappointment, as well as frustrating lapses of time. Because the New Orleans funding efforts needed to respond to federal requirements, state interests, and deep distrust and concern from some about the potential to misuse funds, the mechanisms of financing, and applications for funding are a focal point of this chapter.

While the collaboration and partnerships are critical to forward the closing of these gaps, the work is ultimately realized through the financing. Without funds, supermarkets are not developed or redeveloped. In the New Orleans example, funds for the financing initiative were initially the result of federal disaster recovery monies which were leveraged to create a financing effort for food retailers. Such a mechanism is unique, and raises important questions about sustainability of funds and the extent to which the program will be able to operate over the longer term.

One outgrowth of the FFRI has been the development of other, similar funding mechanisms that have received foundation funding and support through other state or local resources. As such, the New Orleans work has also stimulated other local efforts and additional investments that have broadened capacity for such work regionally. In operation alongside the FFRI are the Baton Rouge Healthy Food Retail Initiative, Deep South Healthy Food Initiative, as well as Louisiana's Healthy Food Retail Program, which are three other efforts funded through private and public monies that are also in operation currently through HOPE Enterprise Corporation's CDFI and offer similar funding opportunities to retailers in the region. In many ways the community, the retailers in it, and the funds that support them are not static and continually evolve, grow, and emerge in different forms. Efforts that begin one way may shift to continue in another; however the work itself is not lost. By stimulating new enterprise, corridors that had deep histories are revitalized and connections between and across funding communities can be established to support current and future efforts.

CRITICAL THINKING QUESTIONS AND EXERCISES

1. How did the natural disaster enable residents to address issues of food equity in New Orleans?
2. What barriers did the program planners face? Could these barriers have been avoided?
3. Go to the HOPE Enterprise CDFI website and examine what programs are available to address issues in healthy food access, and other, related determinants of health.
4. What is meant by retail leakage and what is the impact on underserved communities?
5. How is the New Orleans's Healthy Food Retail Initiative like the FFFI in Pennsylvania described in Chapter 4? And how is it different?

REFERENCES

1. NationSwell. *Grocery to the 9th: One Man's Mission to Rebuild New Orleans's 9th Ward*. 2015.
2. Hardy DJ. The transportation of convicts to Colonial Louisiana. *JSTOR*. 1966;7(2):15.
3. Parry M. How should we memorize slavery? *The Chronicle Review* [Online article]. 2017; https://www.chronicle.com/article/how-should-we-memorialize-slavery/

4. Sullivan J. How to undersign the legacy of racism and redlining that still shapes New Orleans. *The Lens* [Online article]. 2019; https://thelensnola.org/2019/01/18/how-to-undesign-the-legacy-of-racism-and-redlining-that-still-shapes-new-orleans/

5. Gafford DF. It was real village: Community identity formation among black-middle residents in Pontchartrain Park. *Journal of Urban History*. 2013;39(1):36–58.

6. Del Sol D. New Orleans's grocery stores define the fabric of our city. *Preservation Resource Center* [Online article]. 2012; https://prcno.org/historic-groceries-new-orleans/

7. Gibbens S. Hurricane Katrina, explained. *National Geographic* [Online article]. 2019; https://www.nationalgeographic.com/environment/article/hurricane-katrina

8. Mundorf RA, Willits-Smith A, Rose D. 10 years later: Changes in food access disparities in New Orleans since Hurricane Katrina. *J Urban Health*. 2015;92(4).

9. Bodor JN, Rose D, Farley TA, Swalm C, Scott SK. Neighborhood fruit and vegetable availability and consumption: The role of small food stores in an urban environment. *Public Health Nutr*. 2008;11(4):413–420.

10. Bodor JN, Rice JC, Farley TA, Swalm CM, Rose D. The association between obesity and urban food environments. *J Urban Health*. 2010;87(5):771–781.

11. Rose D, B-odor JN, Rice CJ, Swalm MC, Hutchinson LP. The effects of Hurricane Katrina on food access disparities in New Orleans. *Am J Public Health*. 2011;101(3).

12. Committee NOFA. *Building Healthy Communities: Expanding Access to Fresh Food Retail*. New Orleans: Robert Wood Johnson Foundation; 2007.

13. Weinberg Z. *No Place to Shop: The Lack of Supermarkets in Low-Income Neighborhoods*. Washington, DC: Public Voice for Food and Health Policy; May 1995.

14. Ver Ploeg M, Breneman V, Dutko P, et al. Access to affordable and nutritious food: Updated estimates of distance to supermarkets using 2010 data. *Economic Research Service*. 2012;ERR-143.

15. The Reinvestment Fund. *The Economic Impacts of Supermarkets on Their Surrounding Communities*. Philadelphia, PA: The Reinvestment Fund; 2008.

16. The Reinvestment Fund. *The PA Fresh Food Financing Initiative: Case Study of Rural Grocery Store Investments*. Philadelphia, PA: The Reinvestment Fund; 2012.

17. PolicyLink, The Food Trust, the Reinvestment Fund. *A Healthy Food Financing Initiative: An Innovative Approach to Improve Health and Spark Economic Development*. 2009.

18. New Orleans Fresh Food Initiative. In: Eligibility Application.

19. Richard W. Whole Foods part of large redevelopment of our broad street site. *NOLA*. 2013.

20. Sayre K. Whole Foods market opens in mid-city with the hopes of Broad Street revitalization. *Nola.com*. 2014.

21. McNulty I. Circle Food Market, once facing different future, reopens as traditional grocery. *NOLA*. 2020.

6 New York, New York

CONTENTS

INTRODUCTION

Chapter 6 begins with a historic context of the grocery landscape in New York, including early, Black-led efforts to bring food retail to New York City (NYC). Next, a detailed review of the processes undertaken to understand why and how the food retail landscape resulted in gaps in food access is discussed, including the four phases of the Supermarket Campaigns' approach to creating policy change. In the final section of the chapter, the approaches used to receive and distribute funds as part of the New York's Healthy Food, Healthy Community Fund and the FRESH Program Healthy Food, Healthy Communities Fund are described in detail. Finally, the chapter discusses case studies and impactful projects resulting from the establishment of the program. Chapter 6 continues the discussion of state-led initiatives that have increased access to healthy food retail markets in underserved areas throughout the country with a focus on New York, one of the five states selected as an example of success to justify the federal Healthy Food Financing Initiative legislation. The purpose of this chapter is for readers to better understand: (1) the discriminatory policies and practices, such as segregation and redlining, that are associated with fewer banks investing and fewer businesses such as supermarkets operating in low-income and Black neighborhoods in New York; (2) explain who initiated state policy changes to address local food environment disparities; (3) describe the process for developing the Healthy Food, Healthy Communities Fund (HFHC); (4) document how funds were made available through the HFHC, what the status of the program is today, how funds were used and types of projects funded with the HFHC; and (5) articulate how the HFHC impacted underserved areas in New York.

DOI: 10.1201/9781003029151-8

NEW YORK CITY

New York City is the largest city in America, with approximately 8.4 million residents.[1] The city received its current name in 1664, before American independence, after the British captured what was then called New Amsterdam from the Dutch. It wasn't until November 22, 1783, when American troops led by General Washington and Governor Clinton entered New York City that British occupation of the city ended.[2] Throughout the 1800s, the population of New York City grew increasingly diverse, as immigrants from Britain, Ireland, Europe, as well as indentured servants and freed African slaves from across America came to the city to find work and start a new life.[3]

World War I (1914–1918) created a great demand for labor in New York, and as discussed in Chapter 4, it was during this time period (1910–1920), that thousands of African Americans moved from cities and rural areas of the South to northern cities like New York – also known as 'the Great Migration'. One of the largest demographic shifts in American history, it transformed the population of New York City as it became home to 'the largest urban Black population in the world'.[3] Black migrants sought to escape discrimination, violence, exploitation and lack of opportunity they experienced in their southern towns. As Claude Brown wrote in his famous autobiography called *Manchild in the Promised Land*,

> Going to New York was good-bye to the cotton fields, good-bye to 'Massa Charlie,' good-bye to the chain gang, and, most of all, good-bye to those sunup-to-sundown working hours. One no longer had to wait to get to heaven to lay his burden down; burdens could be laid down in New York.[4]

However, after arriving in New York, Black Americans continued to face discrimination. Segregation by race, in employment, schools, and housing were strongly enforced by local and federal policies. In response, Black Americans organized and continued to fight for equality. In addition to advocating for jobs, housing, and health care, activists in New York called for an end to bank redlining as they sought 'full and complete equality in all aspects of life'.[3]

REDLINING IN NEW YORK CITY

Like other U.S. cities, neighborhoods in New York were redlined. As previously described in Chapters 4 and 5, this is the discriminatory practice by which banks, real estate, and insurance companies refused or limited loans, mortgages, and insurance within specific geographic areas, especially targeting black neighborhoods.[5] This led to economic disinvestment, ultimately leading to economic decline, as the housing sector has a strong effect on economic growth and business development in communities. Like other cities in American, the discriminatory practices of the government-sponsored Home Owners' Loan Corporation were used in New York as well. Neighborhoods in New York, such as Bedford-Stuyvesant in Brooklyn, were outlined, colored red on maps, and given a rating of 'D' or 'hazard', eliminating it as a neighborhood where residents could receive government support for housing mortgages. As one government appraiser assessing this Brooklyn neighborhood wrote in the 1930s, 'Colored infiltration a definitely adverse influence on neighborhood desirability'[6] (Figure 6.1). The lack of investment in housing in Black neighborhoods also led to a decline in other businesses. Community members hoping to start their own businesses faced obstacles, as Black homeowners weren't as able to use their home equity for start-up capital as White homeowners could,[7] and Black business owners were not able to access commercial lending. Deborah Young, a long-time resident of Bedford-Stuyvesant explains,

> One of the effects of redlining that you can see to this day is the scarcity of Black businesses in the community. Another effect is that because people could not get regular, conventional mortgages

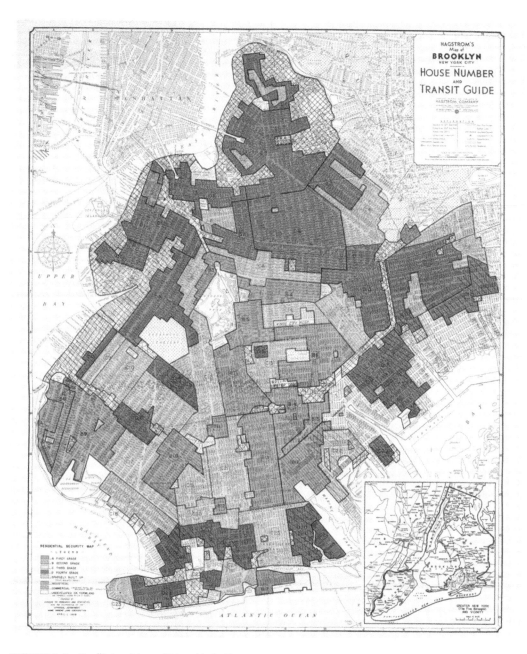

FIGURE 6.1 Redlining Map of New York City, 1938

and they were paying high interest rates, they would have to cut up their beautiful brownstones into rooms, just to be able to make ends meet. And they did that to pass on the legacy to their children. But . . . for so long Bed-Stuy was maligned as this horrible neighborhood where we were . . . shooting each other.[8]

Lack of private bank and government investment in home ownership also contributed to what some have called *supermarket redlining*, described as the avoidance of corporate supermarket chains to locating in predominantly Black areas.[9] For example, among the top factors businesses consider are site location and demographics; a site with a 'D' rating was not considered a viable option. Access to credit is critical to starting businesses like food retail stores, yet, to this day, lending to borrowers in historically redlined communities still dramatically falls behind other areas.[10] In spite of these barriers, as seen in cities across the country, Black New Yorkers came together to create their own financing to support Black-owned businesses, including grocery stores.

BLACK-LED EFFORTS TO BRING FOOD RETAIL TO NYC IN AN ERA OF REDLINING

Marcus Garvey came to New York City in 1916, with the goal to create an American Black nationalist movement and create economic self-sufficiency for Black people.[11] Before arriving in America from London (Garvey was originally from Jamaica), he created an organization dedicated to this effort called the *Universal Negro Improvement Association* (UNIA). When Garvey arrived in New York, most businesses located in Black neighborhoods were owned by Whites. A survey of Black businesses by the *New York Age* (a weekly newspaper focused on racial justice) in 1916 found that Blacks owned only 25% of the 503 businesses in the areas where Blacks lived. Of the identified Black businesses, barbers made up the largest group, followed by grocers, restaurants, beauty salons, real estate offices, and saloons.[12]

Garvey recognized the critical role of financial instruments, such as loans and investments, as the key to supporting business development. As these tools were largely unavailable to Black people in the United States, he established the Negro Factories Corporation as a financing arm to the UNIA.

> Negro producers, Negro distributors, Negro consumers! The world of Negroes can be self-contained. We desire earnestly to deal with the rest of the world, but if the rest of the world desire not, we seek not.
>
> **– Marcus Garvey, 1929**[13]

Through the Negro Factories Corporation, Garvey envisioned Black neighborhoods in New York, like Harlem, with thriving Black-owned businesses supported by Black consumers. By the early 1920s, the UNIA employed hundreds of Black workers and operated several businesses in Harlem including three grocery stores – one on 135th Street and two on Lenox Avenue (Figure 6.2). Despite the efforts of Garvey and others, Black and low-income neighborhoods in New York suffered from a lack of access to affordable, healthy food as many grocery stores followed their middle-class customers to the suburbs in the 1950s and 1960s. As a result, those who remained in the city faced a persisting problem – remaining through the next 50 years – as they had to rely on small independent groceries that charged high prices and offered minimal variety and corner stores selling a limited selection of processed foods.[13] In response, advocates and policymakers knew they needed to come together to find a solution. In response, some residents in New York City came together to organize and create their own neighborhood cooperative stores,[32] including the Harlem Coop Supermarket. Cora Walker, attorney and community activist who was once listed by the New York Times as "one of the most powerful people in Harlem,"[33] explained the food co-op in the following transcript of an excerpt from the documentary called, The Harlem Food Co-op. The entire video can be viewed in the embedded video (https://www.youtube.com/watch?v=2BXMDXPmm4o)[31]:

> *"The idea dawned upon me and really starting in the question of the riots because the riot had hit in '64. That in talking to the people on the street, they felt they didn't have anything. They didn't own anything. Everybody own something, so I then took the co-op concept and went out with them, started out in November of '66 that if they wanted to, they could own something on a cooperative basis.*

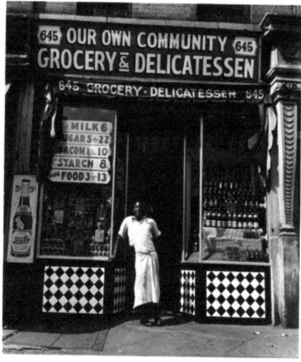

FIGURE 6.2   Harlem, NY Grocery Store, 1940

So, then we took a sound truck, started out 145th Street and 8th Avenue and said, "if you're interested in finding out how you can buy shares in a supermarket that you own" and we were flooded with people.

The store opened June 4th of '68. They voted to name the store Harlem Co-op Supermarket. People used to ride by just to see the store, but . . . the beautiful part was the stockholders. They really loved that store. So, if they came in there and they didn't have salt, they didn't buy salt until we got some.

The first nine months we made two million eight hundred thousand dollars. And it was a threat. It was an absolute threat to our competitors. Nine months after we were there, it arrived, some-body made a decision that we had to be stopped. And they threw around the so-called "picket line" and the picket line, really was not a valid picket line, because it was not our workers who were the backbones of it. Because the co-op really cut into the business of our competitors—that was in the back of it.

But the little people of Harlem kept that store open. They worked in there, they had to go out 'cuz . . . nobody would deliver anything. You couldn't get a loaf of bread. And then we had people who would get in their cars and first they started going to the warehouses and picking it up. Then they [competitors] got word of that and because of threats of retaliation they [the wholesalers] wouldn't sell it to us, so then we developed, would be a young mothers program—any name—but we meet the bread trucks and buy bread from the bread trucks and then they bring it in . . . their cars and then they sell it to themselves.

But we had 16 picture windows and those 16 picture windows were broken 15 times. The police were never able to find anybody, at any time.

Both of my sons at that time were in college and of course when they came home the summer of '69, they were right there at the store helping out whichever way they could. And they came to me and said that they had been told that if they did not convince me to walk away from the supermarket, "they were gonna be without a mother." At that point, the [Black] Panthers . . . were dying, itchin', to retaliate with violence. And some, you know, Black groups, nationalist groups wanted it. My concept was, use, you know, the system of justice that was established and we was gonna get a court order . . . you know . . . I'm sorry they didn't . . . I'm sorry that I didn't let them do their own thing.

But the store closed in March of '76. Because, through all of this, they just, um, were inundated with debt and financial failure . . . not because they couldn't run a store, not because they could not run a supermarket, but because they were not able to deal with the inner workings of the food industry.

I was heartbroken because there was a faith of so many little people, that justice will prevail".

As described by Walker, because of intimidation, discrimination and racism, the Harlem Food Co-op closed in the mid-1970s. Those who remained in the city were left to rely on small independent groceries that charged high prices and offered minimal variety and corner stores selling a limited selection of processed foods.[32] The lack of access to high quality grocery stores also impacted many other neighborhoods in New York City. From the 1980s to the early 2000s, many of the city's grocers, large and small, struggled to survive. This was due in part to high rent, narrow profit margins and increased competition from upscale supermarkets, and drugstore chains that have expanded their wares to include grocery items.[33] In response, advocates and policymakers knew they needed to come together to find a solution.

NEW YORK'S SUPERMARKET CAMPAIGN

ADVOCATING FOR SUPERMARKETS

Michael Bloomberg, mayor of New York City from 2002–2013, and the New York City Council had heard from residents for many years about the need for more supermarkets in their neighborhoods. A strong public health advocate, Mayor Bloomberg was passionate about decreasing obesity rates in NYC and finding ways to increase access to healthy foods. Once in office, Bloomberg immediately launched several initiatives to decrease unhealthy and increase healthy behaviors of New Yorkers. His administration approached the complex problem of obesity by creating multiple new policies while assessing barriers within existing city policies – including those that might create obstacles to new and existing supermarket operators from being successful.[14]

Food policy was a top priority for Mayor Bloomberg and the city council because of its impacts on public health, but also recognized it as a vehicle to address the history of structural racism and its impacts on unequal access to affordable, healthy food in the city. As the New York City Council stated in their report called *Growing Food Equity in New York City*:

In New York City, structural inequities have contributed to neighborhoods that are predominantly low-income communities of color having less access to healthy food and experiencing greater food insecurity and food-related illnesses. These communities have long been on the front lines combatting an unjust food system that harms the environment, negatively affects human health, and contributes to economic inequality.[15]

Building on the food policy work accomplished by the city's existing Food Policy Task Force, multiple organizations, researchers, and policymakers, Mayor Bloomberg worked with his administration to create a number of new programs, including an initiative to increase grocery store access.[14] Through multiple task forces and commissioned reports that engaged stakeholders, the Bloomberg administration identified increasing retail access to healthy foods as one of its top three priorities for food policy. To support his food policy efforts, Mayor Bloomberg created a new government role, a Food Policy Coordinator. The Coordinator was responsible for convening the Food Policy Task Force and coordinating the efforts of City agencies to improve access to healthy food.[16] Ben Thomases, hired for the position, was inspired by the success of the Pennsylvania Fresh Food Financing Initiative and invited The Food Trust and others to help him 'think about how food can be a part of a broader economic development, jobs creation and sustainability initiative'.[17]

A Planned Approach to Creating Policy Change

Working in partnership with Ben Thomases, the Food Bank for NYC, and many others, The Food Trust employed their four-phase approach to developing state and local policies that had succeeded in Pennsylvania. This approach is in alignment with other public health policy processes, including the Centers for Disease Control and Prevention's Policy Process.[18] The approach to creating policy change was a systematic one, following a careful process with multiple phases, ultimately leading to the implementation of policies supporting supermarket development in New York City.

The Food Trust's policy campaign included four phases:[19] (1) conducting mapping research to develop a base of knowledge on the subject and highlight areas in need; (2) engaging a targeted group of leaders to work on the problem; (3) developing a series of recommendations for changes to public policies; and (4) stimulating change by advancing these policy recommendations.

Phase 1: Documenting the Health Impacts of Low Supermarket Access in NYC

One of the first steps in any public health public policy campaign is to clearly state how the problem was created and then share evidence of how the problem affects an identified population's health. This phase is critical, as developing a common understanding of the problem makes it easier to work toward a solution.[20] In the first phase of The Food Trust's approach, a statement on the history of redlining was included, along with maps that demonstrated high rates of diet-related deaths and disease in low-income areas underserved by supermarkets.

After researching successful initiatives to encourage supermarket investment across the country, Food Policy Coordinator Ben Thomases requested that The Food Trust and the Food Bank for New York City work together to document the lack of access to supermarkets in New York, with funding from New York City Council. Using Geographic Information Systems (GIS) software, maps were created to demonstrate that many lower-income communities with poor access to supermarkets also suffered from high rates of diet-related deaths in New York (Figure 6.3). In addition, NYC's Department of City Planning created a Supermarket Need Index (SNI) to determine the areas in the city with the highest levels of diet-related diseases and largest populations with limited opportunities to purchase fresh foods. The index measured the need for supermarkets based on high population density, low household incomes, and low consumption of fresh fruits and vegetables, among other factors. The index showed a high need – that as many as three million New Yorkers live in neighborhoods with high need for grocery stores and supermarkets. City planners also noted that there were approximately $1 billion in lost grocery sales to suburbs and that the lost sales were 'enough to support more than 100 new neighborhood grocery stores and supermarkets'.[21]

Following that research, the Food Policy Coordinator, City Council, the Food Bank, and Food Industry Alliance, with the funding from the Friedman Foundation, asked The Food Trust to assemble the New York Supermarket Commission to educate the public, policymakers, and business leaders about the need for more supermarkets and to develop public policy recommendations intended to reverse the documented diet and health problems.

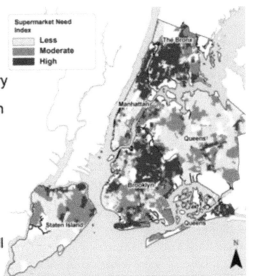

Assessing Need:

- City Planning's assessment of need for new neighborhood grocery stores and supermarkets accounted for the areas in the City that have the highest levels of diet-related diseases and largest populations with limited opportunities to purchase fresh foods

- High need for local grocery stores exists in all five boroughs

FIGURE 6.3   Map of Areas of Greatest Need, New York

Phase 2: Establishment of the New York Supermarket Commission

The second phase aimed to engage and empower and thus a task force was formed. As seen in the examples in Chapters 4 and 5, a group of local leaders from multiple sectors, including nonprofit, business, public health, and finance, plus economic development professionals, were recruited to address the problem. In NYC and other cities, to demonstrate respect and value for their time, leaders were informed that the process would be time-constrained (typically no longer than one year) and require attendance at four meetings, lasting two hours each.

Replicating The Food Trust's task force process in Philadelphia, the commission convened more than forty expert members and included grocery industry leaders, government leaders, financial sector representatives, and children's health advocates. As an important part of the process, well-respected co-chairs were selected to represent both the supermarket industry and the nonprofit sector – in New York, Jennifer Jones Austin of the United Way of New York City and Nicholas D'Agostino, III of D'Agostino Supermarkets served in these roles. The supermarket industry co-chair provides a grounded connection to the challenge of building and operating markets in underserved areas. The second co-chair ensures that task force members hear the community perspective and helps bridge the gap between diverse sectors.

The commission's meetings were focused exclusively on supermarket shortages in underserved communities. This narrow scope, with a limited time frame, helps engage stakeholders such as supermarket operators, who may not typically be involved in broader discussions about public health, food security, or childhood obesity. Focusing on this common goal helps to engage industry leaders and permits task force members to put aside other differences and come together around a shared objective. Through facilitated discussions and presentations from supermarket leaders, real estate developers, and public health and economic development leaders, task force participants build their understanding of the barriers to supermarket development in underserved communities and possible solutions. The goal is to achieve consensus around a set of recommended policy changes to help retailers overcome the barriers to entry and get stores into the areas where people need better access to healthy food the most. Maintaining a clear focus on supermarket development was a critical part of the task force process, as focusing on one issue (with its many facets) helped to facilitate consensus about a set of targeted policy recommendations. Over a six-month period, the commission met and then developed nine policy recommendations that the city and state could implement to stimulate supermarket development while supporting existing stores in underserved areas in New York.

Phase 3: Strategize and Develop Recommendations

In the third phase, the task force came together to strategize and develop recommendations by discussing the problem, sharing their experiences, and considering policy recommendations. For example, a supermarket operator may share obstacles they have faced with land assembly or the cost of training their workforce, while a child advocacy group may stress the need for better public transportation for working mothers to access supermarkets. Task force members then strategize and design a specific set of policy recommendations to promote food retail development in their area.

The New York Supermarket Commission created a set of policy recommendations to incentivize healthy food retail investment in these areas, including the recommendation that a state-wide grocery financing program be created. In April 2009, The Food Trust (with contributions from the New York Supermarket Commission, the Food Industry, Alliance of New York State, and officials from the City and State of New York) released the report called, *Stimulating Supermarket Development: A New Day for New York*.[22] With opening letters of support from Governor Patterson and Mayor Bloomberg, the report detailed recommendations for stimulating supermarket development in New York City, a key to increasing the availability of nutritious, affordable food in underserved communities and to combating obesity, diabetes, and other diet-related diseases. The report highlighted nine recommendations for supermarket development in New York State. The recommendations are detailed in Table 6.1 and cover

TABLE 6.1
New York Supermarket Commission Recommendations

Recommendation	Description
Recommendation #1	State and local economic development programs and public incentives should be targeted to the supermarket industry to maximize their impact on supermarket site location decisions
Recommendation #2	The State of New York should develop a business financing program to support local supermarket development, renovation, and expansion projects
Recommendation #3	State and local governments should streamline the development process to make opening a supermarket more efficient and provide assistance to operators to negotiate the approval process
Recommendation #4	Local governments should give priority to assembling land for supermarket development and make city- and state-owned property available to the industry. Governments should identify targeted areas for investment and promote them to real estate developers and the supermarket industry.
Recommendation #5	City, state, and regional transportation agencies should develop transportation services for shoppers without convenient access to a full-service supermarket
Recommendation #6	State and local governments should employ up-to-date and data-driven market information that highlights unmet market demand for food to the supermarket industry and real estate developers
Recommendation #7	The State of New York and the City of New York should promote green supermarket development and renovation by providing incentives for energy-efficient equipment and systems, and environmentally sustainable building materials
Recommendation #8	The State of New York should require that all projects receiving assistance through a state financing program enroll in the Pride of New York Program. Stores should be encouraged to carry products from farms within 300 miles of their location
Recommendation #9	State and local governments should engage leaders from the industry and civic sector to guide the implementation of these recommendations

these areas: investing in and supporting existing supermarkets and infrastructure, addressing financing and tax barriers for development, providing accurate market research to industry members, and improving transportation for consumers.

A key recommendation was to create a state financing program modeled after the Pennsylvania Fresh Food Financing Initiative to support grocers interested in, or already are, operating in underserved communities. After the policy recommendations were announced, task force co-chair and chairman of the board of the Food Industry Alliance Nicholas D'Agostino III, of D'Agostino Supermarkets Inc. said:

> Our goal was to assure a healthy diet for all of our citizens, especially our children, by recognizing the central role played by neighborhood supermarkets and formulating policy recommendations to encourage and promote their growth in underserved communities. . . . Now it is critical that we all remain engaged in the implementation phase so that our commitment to good health and a healthy retail food sector becomes a reality.[23]

Phase 4: State and City Policy Implementations: HFHC and FRESH

In the fourth phase, a final report is issued with the task force's policy recommendations, and an advocacy campaign is launched aimed to change policy. Task force members are identified who will educate policymakers about the problem, share the report, and advocate for the recommendations (typically there are a total of ten recommendations) with state and local officials.[24] In addition to creating a financing program to support food retailers hoping to operate in underserved areas, recommendations may also include reducing regulatory barriers to the development of stores. Task Force leaders from the supermarket industry, public health, economic development, and civic sectors were all critical to promoting and then successfully creating government programs to support supermarket development in New York City and throughout the state. After a series of meetings at the state and city levels with policymakers, including staff from the governor's office and the office of the First Lady of New York, in 2010 Governor David Paterson launched the Healthy Food and Healthy Communities Fund (HFHC Fund) to improve access to healthy and locally grown foods for residents across the state while Mayor Bloomberg launched a city-focused program called the *Food Retail Expansion to Support Health* (FRESH) program in 2009.

HEALTHY FOOD, HEALTHY COMMUNITIES (HFHC) FUND

AVAILABILITY OF HFHC FUNDS

The Healthy Food, Healthy Communities Fund received $10 million in state funding and $20 million in private investment from Goldman Sachs Bank. In addition, the Fund received operating grants from New York State, the New York State Health Foundation, and Goldman Sachs Urban Investment Group. During the life of the program from 2010 to 2016, the $10 million investment from the State of New York leveraged over $192 million in additional funding.

ADMINISTRATIVE STRUCTURE

Like the Pennsylvania Fresh Food Financing Initiative, the HFHC Fund was an innovative state program designed as a public-private partnership. Public-private partnerships involve collaboration between a government agency and a private-sector company that can be used to finance, build, and operate projects.[25] After an open and competitive process, state funds were granted to and leveraged by a national community development finance institution (CDFI) called the *Low Income Investment Fund* (LIIF). The Food Trust was also contracted to promote the program, help identify eligible grocery projects, and evaluate applications. While LIIF focused on the financing needs of food markets in underserved communities, which often cannot obtain conventional financing for infrastructure costs and credit needs, The Food Trust focused on outreach and marketing to supermarket operators, building relationships with potential applicants and guiding them through the application process.

IDENTIFYING IMPACTFUL PROJECTS TO BE FUNDED BY THE HFHC

The New York Healthy Food & Healthy Communities (HFHC) Fund launched in late 2010 and was open to food retailers throughout the state that were in underserved areas. Underserved was defined as: (1) a low- or moderate-income census tract; (2) a census tract with below average food market density; (3) a food market site with a customer base of 50% or more living in a low-income census tract.[26] From 2010–2016, the HFHC Fund provided grants and loans to twenty-five diverse projects in urban and rural communities throughout the state, both in New York City and many upstate cities and rural towns, such as Buffalo, Syracuse, Mount Vernon, Red Creek, Highland Falls, Poughkeepsie, Rochester, Hudson, and Broome County. Projects included new and expanded or renovated grocery stores, mobile markets, farmers markets, and corner stores. In total, 200,130 square feet of healthy food retail space was created or preserved in addition to 1,450 direct permanent and construction jobs that were created or preserved. Local farmers and producers were also supported through the HFHC, with ten recipients of financing participating in the New York Department of Agriculture and Markets' Pride of New York program. LIIF, the lead administrator of the HFHC program, was charged with disbursing a total of $30 million, including $26.6 million in loans and $3.4 million in grants. In addition, some projects based in New York City also received tax incentives through city-focused FRESH (Food Retail Expansion to Support Health).[27] Selected projects funded by the HFHC are described on Table 6.2.

HFHC CASE STUDIES: FINE FARE AND KEY FOOD SUPERMARKETS

LIIF provided Triangle Equities with a $10 million allocation of New Markets Tax Credit and a $5.75 million leverage loan through the HFHC Fund as part of a $36 million transaction. The new development was in a highly distressed area of the South Bronx with little access to healthy food, poverty rates greater than 30% and unemployment levels at 1.5 times the national average. Triangle Equities transformed an underutilized lot into an 86,000-square-foot mixed-use, transit-oriented facility anchored by a full-service supermarket and an accredited college for working adults. The mixed-use facility created 188 permanent jobs, as well as 117 construction jobs. At the opening of the Fine Fare Supermarket in July 2016, Borough President Ruben Diaz, Jr said,

> I am very proud of this beautiful facility – for the fact that it has created economic opportunities, educational and social services and provided this area with a much needed supermarket – an area that has been a food desert for years.[28]

Fine Fare is a 14,500-square-foot supermarket that has created 188 permanent jobs. It has LEED Silver certification and offers commercial space to be solicited to minority and women owned businesses.

The second project highlighted is the Key Food supermarket in Staten Island, which was a vacant 6,000-square-foot building located about a mile from the nearest supermarket. The store's owner, Joe Doleh, head of Kingdom Castle Food Corp., Staten Island, NY, which runs three other Key Food locations, received $3.78 million in HFHC financing. He said,

TABLE 6.2
Selected Projects Financed by the New York HFHC Fund

Project Title	Location in NY	About	FFFI Grant/ Loan Amount Awarded*	Partnerships	Fund Use	Intended Community Outcome
Reliable Market	Conklin	A second-generation family-owned grocery and deli since 1964, serving a low-to-moderate income area with fresh produce, meats, dairy, and deli items	n/a	Low-Income Investment Fund (LIIF)	A pre-development grant to initiate plans to double the size of the existing store	n/a
Food Town	Mount Vernon	A full-service supermarket located in downtown Mount Vernon, New York, a densely populated, lower-income neighborhood where more than half of schoolchildren qualify for free or reduced-price school meals	n/a	Empire State Development Goldman Sachs Group, Inc., New York State Department of Agriculture and Markets, New York State Health Foundation The Reinvestment Fund, The Food Trust, LIIF	A full renovation of the store, including installation of energy-efficient lighting and equipment and an expansion of perishable departments by 3,000 square feet to accommodate a greater variety of produce, fish, and meat to cater to the diverse preferences of local residents	18,000 square feet of improved/ expanded healthy food retail space 6,000 people served 50 permanent jobs created or preserved
Food Dynasty	Queens	Opened as part of the Key Food Cooperative in 2011, providing fresh, healthy food in a community where 25% of families live in poverty and residents are affected by high rates of diet-related diseases, including heart disease, diabetes, and obesity	$250,000 term loan	LIIF	Hurricane Sandy hit the community hard and caused power outages that lasted more than 15 days, forcing Food Dynasty to close. The owners lost an estimated $500,000 due to spoilage, loss of business and fuel expenses to run a generator. The funds covered expenses and losses incurred during the storm	23,000 square feet of healthy-food space preserved
My Town Marketplace	Highland Falls	A supermarket in the village of Highland Falls in New York's mid-Hudson region, home to a large population of seniors and families	n/a	n/a	Reestablishment of a previously closed grocery store in the community	Eight full-time and 19 part-time employees. The store is registered to participate in the 'Pride of New York' local agriculture promotion program

Name	Location	Description		Partners	Project	Outcomes
Morris's Discount Supermarket	Brooklyn	A full-service supermarket offering quality, low-cost food to a low-income, underserved neighborhood	n/a	Empire State Development, Goldman Sachs Group, Inc., New York State Department of Agriculture and Markets, New York State Health Foundation, The Reinvestment Fund, The Food Trust	Renovations of a 50-year-old, overcrowded facility to double its size, including the purchase of equipment for the store's significantly expaded departments	20 new full-time and 25 new part-time jobs while retaining its existing 40 full-time and 30 part-time employees; 15,000 square feet of improved/expanded healthy food retail space; 5,000 people served; 87 permanent jobs created or preserved
Buffalo Grown Mobile Market	Buffalo	Delivers organic, locally grown, affordable produce to Buffalo's low-income, food insecure neighborhoods, traveling regularly to drop-off sites to sell fresh fruits, vegetables, and bulk items. The group grows most of its produce on an urban farm and offers on-site nutrition education for market patrons	n/a	Empire State Development, Goldman Sachs Group, Inc., New York State Department of Agriculture and Markets, New York State Health Foundation, The Reinvestment Fund, The Food Trust	The purchase and retrofitting of a new vehicle	1 mobile market vehicle; 1,500 people served; 2 jobs created or preserved
A & D Market	Red Creek	An independently owned market in a low-income, rural community which previously had no full-service grocery store	n/a	Empire State Development, Goldman Sachs Group, Inc., New York State Department of Agriculture and Markets, New York State Health Foundation, The Reinvestment Fund, The Food Trust	Expansion of the store's perishables department, including hiring a local butcher and opening a creamery operated by a local dairy	4,000 square feet of healthy food retail space; 1,300 people served; 2 permanent jobs created or preserved
Key Food	Staten Island	A grocery store located on the border between low- and moderate-income neighborhoods, which serves residents of both areas who have limited access to fresh, healthy-food retail nearby	n/a	Tax incentives from the NYC Industrial Development Agency, Empire State Development, Goldman Sachs Group, Inc., New York State Department of Agriculture and Markets, New York State Health Foundation, The Reinvestment Fund, The Food Trust	Vacant building acquisition, renovations, and equipment for the space, including construction for 9,000 square feet of new food retail space	9,000 square feet of new healthy food retail space; 3,000 people served; 33 new permanent jobs created

(Continued)

TABLE 6.2 (Continued)
Selected Projects Financed by the New York HFHC Fund

Project Title	Location in NY	About	FFFI Grant/Loan Amount Awarded*	Partnerships	Fund Use	Intended Community Outcome
Triangle Plaza Hub	South Bronx	A new development located in a highly distressed area of the South Bronx with little access to healthy food, poverty rates greater than 30% and unemployment levels at 1.5 times the national average	LIIF provided Triangle with a $10 million allocation of New Markets Tax Credit and a $5.75 million leverage loan as part of the $36 million transaction LIIF's leverage loan was funded by the New York Healthy Food Healthy Communities Fund	Empire State Development, Goldman Sachs NYC Economic Development Corporation, United Fund Advisors Triangle Development	Triangle Equities (Triangle) is transforming an underutilized lot in the South Bronx into an 86,000-square-foot mixed-use, transit-oriented facility anchored by a full-service supermarket and an accredited college for working adults The new two-story facility will also house retail and office space and a public plaza	14,500-square-foot supermarket 188 permanent jobs created LEED Silver certification Accredited college serving over 500 working adults Commercial space solicited to minority- and women-owned businesses 188 permanent jobs, 50% of which will be targeted toward individuals who earn up to 80% of AMI. 117 construction jobs
Nojaim Supermarket	Syracuse	Supermarket owned and operated by the third generation of the Nojaim family. The store is an anchor in a severely distressed community, where residents have limited access to healthy food	$2.23 million construction loan and $400,000 grant through the New York Healthy Food and Healthy Communities (HFHC) Fund	St. Joseph's Hospital, Syracuse University Onondaga, Department of Health on several initiatives to help link primary care with nutrition and healthy food access	A complete renovation of a 50-year-old building including new equipment and a 3,000-square-foot expansion	24,300 square feet of healthy food space preserved Store rewards program which incentivizes healthy food purchases Joint nutrition programming with community health clinic 17 construction jobs 51 permanent jobs in the local community

I would probably have walked away from the project without the HFHC funds, It's tough to get financing from banks these days. The interest rate on the HFHC loan is a little lower than that of a commercial bank loan.[27]

Kimberly Latimer-Nelligan, LIIF's chief operating officer and executive vice president of community investments and programs also expressed enthusiasm for the Key Food project.

The recent financing for . . . the Key Food in Staten Island is the type of project the New York Healthy Food & Healthy Communities Fund was created to support. They are providing residents with access to fresh, healthy food options and creating jobs for New Yorkers. We are excited to continue to work across the state to invest in more projects like this going forward.

Through the FRESH program, Doleh also received tax breaks on equipment and construction costs as well as a tax abatement on the property for ten years. He also invested $2 million of his own money in the project.[27]

New York City's FRESH Program

The Bloomberg administration acted on the New York Supermarket Commission's recommendations by creating the FRESH Program (Food Retail Expansion to Support Health) to encourage healthy food retail development in underserved areas throughout New York City. Launched in the summer of 2010, the FRESH Program (1) provided tax incentives to healthy food retailers, (2) created incentives in the zoning code for real estate developments that incorporate healthy food, and (3) created a single point of access for supermarket operators to interface with city government. Like the HFHC Fund, FRESH was established to encourage grocery store openings and retention in the identified 'eligible' (i.e., underserved) neighborhoods through financial and zoning initiatives. The program used a variety of tax incentives and zoning enhancements, such as real estate tax reductions, density bonuses, sales tax exemptions and as-of-right development in manufacturing districts. These targeted incentives were available to supermarkets investing in lower income, underserved neighborhoods across the city.

FRESH provided tax breaks for supermarket operators and developers seeking to build or renovate new retail space to be owned or leased by a full-line supermarket operator. Some examples include: (1) building taxes that could be stabilized at pre-improvement real estate tax amounts for up to 25 years; (2) land taxes that could be fully abated for up to 25 years; (3) sales taxes (city and state) that could be waived on materials used to construct, renovate, or equip facilities; and (4) mortgage recording taxes that could be reduced from 2.8% to 0.3% for project mortgages.[29] After launching in 2009, twenty-two projects were approved for FRESH tax incentives across five boroughs. These supermarkets represent over 700,000 square feet of new or renovated space, created over 1,000 new jobs, retained more than 600 jobs, and contributed to an investment of $100 million into New York City's economy.

CONCLUSION

New York State's HFHC Fund is no longer active; however, LIIF continues to support healthy food retail projects through the federal Healthy Food Financing Initiative. After the federal program launched in 2010, LIIF utilized the federal dollars to further support HFHC efforts, and once the state program ended, sustained investment exclusively with federal support. For example, in 2019, the LIIF announced the investment of $750,000 into Healthy Food Financing Initiative (HFFI) for the fit-out of a new 7,300-square-foot, full-service supermarket on the ground floor of a 75-unit affordable housing development known as The Frederick in Central Harlem. The market expands healthy food options for a neighborhood with twice the national poverty rate and was previously underserved by grocery stores.[30]

The negative effects of racism, redlining, and segregation continue to this day – and are largely responsible for creating the food access problem in urban and rural areas in New York and throughout America. Deliberate disinvestment practices in New York City (NYC) have contributed to persistent disparities in health and socioeconomic status across the city.[5] In response, community members, nonprofit groups, community development banks, grocers, and policymakers came together to bring needed services, and critical businesses, like supermarkets, to underserved neighborhoods New York City (NYC).

Nonprofit groups such as The Food Trust and the Food Bank for New York City, Low Income Investment Fund, and policymakers like former Governor Patterson and Mayor Bloomberg joined together to create the Healthy Food, Healthy Communities Fund and the FRESH program to increase investment in formerly redlined areas and bring high-quality grocery stores back to urban and rural areas throughout the state and New York City. The successful replication of Pennsylvania's Fresh Food Financing Initiative in New York paved the way to the creation of the federal Healthy Food Financing Initiative, which continues to this day and supports healthy food retail in underserved areas throughout the country.

CRITICAL THINKING QUESTIONS AND EXERCISES

1. In what ways does the Supermarket Campaign Approach incorporate stakeholder feedback?
2. Another approach to addressing food security needs in communities is called a *Food Policy Council*. Examine how Food Policy Councils works and compare and contrast their approach to that of the Supermarket Campaign.
3. What was unique about the NY approach as compared to the PA FFFI described in Chapter 4? How do the kinds of projects funded in New York differ, or not, because of the way the funding is structured?
4. Draw a timeline outlining critical factors that contributed to the development and funding of food retail efforts in New York. Discuss how long certain phases took and reflect on the time frame for the policy effort and funding distribution to store openings, including the implications of the time frame for stakeholders and evaluation efforts.

REFERENCES

1. US Census Bureau. Quick Facts: New York, New York. 2019; www.census.gov/quickfacts/newyork citynewyork.
2. George Washington's Mount Vernon. British Occupation of New York City. www.mount vernon.org/library/digitalhistory/digital-encyclopedia/article/british-occupation-of-new-york-city/. Accessed July 7, 2021.
3. History and Role of Immigration and Migration in New York. 2021; https://study.com/academy/lesson/history-role-of-immigration-migration-in-new-york.html#:~:text=This%20new%20wave%20of%20immigrants,neighborhoods%20around%20New%20York%20City.
4. Black New Yorkers. WWII, Housing, and Politics. 2017; https://blacknewyorkers-nypl.org/education/. Accessed July 6, 2021.
5. Primary Care Development Corporation. New Findings: Historic Redlining Drives Health Disparities for New Yorkers. 2020; www.pcdc.org/new-findings-historic-redlining-drives-health-disparities-for-new-yorkers/. Accessed July 7, 2021.
6. Badger E. How redlining's racist effects lasted for decades. *New York Times*. 2017;Up Shot.
7. Masunaga S, Avery T. Black-owned businesses face a system set up against them. COVID-19 makes it worse. *Los Angeles Times*. June 20, 2020;Business.
8. The Red Line Archive Project. 17-deborah-affects [sic] of redlining [Internet]. *SoundCloud*. 2016. Podcast: 1:49; https://soundcloud.com/user536264376/17-deborah-young-affects-of-redlining.

9. Meyersohn N. How the rise of supermarkets left out black America. *CNN Business*. 2020.

10. Lee A, Mitchell B, Lederer A. *Disinvestment, Discouragement and Inequity in Small Business Lending*. Washington, DC; 2017; https://ncrc.org/dWoSnvestment/.

11. The Editors of Encyclopedia Britannica. Marcus Garvey. *Encyclopedia Britannica*. 2021; www.britannica.com/biography/Marcus-Garvey.

12. Robertson S. Black businesses in 1920 Harlem. *Digital Harlem: Everyday Life 1915–1930*. 2018: Digital Harlem Blog; https://drstephenrobertson.com/digitalharlemblog/maps/black-businesses-in-1920s-harlem/.

13. PBS. People & events: The negro factories corporation. *American Experience: Marcus Garvey*. www.shoppbs.pbs.org/wgbh/amex/garvey/peopleevents/e_factoriescorp.html. Accessed July 5, 2021.

14. Gearing M, Anderson T. *Innovations in NYC Health & Human Services Policy: Food Policy*. Washington, DC: Urban Institute; 2014.

15. New York City Council. Growing Food Equity in New York City. https://council.nyc.gov/data/food-equity/. Accessed July 20, 2021.

16. Office of the Food Policy Coordinator. CEO Internal Program Review Summary. 2007:17; www1.nyc.gov/assets/opportunity/pdf/fpc_prr.pdf.

17. Cardwell D. Food policy chief leaves job city seeks successor. *New York Times*. July 14, 2010; www1.nyc.gov/assets/opportunity/pdf/fpc_prr.pdf.

18. Centers for Disease Control and Prevention. The CDC Policy Process. www.cdc.gov/policy/polaris/policyprocess/index.html. Accessed July 5, 2021.

19. Karpyn A, Manon M, Treuhaft S, Giang T, Harries C, McCoubrey K. Policy solutions to the "Grocery Gap". *Health Affairs*. 2010;29(3):473–480.

20. Centers for Disease Control and Prevention. POLARIS Policy Process Problem Identification. www.cdc.gov/policy/polaris/policyprocess/problem_identification.html. Accessed July 5, 2021.

21. New York City Department of City Planning. Going to Market: New York City's Neighborhood Grocery Store and Supermarket Shortage. October 29, 2008; www1.nyc.gov/assets/planning/download/pdf/plans/supermarket/supermarket.pdf.

22. The Food Trust. *Stimulating Supermarket Development: A New Day for New York*. Philadelphia, PA: The Food Trust; April 2009.

23. The Progressive Grocer. New York supermarket commission issues recommendations. *Progressive Grocer*. 2009.

24. Lang B, Harries C, Manon M, et al. The Healthy Food Financing Handbook. 2013; http://thefoodtrustorg/uploads/media_items/hffhandbookfinaloriginalpdf.

25. The Investopedia Team. Public-private partnerships. *Fiscal Policy Government Spending & Debt*. 2021; www.investopedia.com/terms/p/public-private-partnerships.asp. Accessed July 7, 2021.

26. New York State Empire State Development. New York Healthy Food & Healthy Communities Fund. 2021; https://esd.ny.gov/businessprograms/healthyfoodhealthycommunities.html. Accessed July 7, 2021.

27. Garry M. N.Y. Food Desert Fund Distributes $6 Million. April 16, 2012.

28. Goodstein S. Triangle plaza hub officially opens. *Bronx Times*. July 21, 2016.

29. NYCEDC. Finance Solutions: Food Retail Expansion to Support Health (FRESH). https://edc.nyc/program/food-retail-expansion-support-health-fresh.

30. Low Income Investment Fund. LIIF provides healthy food financing loans in Maryland & Harlem food deserts. *LIIF News*. October 16, 2019.

31. Harlem Food Co-op. YouTube, uploaded Nov. 26, 2016, https://www.youtube.com/watch?v=2BXMDXPmm4o.

32. Flournoy R, Treuhalt S. Healthy Food, Healthy Communities: Improving Access and Opportunities through Food Retail, PolicyLink 2005. https://www.poilylink.org/sites/edfault/HEALHYFOOD.PDF. Accessed July 19, 2021.

33. Kaysen R. Where did my supermarket go? New York Times, November 4, 2016. https://www.nytimes.com/2016/06/realestate/new-york-city-small-supermarkets-are-closing.html, Accessed July 19, 2021.

7 Denver, Colorado

CONTENTS

INTRODUCTION

Chapter 7 provides a review of the mechanisms by which the Colorado Fresh Food Financing Fund (CO4F) was established. In addition to providing a context for the work, including a review of the role of redlining, the chapter documents how funds were made available through the CO4F, what the status of the program is today, how funds were used, and the types of projects funded with the CO4F. Finally, the chapter concludes with a case study of a new Save-A-Lot store and a summary of how the CO4F impacted underserved areas in Colorado.

Colorado was one of the first states to launch a supermarket financing program with initial investment from a private foundation, the Colorado Health Foundation. Readers will understand how the discriminatory policies and practices that have occurred in other areas of the United States has also impacted Colorado, also creating underserved areas. The chapter aims to describe how groups of Americans migrated to Colorado, and many Black, Indigenous, and People of Color (BIPOC) groups experienced redlining, which has impacted the economic growth of these communities. The story told about Colorado is similar to those told in previous chapters, but the initiation of the Supermarket Campaign without state support makes this a unique case study of statewide food environment modifications. Also unique to this chapter is the story of the Leever family, who brought one of their Save-A-Lot supermarkets to an underserved area. What makes this a particularly unique story is the business model of the supermarket; Save-A-Lot recently became an employee-owned company, allowing full- and part-time workers to be given annual stock in the company, increasing their opportunities for personal wealth as well as access to healthy foods.

DENVER, COLORADO

The city of Denver, founded in 1858, attracted residents hoping to find greater economic opportunity and freedom. In the 1860s, thousands of workers came to Denver to help extend

DOI: 10.1201/9781003029151-9

the reach of the Union Pacific and Central Pacific railroads. Denver's railroad construction attracted workers from a wide variety of cultural and racial backgrounds. Denver's residents included Europeans (Swedes, Italians, Irish, Greeks, Poles, and other Eastern Europeans), Black Americans, Jews, Chinese, Japanese, and Latinx who also came to the city to work in transportation, mining, agriculture (including sugar production which was the largest employer of Mexican/Latinx workers in Colorado[1]), retail, brickyard, flour-milling, and canning centers[2] in the city known, from as early as 1906, as the capital of the Rocky Mountain Empire.[3]

From its inception, Denver neighborhoods were segregated by race and ethnicity, and Black, Indigenous, and People of Color (BIPOC) groups experienced intense discrimination and racism. The first race riot in Denver occurred on Halloween day in 1880, in Chinatown, destroying the neighborhood. Chinatown at its height offered groceries and mercantile houses that stocked ginger, preserved fruits, teas, relishes, and other imported foodstuffs,[2] offering community to workers who were forced out from nearby mining towns and discharged from the railroads once the work was completed (Figure 7.1).[4]

By the early 1920s the population of Auraria, one of Denver's oldest neighborhoods, shifted from a White European immigrant community to a Mexican American/Latinx neighborhood. Many Latinx residents came to Denver from southern Colorado and northern New Mexico, and Mexico.[5] Latinx residents also found a home in Denver's Five Points neighborhood.[6] Black Denverites were primarily segregated in the Five Points neighborhood, as the Great Migration[7] brought a wave of new Black workers to the city. The Five Points community developed its own business district, and for many years the neighborhood offered a rich nightlife with over fifty bars and clubs where many of the greatest American musicians performed, including Louis Armstrong, Billie Holiday, Dinah Washington, Duke Ellington, and Miles Davis.[8] 'From the 1920s to the 1960s is when we were considered Harlem of the West, with the jazz history, with the businesses and

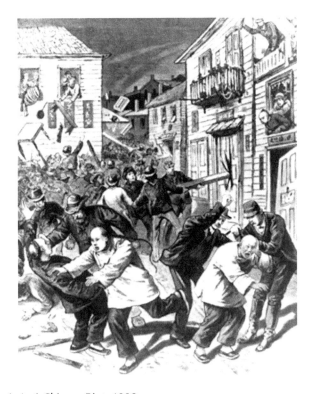

FIGURE 7.1   Denver's Anti-Chinese Riot, 1880

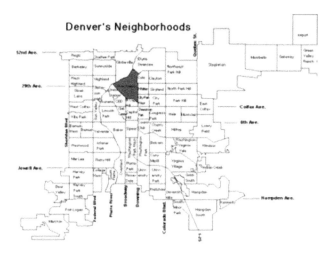

FIGURE 7.2   Denver's Neighborhoods

along the Welton Street Corridor', Terri Gentry, docent with the Black American West Museum said. However, it is well-documented that Black families in this vibrant community faced racial discrimination, and they, along with Mexican Americans, Native Americans, and other immigrants suffered from attacks from the Ku Klux Klan (Figure 7.2).[9]

REDLINING IN DENVER

Denver, as is the case with every city across the United States, has a history of redlining. As discussed in previous chapters, starting in the 1930s the Federal Housing Administration drew up maps of major metropolitan areas around the country. Redlining securely reinforced racial segregation in American cities like Denver, and today, 64% of redlined neighborhoods are still primarily BIPOC communities.[10] As Terri Gentry further explained, 'Redlining goes way back, to part of a process of . . . perpetuating segregation, and the folks that have versus the have nots'.[11] As described in previous chapters, government housing agencies assigned a grade to different neighborhoods in Denver. Black, Latinx, and Asian residents lived in areas that received a poor grade of 'C' or 'D', and as a result, were not able to purchase homes. Redlining hurt their ability to qualify for loans and in turn greatly diminished their opportunity to build wealth.[10] Denver neighborhoods colored in red in the map (Figure 7.3, center sections D.12 and D13) represent areas that received a poor grade, and these neighborhoods still experience the highest inequity in the city today.[12]

BLACK-LED EFFORTS TO BRING FOOD RETAIL TO DENVER IN AN ERA OF REDLINING

Unable to access support from banking institutions, Black community members joined together to provide financing and support Black-owned businesses, including food retail establishments in Denver. Black leaders helped those in Five Points own their own home and start businesses.

> We had the Cousins family, Charles and Alta Cousins. We had the Colored American Loan Company. There were several folks in this neighborhood who made sure people had resources, places to live, money to utilize for those homes, money to utilize for businesses.
>
> – Terri Gentry[11]

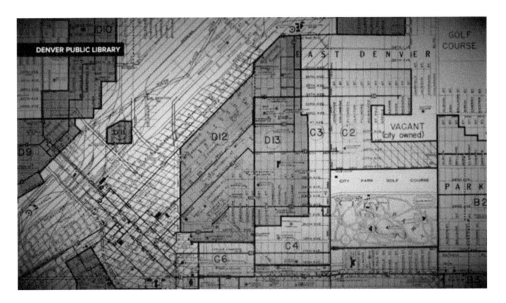

FIGURE 7.3   Redline Map, Denver

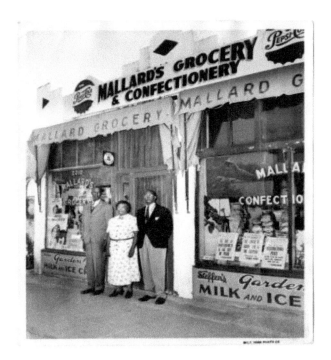

FIGURE 7.4   Mallard's Grocery & Confectionery

One of those community leaders was Reverend David West Mallard. After his retirement as a railroad employee, he became a Five Points entrepreneur, owning several businesses including a restaurant, a cleaning business, and Mallard's Grocery and Confectionery. which opened in 1933 (Figure 7.4). Historically, Black Denverites 'could not go to a local doctor, or a local bank, or a local liquor store, so they had to create their own', says Olivia Omega, representative of the Five Points Business Improvement District.[13] Mallard's

Grocery and Confectionery operated through the 1940s but eventually fell to the pressure of new supermarket chains opening in the area. Denver was not unique to this phenomenon – starting in the 1950s and 1960s, the country witnessed the fast-paced rise of supermarket chains and their eventual domination of the food retail market. In 1950, supermarket chains brought in about 35% of the national food-retailing dollar, and just ten years later by 1960, that market share jumped to 70% of the food retail business.

Nationally and in Denver, the growing physical size of supermarkets allowed for a greatly expanded number of food offerings and other essential products in the stores. As described in Chapter 2, supermarket spaces grew from 10,000–15,000 square feet to a current average of approximately 45,000 square feet.[14] More space allowed for more product choices, up from approximately 9,000 products in the mid-1970s to more than 47,000 in 2008.[15] Supermarkets became 'superstores' where customers could also fill a prescription, drop off dry cleaning, and buy items like cards, toys, and flowers. Supermarket chains and other grocers opened and/or moved operations to the surrounding suburbs, departing Denver's low-income neighborhoods. Consequently, many neighborhoods were left with smaller stores that were generally unable to provide both the quality and variety of foods residents desired.

Residents of Five Points and other underserved communities in Denver continued advocacy efforts to improve their neighborhoods and increase access to basic services, including access to high-quality grocery stores, eventually catching the attention of private foundations and policymakers.

COLORADO'S SUPERMARKET CAMPAIGN

In 2007, the Colorado Health Foundation identified obesity as a major health issue for Coloradans and as a result, dedicated resources to increase access to healthy foods and support healthy eating. After careful planning, the foundation identified measurable goals to help it achieve its vision to make Colorado the healthiest state in the nation, including increasing the number of underserved Coloradans who have convenient access to fruits and vegetables. To help achieve its goal to make produce easily accessible to all Coloradans, the foundation commissioned The Food Trust and the University of Colorado to conduct a study on supermarket access in the state, with special focus on underserved communities in the city of Denver.

In late 2009, The Food Trust in partnership with the University of Colorado released a report titled, *The Need for More Supermarkets in Colorado.*[16] The report mapped lower-income areas with residents suffering from high rates of diet-related deaths that were also underserved by fresh food retailers in Denver, similar to what The Food Trust has documented in other areas of the United States.[17] The report concluded that: (1) access to food was not evenly distributed in Colorado; (2) many people had to travel excessive distances to buy food at a supermarket; (3) the uneven distribution of food in Colorado disproportionately affected large numbers of lower-income people; and (4) aggregately, there was a connection between diet-related disease and lack of supermarket access (Figure 7.5).

DOCUMENTING THE PROBLEM

As previously mentioned, starting in the late 1960s, older supermarkets and grocery stores located within the city of Denver began to close, while bigger, newer supermarkets opened in the suburbs. This left a number of communities within Denver without a nearby place to shop for high-quality groceries. As documented in the report *Healthy Food for All: Encouraging Grocery Investment in Colorado,* several BIPOC communities and lower-income neighborhoods in Denver had low supermarket sales, including Westwood, Barnum, Barnum West, Villa Park, Sun Valley, East Colfax, Elyria Swansea, Clayton, Cole, Globeville, Five Points, Montbello, North Park Hill, and Northeast Park Hill.[17]

Supermarkets hard to find, harder to get to

A survey of 21 metro areas nationwide looked at the number of supermarkets per 10,000 residents in every ZIP code and found low-income areas had 30 percent fewer stores than the highest-income areas. Colorado has many low-income and rural communities where access to the kinds of foods needed for a healthy diet is limited. Worse, low-income households are less likely to have automobiles, making it difficult to reach adequate grocery shopping.

High sales/high income: More supermarkets and more vehicle owners who can drive to supermarkets.

Low sales/low income: Fewer supermarkets and low auto-ownership rates.

High sales/low income: Typically rural communities, where people travel from surrounding areas to shop.

Low sales/high income: Fewer markets, but high vehicle-ownership rates allowing people to drive to shop.

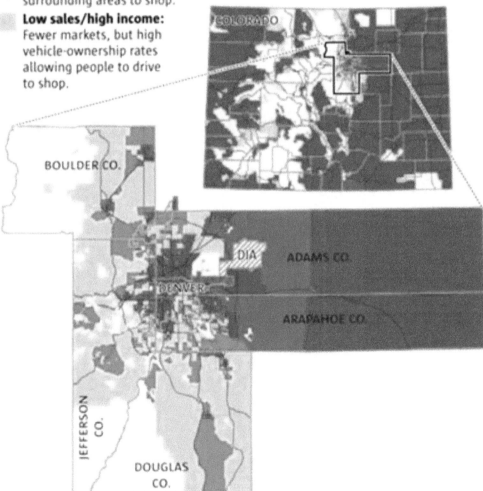

FIGURE 7.5 Map of Areas of Greatest Need, Colorado

(From Trade Dimensions Retail Database, 2008: U.S. Census Bureau, 2008; Jeff Goertzen, *The Denver Post*.)

The North Park Hill and Northeast Park Hill neighborhoods had been without a local gro-cery store since the 1970s when King Soopers and Safeway both closed. These communities were left with two convenience stores for those who needed a nearby location to buy food. As voiced by an affected community member in a *Denver Post* article,

> One [convenience store] is a market across from Holly Square, a shopping center that was a gang hangout before it burned down in a battle between feuding factions. The other is Fairfax Market, at the intersection of Fairfax Street and East 28th Avenue, where people such as C. Logan buy dish soap, Crisco, soda and Doritos and other items because they need something quick and don't have time to catch a bus or two, to shop at a grocery store with lower prices.[18]

The North Park Hill and Northeast Park Hill neighborhoods were not the only communi-ties in Denver or in Colorado suffering from this problem. Moreover, The Food Trust's report concluded what many were already aware of, that access to supermarkets is a problem in many Colorado neighborhoods but exceedingly so in lower-income, inner-city and rural communities. These areas also carried a greater burden of diet-related diseases. The report concluded that the public sector has a responsibility to help provide a safe and nutritious food supply in underserved communities in order to safeguard the public's health and pro-mote economic development in these neighborhoods.[16] In response, the Colorado Health Foundation and the Office of former Mayor John Hickenlooper convened a task force to address the problem. With their support, The Food Trust and the Denver Department of Environmental Health, Denver Healthy People Program worked to bring together the needed stakeholders to ensure equitable access to healthy, affordable food for all Denver residents.

ESTABLISHMENT OF THE DENVER FOOD ACCESS TASK FORCE

The Denver Food Access Task Force included a broad group of members that was com-prised of civic leaders, child advocates, public health advocates, redevelopment agencies, local philanthropic foundations, community development groups, and finance experts to develop a series of recommendations to increase access to grocery stores.[19] Importantly, of the thirty-eight representatives, several members were also experienced at operating local supermarkets and grocery stores – representing King Soopers and City Market, Downing Supermarket and Know Court Market, Mi Pueblo, Safeway, Leevers Companies/Save-A-Lot Stores, and Marczyk Fine Foods (Table 7.1). The inclusion of task force members from the

---

TABLE 7.1
Denver Food Access Task Force Members[17]

Member	Professional Affiliation
Stephanie Adams	Manager of Performance Initiatives, Denver Office of Budget and Finance
Alfonso Avila	Real Estate Director, Mi Pueblo
Cameron Bertron	Senior Redevelopment Manager, Denver Urban Renewal Authority
Alisha Brown	Director, Be Well Health & Wellness Initiative, Stapleton Foundation
William Burman	Director, Denver Public Health, Denver Health and Hospital Authority
Emily Bustos	Director, Denver Early Childhood Council
Mary Lou Chapman	President, Rocky Mountain Food Industry Association
Timothy Dolan	Senior Commercial Lender, Colorado Housing and Finance Authority
Crissy Fanganello	Director of Policy & Planning, Denver Department of Public Works

(Continued)

TABLE 7.1 (Continued)
Denver Food Access Task Force Members

Member	Professional Affiliation
David Fine	City Attorney, Denver Department of Law
Howard Gerelick	Vice President, Real Estate, Safeway
Steve Gordon	Development and Planning Supervisor, Denver Department of Community Planning and Development
Thomas Gougeon	Executive Director, Gates Family Foundation
James O. Hill	Director, Center for Human Nutrition, University of Colorado Health Sciences Center
Patrick Horvath	Director of Strengthening Neighborhoods, The Denver Foundation
Jim Koch	Former owner, Downing Supermarket and Knox Court Supermarket
Kay Koch	Former owner, Downing Supermarket and Knox Court Supermarket
John Leevers	President, Leevers Companies/Save-A-Lot Stores
Pete Marczyk	Owner, Marczyk Fine Foods
James Mejia	Interim President & CEO, Denver Hispanic Chamber of Commerce
Michael Miera	Community Development Specialist, Denver Office of Economic Development
Meredith Miller	Chief of Staff, Piton Foundation
Aaron Miripol	President & CEO, Urban Land Conservancy
Christopher Parr	Development Director, Denver Housing Authority
Joshua Phair	Senior Manager, Public Affairs and Government Relations – Mountain Division Walmart Stores, Inc.
Susan Powers	President, Urban Ventures, LLC
David Roberts	Chief Services Officer, Office of Denver Mayor John W. Hickenlooper
Kevin Seggelke	President & CEO, Food Bank of the Rockies
Nancy Severson	Manager, Denver Department of Environmental Health
Alyson Shupe	Chief, Health Statistics Section, Colorado Department of Public Health & Environment
Jeff Siefried	Executive Director, Mile High Community Loan Fund
Jerry Spinelli	Owner, Spinelli's Market
Jamie C. Torres	Director, Office of Community Support Agency for Human Rights and Community Relations
Kathy Underhill	Executive Director, Hunger Free Colorado
Charlie Walling	General Manager, Robinson Dairy
Lisa Walvoord	Policy Director, LiveWell Colorado
Chris Watney	President, Colorado Children's Campaign
Randy Wright	Real Estate Director King Soopers & City Market

grocery industry was essential in order to hear directly from business owners what the barriers were to operating in underserved areas of Colorado.[20]

Developing Recommendations

In fall of 2011, the Denver Food Access Task Force released its policy recommendations to improve access to affordable, healthy food and stimulate economic development in Denver and throughout Colorado.[21] The task force found the need for improved grocery store access in several lower-income neighborhoods in Denver, as well as more rural parts of Colorado, and offered as one solution the creation of a statewide healthy food financing initiative, with recommendations based on the Pennsylvania Fresh Food Financing Initiative (Table 7.2).

TABLE 7.2
The Denver Food Access Task Force Recommendations[17]

	Description of Recommendation
Recommendation #1	Members of this task force from the grocery retail industry, state and local government, and the nonprofit and civic sectors will guide the implementation of these recommendations, which we believe to be imperative to support the comprehensive development of communities and to ensure the health of families. City and County of Denver – Systems
Recommendation #2	We recommend that in partnership with the task force, the City and County of Denver prioritize food retailing, work with grocers to navigate the development review process and explore ways to expedite the opening of new stores
Recommendation #3	With support from Colorado's philanthropic community, we recommend that local economic development agencies within the City and County of Denver employ innovative, data-driven market assessment techniques to identify unmet market demand in Denver's neighborhoods and to highlight information that would support successful grocery retail projects in underserved areas. Such research should also gather input from communities around the city advocating for better access to healthy, affordable food
Recommendation #4	In partnership with the leadership of the city's economic and community development agencies, we recommend that the City and County of Denver create and aggressively market economic development programs designed for the grocery retail industry in identified high-need areas
Recommendation #5	We recommend that the City and County of Denver establish a single point of contact for the grocery retail industry that coordinates city departments and services for grocery retail development
Recommendation #6	In partnership with local transit agencies, we recommend that the City and County of Denver take steps to promote safe, affordable, and efficient transportation services for neighborhoods lacking healthy food retailers. State of Colorado and Private Foundations – Fresh Food Financing Fund
Recommendation #7	The task force calls upon Colorado foundations and state and local governments to seed a development and business financing program for grocery retail development projects and seek to leverage seed capital with additional public and private loan fund capital investments. The program should work in concert with the tools described in Recommendation #4
Recommendation #8	A task force subgroup, with representatives from state and local government, redevelopment and financing authorities, foundations, and local Community Development Financial Institutions, should be convened to define the goals, policies, guidelines, and delivery model needed to effectively manage the fund and attract private investment. City and County of Denver and State of Colorado – Supplemental Nutrition Assistance Program (Food Stamp) Enrollment
Recommendation #9	In partnership with hunger advocates, members of the Denver supermarket and grocery business, and the Office of Economic Development, the task force calls upon the leadership of Denver Human Services to prioritize increasing the rate of enrollment in the Supplemental Nutrition Assistance Program (SNAP). To bring about this change, the City of Denver needs to work with the state to ensure effective infrastructure exists to administer the program

IMPLEMENTING THE COLORADO FRESH FOOD FINANCING FUND (CO4F)

The creation of a financing program focused on increasing healthy foods in Colorado received enthusiastic support from task force members and policymakers, and in 2012, the Colorado Fresh Food Financing Fund (CO4F) was launched. Modeled after the Pennsylvania Fresh Food

Financing Initiative and aligned with the federal Healthy Food Financing Initiative, CO4F from its very beginnings was designed to improve retail access to fresh and healthy foods and remove financial barriers from the construction, expansion, and renovation of grocery stores in underserved areas in Colorado.

Availability of Funds

The Colorado Fresh Food Financing Fund (CO4F) was seeded with a $7.1 million investment from the Colorado Health Foundation. The fund was the first in the country created with support from a private foundation and soon became a model for other states such as California and New Jersey. Like Pennsylvania, the fund was structured as a public-private partnership and receives funding through government sources. Colorado Enterprise Fund also directly receives grants, from sources such as the Healthy Food Financing Initiative (HFFI) – the federal program described in Chapter 3, with the goal to increase access to healthy food throughout the United States.

Administrative Structure

The administrative structure of the CO4F fund includes three organizations: a lead administrative organization, a financial organization, and an organization responsible for community outreach. The Colorado Housing and Finance Authority (CHFA), which has a mission to strengthen Colorado by investing in affordable housing and community development, served as the CO4F fund administrator and managed the allocation of grants and loans. From the very start, the CHFA knew they wanted to partner with a community development finance institution (CDFI) and chose to work with the Colorado Enterprise Fund (CEF) because a CDFI, 'offers lower rates and more "patient" capital than traditional lenders'. As Alan Ramirez, CEF's Director of Lending explained, 'As a CDFI that's what you do. You try to be as flexible as you can, especially when you know these deals have a good impact in these communities'.

CO4F also partners with Progressive Urban Management Associates (P.U.M.A.) which serves as the Food Access Organization for the fund. In this role, P.U.M.A. conducts the initial screening of applicants and provides general information to prospective borrowers, like the process used at The Food Trust in Chapter 4. Briefly, the first step in screening is to review applications to ensure that the location and type of store would meet program guidelines and would be eligible to apply for funding. Criteria that may play a role in determining eligibility include assessing if the project supports local job creation, has support from the community it would serve, is accessible to public transit, and/or can demonstrate other positive impacts on the community. Once an applicant is deemed eligible, they are then able to move ahead to step two, the financial application, which is reviewed by CEF.

Supporting Healthy Food Financing Projects throughout Colorado

Since the creation of CO4F, CEF has provided financing to multiple food access projects that serve communities in urban and rural Colorado. This includes full-service grocery stores, urban farms, mobile markets, food distributors, value added production, restaurants, food trucks, food production (e.g., a loan to Jumpin' Good Goat Dairy) and more. See Table 7.3 for a selected list of funded food retail projects (e.g., supermarkets, grocery stores, superettes, corner stores, and a butcher shop).

CO4F and other healthy food financing programs have been successful, but it is important to note that investments can also be incredibly challenging for CDFI lenders. As Ceyl Prinster, CEO of Colorado Enterprise Fund explains, 'It's a risky industry. The margins are so thin, and the collateral is so weak – especially if you don't have real estate'. While not every community in

TABLE 7.3
Selected CO4F and Healthy Food Financing Projects – Food Retail[24]

Store	Location	Description
Accra Kumasi African Market	Aurora	Retail, superette
Crunchy Grocer	Loveland, urban	7,620 sq. ft. food retail space created; new grocery store created
New Discount Store	Aurora, urban	2,300 sq. ft. food retail space created; new grocery store serving Somalian and Ethiopian communities
Fairfax Market	Denver, urban	14,000 sq. ft. food retail space preserved; existing corner store expanding sale of healthy food in low food-access area
The Kitchen Pantry	Canon City, urban	180 sq. ft. additional food retail space created for a total of 630 sq. ft. food retail space; new fresh produce retail space in existing commercial kitchen in downtown
Hardin's Natural Foods	Hotchkiss, rural	1,500 sq. ft. food retail space preserved; existing rural, natural foods store, provides a low-cost buying club option for community
Fort Market	Fort Garland, rural	4,500 sq. ft. food retail space preserved; existing store, working to upgrade inefficient equipment and refresh old store interior/ exterior; located in a food desert in a county with persistent poverty
Dia International Market	Aurora	1,168 sq. ft. food retail space expanded; existing African market expanding fresh food and meat offerings to immigrant community
Max Market	Denver, urban	2,800 sq. ft. food retail space created; new store created in a low food-access area
Franko's Food Mart	Denver, urban	4,000 sq. ft. food retail space created; existing superette switching ownership and expanding healthy food options
The Local Butcher	Denver, urban	488 sq. ft. butcher shop created; expanding access to fresh, local meat as part of a larger indoor market
Aladdin Market	Aurora, urban	3,500 sq. ft. food retail space expanded; existing African market expanding fresh food and meat offerings to immigrant community
Thrive	Boulder	Restaurant and retail
Save-A-Lot	Denver, urban	26,000 sq. ft. food retail created; first grocery store in 3 years in Montebello neighborhood. Includes community room and teaching kitchen
Asian American Market	Aurora, urban	2,600 sq. ft. food retail space created; new market serving Thai and Burmese products for surrounding community
Valley Food Co-op	Alamosa, rural	700 sq. ft. food retail space preserved; co-op providing local and healthier options for community
Re:Vision	Denver, urban	Local nonprofit incubating a community-owned grocery store in a food desert
Noco Farms	Loveland	Retail, farmers market
Morrow Ventures	Denver	Retail, superette
Stop and Shop Supermarket	Limon	Retail, full-service supermarket

Colorado offered enough of a market opportunity for larger supermarkets, CEF saw superettes (stores with less than $2 million in sales) as a viable alternative. Anne Misak, CEF's Healthy Food Program Manager explained, 'We're focused on making sure areas that don't have full-service grocery stores have better options. . . . Our small ethnic markets and corner stores don't solve everything, but at least they provide options'. Colorado Enterprise Fund's dedication and commitment to increasing food access has resulted in several small retailers receiving support in the city of Denver, as well as larger retailers like Save-A-Lot.

CO4F Case Study: Save-A-Lot

The Montbello neighborhood in Denver had been lacking a grocery store for many years. After the closing of a Safeway supermarket, residents rallied to get another supermarket chain in the neighborhood. A racially diverse area, with approximately 54% Hispanic/Latinx and 43% Black residents, it is also a low-income community with at least one-fifth of Montbello residents living in poverty. Chris and John Leevers were committed to bringing their employee-owned supermarket, Save-A-Lot, into the neighborhood. The Leevers already had some bank funding for the project (a $4.9 million loan from Wells Fargo & Company Bank), but it only covered about half of the total project costs. John Leevers had served on the Denver Food Access Task Force and saw a renewed opportunity with the creation of the CO4F. The Colorado Enterprise Fund was able to fill their funding gap by working as the lead lender on the project and assembling additional nonprofit lending partners such as the Colorado Trust and the Colorado Housing and Finance Authority, who contributed $1 million and $1.5 million, respectively.

All Colorado Save-A-Lot stores fall under the umbrella of Leevers Supermarkets, an eighty-year-old company that was owned by three generations of Leevers before it became employee-owned five years ago. Employees over the age of 21 with at least one year of working at the store and an average of twenty work hours a week are given annual stock in the company. The grocery store also includes a community room with a kitchen that is used for cooking and nutrition classes, community meetings and health screenings. 'We try to go one step further by working with customers to build healthier families and communities', said John Leevers, president of LSI. 'The hope is that our large assortment of produce, cooking and nutrition classes, and having tenants that promote active and healthy living will achieve that'.[22]

With support from the Colorado Health Foundation, the Sarah Samuels Center for Public Health Research and Evaluation was contracted to conduct an evaluation of the financing program. Findings indicated that 'most shoppers had difficulty accessing healthy food before the CO4F investment' in their community. However, after a store received investment through CO4F, 'shoppers reported having better access to healthy food, and have increased their purchase of healthier items, particularly those in the lowest income group and those living in rural areas'.[23] The evaluation also documented the creation of hundreds of jobs as well as 134,000 square feet of retail space.

CONCLUSION

Redlining and segregation led to divestment in BIPOC communities and low-income areas of Denver as well as other areas in Colorado. Like other areas discussed in this book, deliberate disinvestment practices in Denver and throughout the state have contributed to a lack of businesses offering healthy foods, leading to persistent disparities in health and socioeconomic status across the city.[12] In response, the Denver Food Access Task Force was formed and offered public policy recommendations to help remedy the problem. Community members, nonprofit groups, community development banks, grocers, and policymakers came together to bring needed services, and critical businesses, like supermarkets, to underserved neighborhoods throughout the city of Denver. The Colorado Fresh Food Financing Fund brings increased investment in formerly redlined areas and has brought high-quality grocery stores back to urban and rural areas throughout the state of Colorado. The creation of this successful program in Colorado paved the way for private foundations to invest in similar programs in additional states such as California, Michigan, and New Jersey, which continue to this day.

CRITICAL THINKING QUESTIONS AND EXERCISES

1. What role did philanthropy play in developing the CO4F program in Colorado? How is it different than state-led efforts described in previous chapters both in relation to start-up funds and sustainability of the program?

2. Review the recommendations issued by the Task Force and critically reflect on their causes.
3. What are the differences in the ways that the CO4F program operated, and distributed funds as compared to other programs discussed in this text?
4. Part of the task force process is hearing from retailers what the barriers to operating in lower income communities are. What barriers did the retailers in Colorado report, and what barriers were and were not addressed through the financing program?
5. How are the funded projects different in Colorado compared to those funded in Pennsylvania, New Orleans, or New York?
6. Describe the process for developing the Colorado Fresh Food Financing Fund (CO4F).
7. Document how funds were made available through the CO4F, what the status of the program is today, how funds were used.
8. Articulate how the CO4F has impacted underserved areas in Colorado.

REFERENCES

1. Chase GT. Hispanic Migration to Northeastern Colorado During the Nineteen Twenties: Influences of Sugar Beet Agriculture. *Electronic Theses and Dissertations*. 2011;777. https://digitalcommons.du.edu/etd/777.
2. Philpott W. More than meat and potatoes: The forgotten history of Denver food. *Perspectives on History*. 2016; www.historians.org/publications-and-directories/perspectives-on-history/december-2016/more-than-meat-and-potatoes-the-forgotten-history-of-denver-food.
3. Cherland SM. *No Prejudice Here: Racism, Resistance, and the Struggle for Equality in Denver, 1947–1994*. UNLV Theses, Dissertations, Professional Papers, and Capstones. 2526, University of Nevada, Las Vegas; 2014.
4. Fulcher MP. On Halloween nearly 150 years ago, an Anti-Chinese riot broke out in Denver: It was the city's first race riot. *CPR News*. Vol. 2021. 2019; www.cpr.org/2019/09/02/on-halloween-nearly-150-years-ago-an-anti-chinese-riot-broke-out-in-denver/.
5. Denver Public Library. Auraria Neighborhood History. *Genealogy, African American & Western History Resources*. 2021; https://history.denverlibrary.org/auraria-neighborhood#:~:text=By%20the%20early%201920s%2C%20the,to%20a%20distinctly%20Hispanic%20neighborhood. Accessed July 7, 2021.
6. Denver Public Library. Five Points-Whittier Neighborhood History. *Genealogy, African American & Western History Resources*. 2021; https://history.denverlibrary.org/five-points-whittier-neighborhood-history. Accessed July 7, 2021.
7. The Editors of Encyclopaedia Britannica. Great Migration African American History. 2021; www.britannica.com/event/Great-Migration. Accessed July 7, 2021.
8. Five Points Business Improvement District. Five Points History & Culture. 2021; www.fivepointsbid.com/history-culture. Accessed July 7, 2021.
9. Colorado History Detectives. Who Fought for Equality in Colorado? 2021; https://coloradohistorydetectives.pressbooks.com/chapter/who-fought-to-belong-in-colorado/. Accessed July 7, 2021.
10. Denver Metro Chamber Leadership Foundation. The Lasting Impact of Redlining in Denver. *Virtual Voices*. 2020; https://denverleadership.org/the-lasting-impact-of-redlining-in-denver/, Accessed June 20, 2021.
11. Porter J. Redlining: How the Five Points Neighborhood Formed Amid Racist Practices in the 1930's. 2019. www.thedenverchannel.com/news/black-history-month/redlining-how-the-five-points-neighborhood-formed-amid-racist-practices-in-the-1930s. Accessed July 4, 2021.
12. Kauffman M. Denver Neighborhood Equity Index in Relation to Historical Redlining Grades. 2019; www.denvergov.org/content/dam/denvergov/Portals/771/documents/CH/health-equity/RedliningAnd%20EquityInDenver_9.20.19.pdf. Accessed July 8, 2021.
13. Salzman N. In: Five Points, Change Comes at the Community Level. 2020.
14. FMI Information Service. Supermarket Facts: Median Total Store Size–Square Feet. n.d.; www.fmi.org/our-research/supermarket-facts/median-total-store-size-square-feet. Accessed July 8, 2021.
15. Consumer Reports. What to Do When There Are Too Many Product Choices on the Store Shelves? 2014; www.consumerreports.org/cro/magazine/2014/03/too-many-product-choices-in-supermarkets/index.htm. Accessed July 8, 2021.

16. Karpyn A, Weidman J, Lang B, Thomas D. The need for more supermarkets in Colorado. *Healthy Food, Healthy Coloradans.* 2009; https://coloradohealth.org/sites/default/files/documents/2017-01/Food_Trust_Rpt-Colorado-Special%20Report%20the%20Need%20for%20More%20Supermarkets%20in%20CO.pdf. Accessed July 8, 2021.

17. Lang B, Kim E, Weidman J, McConlogue S. Healthy Food For All: Encouraging Grocery Investment in Colorado. 2011; Accessed July 8, 2021. www.policylink.org/resources/library/healthy-food-for-all-encouraging-grocery-investment-in-colorado.

18. O'Connor C. Park Hill hoping to satisfy hunger for grocery store. *The Denver Post.* 2016.

19. The Food Trust. HFFI Impacts: Case Studies–Colorado. n.d.; http://thefoodtrust.org/administrative/hffi-impacts/hffi-impacts-case-studies/colorado. Accessed July 8, 2021.

20. Lang B, Harries C, Manon M, et al. The Healthy Food Financing Handbook: From Advocacy to Implementation. 2013; http://thefoodtrust.org/uploads/media_items/hffhandbookfinal.original.pdf. Accessed July 9, 2021.

21. chfa. Colorado Fresh Food Financing Fund. 2021; www.chfainfo.com/CO4F/. Accessed July 9, 2021.

22. Mendoza M. Colorado enterprise fund makes biggest-ever commercial-project loan. *Denver Business Journal.* 2018.

23. The Sarah Samuels Center for Public Health Research & Evaluation. Colorado Fresh Food Financing Fund: Evaluation Findings. 2017; www.chfainfo.com/business-lending/BusinessLenderForms/CO4FEvalution.pdf. Accessed July 9, 2021.

24. Reinvestment Fund. Linking the Network: Colorado Enterprise Fund's Partnerships to Improve Colorado's Food System through Healthy Food Financing to Small Businesses: HFFI CDFI-Financial Assistance Program; Fiscal year(s): 2012, 2013, 2016.

8 Detroit, Michigan

CONTENTS

INTRODUCTION

Chapter 8 provides an overview of the history, context, and processes undertaken to establish a Green Grocer Project in Detroit and a Good Food Fund in Michigan. The chapter examines several examples of the Michigan food access movement, featuring key leaders such as Oren Hesterman and Malik Yakini. The mechanisms by which the programs were built and operate, as well as the outcomes, are discussed. The chapter highlights and emphasizes the unique ways that Michigan has structured its multiple mechanisms of funding, including the Good Food Charter, which has worked to elevate the importance of local food and to address needs across the food system beyond grocery retail alone. The chapter concludes with a reflection of how the historic context and community-engaged efforts supported increased access to healthy food retail.

More specifically, the Detroit's Green Grocer Project and Michigan's Good Food Fund (MGFF) initiatives to boost financing to projects that seek to improve food access efforts across the state are discussed. Michigan is a state well-known for its agricultural traditions and in the last several decades has been recognized for its progressive approach to addressing inequities in food access across the food system. Readers will learn the cultural and historic context that fostered poor access to food in low-income areas across Michigan and understand how the Green Grocer and MGFF operates and how its operations differ from other states, such

DOI: 10.1201/9781003029151-10

as Pennsylvania. Most uniquely, the chapter describes how the Michigan task forces looked beyond food retailing in underserved areas and considered the impact of projects through the whole food system as mechanisms to address food access disparities in Detroit and the state.

A BRIEF HISTORY OF MICHIGAN

Michigan is a state long-known for agriculture, an industry that contributes $101.2 billion to the state's economy. It is also a state where local food movements have taken shape, giving rise to terms such as 'good food', which seek to elevate efforts to establish fair and equitable strategies to ensure that food is healthy, green/environmentally sustainable, fair (no one has been exploited in its creation), and affordable. Michigan is home to many important industrial developments as well. For example, Detroit was the birthplace of Henry Ford's moving assembly line, the first mile of paved road, the first stoplight, and the first urban highway. Historically, many Black Americans in Detroit and surrounding areas moved to Michigan in hopes of escaping the harsh conditions of the South, setting their sights on new opportunities. The boom of Detroit's motor industry and related businesses and services offered many former agricultural workers new industrial working-class jobs.

Yet, while new opportunities were present, discriminatory hurdles persisted for many Black Americans in Michigan. Northern racism still subjected Black residents to the inability to vote, menial jobs, lack of access to public schools, systematic segregation, and unequal treatment in everyday life. Black Americans, for example, were regularly charged more than Whites for the same products, a practice that lasted well into the 1930s. As one resident living during the time recalled, 'In June 1930 the White owner of a tavern and grocery store charged two Black men in his tavern 75 cents for two bottles of beer, which he sold to White customers for 15 cents'.[1]

By the 1930s, chain supermarkets had opened stores in predominately Black Detroit neighborhoods, although unlike many cities across the United States, Detroit remained balanced in terms of the presence of chain versus independent grocers. Amidst the shifting retail structures came many reports of stores perpetuating discriminatory practices; A&P, for example, initially forbade the hiring of Black residents as store managers. So, while the business community recognized the importance of the growing Black consumer market, retail practice did not always justly serve the community. These and other injustices saw strong resistance at the time and seeded tensions which would erupt in protest for many years to come.

REDLINING IN MICHIGAN

Redlining, as described elsewhere in this text, was a practice undertaken by the federal government in the 1930s, whereby neighborhood race and ethnicity data were used to determine which neighborhoods and families were eligible for government-backed loans. The practice designated predominately White neighborhoods as investment-worthy and designated minority neighborhoods as hazardous areas for investment.[2] The practice mimicked earlier efforts to use racial or economic zoning as a mechanism for segregation, such as that used in Baltimore in 1910. The mayor at the time reported the rationale for the changing zoning ordinances that would work to separate White residents from Black and other minority residents as: 'Blacks should be quarantined in isolated slums in order to reduce the incidence of civil disturbance, to prevent the spread of communicable disease into nearby White neighborhoods, and to protect property values among the White majority'.[3] Such practices were not illegal, and, as they expanded, were tested in the Supreme Court in cases like *Corrigan v. Buckley*, 1926. The case ultimately upheld those covenants where Black residents were restricted by an agreement made by residents of a specific neighborhood or area and found that private contracts were not to be subject to the Constitution; this even though these so-called private contracts would have to be upheld by the state, who would have to use their power for enforcement. It would not be until 1948 in the case *Shelley v. Kramer* that restrictive covenants would be struck down and made illegal. However, even then, Black residents were often not welcomed into White neighborhoods and were met with violence, isolation, and fear tactics. Such tactics too were often ignored by police or met with delayed response with few or no arrests.[4]

Michigan neighborhoods in Kalamazoo, Detroit, Battle Creek, Flint, and Pontiac in the 1930s claimed that Black American homeowners were bad for real estate; that mixing races hurt home values; and those all-White neighborhoods needed protection from the 'lesser' minority population. During the post–World War II rise in the housing market and the creation of the suburbs, Black Americans received 2% of all loans in Michigan despite representing 10% of the population. The Detroit redlined map from 1939 is presented in Figure 8.1.

Like much of the nation, the redlining that instituted housing discrimination contributed also to job discrimination, interpersonal racism, and continued racial inequity of opportunity. While our focus in this text is on food access, it is imperative that the reader recognize that food systems are part of a larger web of community infrastructure, heavily influenced by policies from

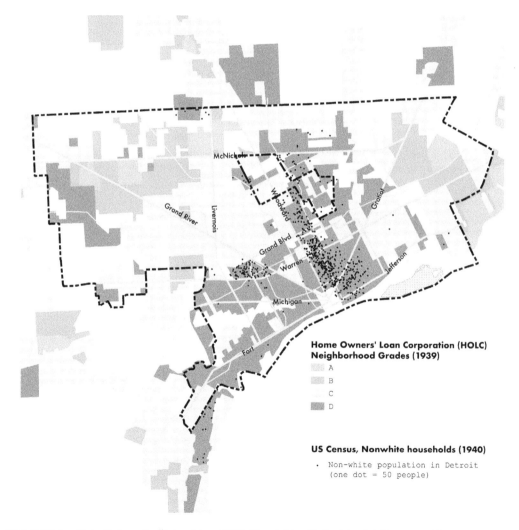

FIGURE 8.1 Detroit Area Redlining Map, 1939, Overlaid with Residential Demographics

(From Mapping Inequality, University of Richmond Digital Scholarship Lab; IPUMS NHGIS, University of Minnesota, www.nhgis.org.)

other sectors, including housing and educational policy. For example, in the 1970s, a lawsuit was filed against Detroit and the state of Michigan by the NAACP (*Milliken v. Bradley*), which argued against the repeal of desegregation of Detroit's high schools. In so doing it meticulously documented the close ties that housing segregation has on educational segregation. Studies looking at the relationship between housing segregation and food access are emerging.

In many places the redlined areas of the 1930s continue to have lower property values today than similar neighborhoods.[5] Racial housing segregation in America has deep ties to a persons' ability to accumulate wealth, and when a neighborhood is systematically devalued, prohibits the appreciation of home values in predominately Black neighborhoods. Homes are often a person's largest asset, and the ability to finance and grow the value of such an asset is integrally tied to one's own and their family's wealth. The development of the redlined maps however may not be the sole cause of perceptions of devaluation but rather both a symptom of predominant views of the worth of predominately Black neighborhoods as well as a perpetuating factor for segregation. A study of racial beliefs and segregation found, for example,[6] that White study participants consistently viewed predominately Black neighborhoods as less desirable and less safe than White neighborhoods, even when all other housing and community factors were kept identical. The lack of opportunity to purchase and grow wealth through the ownership of homes explains in part how the wealth gap between Black and White America has grown so large.[7] Housing discrimination later took the form of efforts labeled 'urban renewal' in the 1960s, which displaced thousands of Black residents to public housing complexes. With the shift in housing too came segregation in the educational system in the 1980s. Gentrification also plays a significant role in determining a community's resources and resident access to food. One study that examined the impacts of redlining found that it was also closely associated with gentrification and ultimately better food access.[8]

While redlining set the stage for housing discrimination, other ways to discriminate neighborhoods persisted across the country, even after the institution of Fair Housing was legislated in 1968. One such practice is called *blockbusting*, whereby unscrupulous real estate agents would capitalize on the racist fears of White homeowners by telling them that Black residents were moving into the neighborhood. Then would offer to buy their home at a low price before it was 'too late'. Once purchased at low prices, the agents would then flip the homes and sell to Black residents who suffered from few options, at much higher prices, often with financially stringent terms.[9] *White flight*, as it is commonly called, then ensued, resulting in massive disinvestment of what are now communities of color. Recent research looking at the relationship between redlining and other forms of discrimination, including blockbusting, reveals that there is a strong association between blockbusting and food access and has called for more attention to be paid to the practice.[8]

THE DETROIT FRESH FOOD ACCESS INITIATIVE (DFFAI)

FOOD RETAIL IN DETROIT

The Detroit food retail landscape continues to suffer from many years of inequity and disinvestment and sits squarely in the shadow of housing discrimination. In the past 100 years only a handful of Black owned grocery stores have operated in the city of Detroit. However, the story of food retail in Detroit would be remiss not to recognize the Booker T. Washington Grocery Store, which was owned and operated by Berry Gordy Sr., the father of Berry Gordy Jr., founder of Motown Records, one of the most important independent record labels of the 1960s.[10] That aside, there were no Black-owned stores between 2017 and 2019 in a city where 80% of residents today are Black.

The reasons for the lack of diversity in the industry are multifaceted but can be traced to inadequate networks, technical assistance to support business development administrative requirements, and the capital needed to access financing. Charles Walker is one of the few Black supermarket owners in Michigan's history. He has been open about his experience in starting and operating a Sav-A-Lot store, as well as the struggles that such an effort has presented. In an interview he shared some of the operational realities and the factors that have contributed to a lack of Black ownership in the industry:

> With grocery stores or in any industry, you have to have some experience to be able to own one. We are working in grocery stores, but, especially at the independent stores, we are not in management positions, so we can't understand the leadership of it. We are stock clerks, cashiers, but the everyday running of the business – we don't get that experience . . . just the basic parts, the menial jobs.[11]

Begun in 2004 with optimism that the newly renovated plaza, which was also home to other social services, a popular flea market, and across the street from a Chrysler factory would flourish and bring needed food to a community, it ultimately fell victim to a fire and layoffs at the factory, closing its doors in 2010.

Another iconic Black-owned store tells a story of both struggle and how access to capital is a critical factor in the viability of local minority owned retail. The Detroit store which became Metro Foodland, was initially a Kroger. Kroger was a store that embraced the hiring of local residents, including Mr. James Hooks, who began working at the store in 1969 at the age of 16. Because of his experience in retail and the opportunities he had to move into higher levels of leadership, he became interested in purchasing the Kroger store when the retailer no longer sought to operate it under their banner. In an article published in 2012 about the store, James Hooks commented,

> I think there should be more Black American-owned-and-operated stores so we can do a better job of serving our folks and showing young people that you can run a store, you can run any kind of business. . . . If you don't see us doing it, why would you think to be involved in that industry, or aspire to be a retailer or grocery retailer or something like that? That's not something you would think about. Right now, what we see is people playing basketball, or people doing whatever people do, things you see Black folks get involved in a lot of. It ain't good. To me it just seems like we're missing the boat.[12]

In response, the Kroger Corporation offered to sell the store to him and helped him directly to obtain the needed financing to operate the store independently. For twenty-nine years Mr. Hooks owned and operated Metro Foodland in the Detroit community, and during that time inspired others, like Mr. Walker to open stores. When word of the stores' struggle to stay in business hit the street in 2013, outspoken community support followed, including from coalitions such as the Nation of Islam who called its members to support the Black-owned store. One member, Reed, at the time shared with the press the importance of the store for the community:

> The importance is, when you own businesses in the community, that allows you to build an economy that will enable you to do for the community that you are a part of. When you have other people who are not a part of your community owning the businesses, making money from the community and taking it outside of the community, then that's when the community becomes depleted and destitute, as Detroit is right now, today.[12]

Yet, despite community support from Reed and others, Metro Foodland closed in 2014 following the economic downturn. The store closing is one of several examples that demonstrates the challenges associated with owning and operating independently owned stores in moderate income communities. Some also blame competition from stores like Meijer. Meijer is a national chain with strong Midwest operations that had begun to operate within Detroit city-limits and was rumored to have plans, at the time, to open near the Metro Foodland store. While some welcomed the national retailer to the community, others were very resistant, threatened by the retailer's size, vertical integration, and large network of suppliers that enabled the store to sell high volumes of a wide variety of products at lower prices than independent retailers cold offer since they cannot move the same volume, factors discussed as part of the supermarket industry in Chapter 2. A 20-year-old store employee at Metro Foodland explained his concerns as going beyond his own store to affecting the larger community of locally owned stores.

> Not only will it affect us, but it will affect the other independents too – the hardware stores, 'cause they sell tools. They sell gas, so the gas stations too. They sell plants, so the flower shops too. The liquor stores, 'cause they sell beer and wine. So small independents, they won't have a chance if that guy gets up here. You can't compete with that.[12]

When stores cease to exist, residents too are presented with a food access dilemma: to get good food, one must travel to the suburbs. In Detroit alone, residents who have to drive to the suburbs to purchase their food, either because no local store is available, or because the stores that are available have unappealing or inadequate offerings, such as the practice of relabeling food that has expired or showing a lack of respect to customers, has pushed about $200 million annually out of local neighborhoods,[13] to the suburbs where many grocery stores are located. Shopping outside of the neighborhood, while inconvenient, also perpetuates community disinvestment, and extracts needed tax dollars, jobs, and other retail which are anchored by a large store like a grocery store.

While it's clear that larger retailers are disproportionately located outside of the city of Detroit than within the limits, some have persuasively argued that there are many access points for good food across the city, including many smaller, community-based resources that might not be recognized as grocery stores or listed in larger secondary datasets.[14]

FOOD ACTIVISM IN DETROIT

Given its history, it should be no surprise that Detroit has become home to a dedicated and progressive food access movement, with many diverse tentacles of interests, grounded in very different theoretical underpinnings. For example, on one end of the spectrum are efforts that believe in, and advocate for, a market-driven approach to food retail, while others are rooted in the belief that food sovereignty is the best way to empower communities. The city is internationally known for its advances in urban agriculture and is home to some of the most established food policy councils in the country, groups that do not hesitate to actively share their voice to City Councils and other legislative bodies. Other strong efforts, for example, the Detroit Food Justice Task Force and members of the Detroit Community Markets (farmers markets) have also played critical roles in advancing food access, policy, and critical dialogue across the city. The Black Farmer Land Fund, Oakland Ave Urban Farm, Keep Growing Detroit, Church of the Messiah, and Detroit Neighborhood Grocery actively operate to change the food access landscape and dialogue in the city. Malik Yakini is the Executive Director of the Detroit Black Community Food Security Network, an organization founded with a mission to:

> "ensure that Detroit's African American population participates in the food movement and, because we are the vast majority of the population in Detroit, that we are in the leadership on that movement locally".[15]

Besides running a farm, providing educational and youth programs, and operating the Detroit People's Food Co-Op, the organization has provided valuable commentary and insight into the food movement. Mr. Yakini has called to question the commonly used term 'food desert' as a term that lacks cultural humility. He argues it reduces underserved communities to the issue of poor food access only, diverting attention from these larger issues that have supported the development of economically underserved communities.[16,17] In his words,

> 'Public policy and economic practices have created these areas that have low access to foods, and food desert does not speak to that intentionally'. Yakini goes further to say,[16] 'The struggle for food justice has to be tied to the struggle for economic justice'.

A similarly minded activist named Dara Cooper, has introduced the term *food apartheid* as a better description of the problem. She describes food apartheid as the,

systematic destruction of Black self-determination to control one's food, hyper-saturation of destructive foods and predatory marketing, and blatantly discriminatory corporate controlled food system that results in [communities of color] suffering from some of the highest rates of heart disease and diabetes of all time.

THE DFFAI TASK FORCE AND ADMINISTRATIVE STRUCTURE

Another example of activism in Detroit is captured by The Detroit Fresh Food Access Initiative (DFFAI). Like other task forces described in other cities and states in this book, the DFFAI consisted of a member group and co-chairs. The DFFAI was led by three co-chairs and a forty-six--member committee that represented a range of industry leaders, including local food retailers, and distributers, grocers, national grocery retail development experts, banks, philanthropy and academics (Table 8.1).[18] The task force specifically sought to address the role of traditional food retail outlets in fresh food access and to recommend ways to strengthen the overall grocery industry as a delivery mechanism for fresh and healthy foods.[18] They worked strategically to

TABLE 8.1
Detroit Fresh Food Access Initiative Membership

Member	Professional Affiliation	Contribution and Development Specialty
Jane Shallal (Co-Chair)	President, Associated Food and Petroleum Dealers	Grocery
Warren Sisch (Co-Chair)	Regional VP, Market Development SUPERVALU	Grocery
Olga Savic (Co-Chair)	Acting VP, Business Development, Detroit Economic Growth Corporation	Community Development
Edward Deeb	President, Michigan Food and Beverage Association	Association, Grocery
Kirsten Simmons	Executive Coordinator, Michigan Food Policy Council	Association, Policy and Local Food
Linda Gobler	President, Michigan Grocers Association	Association, Grocery
Glenn Lapin	Director, Planning and Development, Detroit Renaissance	Association, Community Development
Jim Sutherland	Director of Operations, Eastern Market Corporation	Independent Food Retailer, Local Food
Kim Hill	Director, Outreach & Community Relations, Eastern Market Corporation	Independent Food Retailer, Local Food
Joe Grappy	Vice President Gigante Prince Valley Super Mercado	Independent Grocer
Najib Attisha	Owner, Indian Village Market	Independent Grocer
James Hooks	Owner, Metro Foodland	Independent Grocer
Charles Walker	Owner, Save-A-Lot	Independent Grocer
Norman Yaldoo	Owner, University Foods	Independent Grocer
Terry Farida	Owner, Value Center Market	Independent Grocer
David Kapusansky	Director of Real Estate, ALDI	National Retailer, Grocery Development
Scott Nowakowski	Director of Real Estate, Meijer	National Retailer, Grocery Development
Rick Ragsdale	Director of Real Estate, Michigan, The Kroger Company	National Retailer, Grocery Development
Michael Curis	President, Curis Enterprises, Inc.	Economic Development

(Continued)

TABLE 8.1 (Continued)
Detroit Fresh Food Access Initiative Membership

Member	Professional Affiliation	Contribution and Development Specialty
Ted Simon	Grand Sakwa Properties	Economic Development
Mike Dikhow	Owner, Liberty International	Wholesale Food Distribution
Joseph Kuspa	Owner, Metro Produce	Wholesale Food Distribution, Produce
Jim Gohsman	Manager of New Business Development, Spartan Stores	Wholesale Food Distribution Development
Dave Blaszkiewicz	President, Detroit Investment Fund	Finance, Economic Growth and Development
Dennis Quinn	Regional President-SE Michigan, Great Lakes Capital Fund	Finance, Economic Growth and Development
Deborah Younger	Executive Director, LISC	Finance, Economic Growth and Development
Rita Hillman	Director, Community Development Michigan Interfaith Trust Fund	Finance, Economic Growth and Development
Ray Watters	Executive Director, Shorebank/Detroit Community Loan Fund	Finance, Economic Growth and Development
Anika Gross-Foster	Director Philanthropic Affairs and Next Detroit Initiative, City of Detroit Mayor's office	Regulatory, Planning and Economic Development Agencies
Bill Ridella	Deputy Director, City of Detroit Health Department	Regulatory, Planning and Economic Development Agencies
Douglass Diggs	Director, City of Detroit Planning and Development	Regulatory, Planning and Economic Development Agencies
Marja Winters	Director, Mayor's Office of Neighborhood Commercial Revitalization	Regulatory, Planning and Economic Development Agencies
Kathy Fedder	Director, Food and Dairy Division, Michigan Department of Agriculture	Regulatory, Planning and Economic Development Agencies
Karen Butler	Regional Supervisor, Michigan Department of Agriculture	Regulatory, Planning and Economic Development Agencies
Nancy Cappola	Deputy Director, Business Development, Wayne County Economic Development	Regulatory, Planning and Economic Development Agencies
Mike Hamm	C.S. Mott Professor of Sustainable Agriculture, MSU Mott Group for Sustainable Agriculture	Academia
Kami Pothukuchi	Department of Geography and Urban Planning, Wayne State University	Academia
Susan Goodell	Co-Chair of Food Systems Sub-Committee and Executive Director, Forgotten Harvest, Detroit Food and Fitness Initiative	Academia, Healthy Communities
Nikita Buckhoy	City Connect Detroit Project Partner	Academia
Rob Grossinger	Senior VP & Community Impact Regional Manager, La Salle Bank (now Bank of America)	Banking, Finance
Tosha Brown	Assistant VP, Market Development Specialist, La Salle Bank (now Bank of America)	Banking, Finance
Tiffany Douglas	VP, Market Development Manager, La Salle Bank (now Bank of America)	Banking, Finance
Chris Smith	Program Officer, Community Foundation for Southeast Michigan	Philanthropy
Ed Egnatios	Senior Program Officer, The Skillman Foundation	Philanthropy
James Johnson-Piett	Program Coordinator, The Food Trust	Consultants, Technical Assistance
John Talmage	President and CEO, Social Compact	Consultants, Technical Assistance

examine issues of grocery retail access in the city and conducted several structured convenings of leaders and key stakeholders to discuss needs and solutions to challenges.[18] The formation of the DFFAI Task Force was established in October 2007 and was in response to many of the efforts discussed here as well as other related efforts happening across the nation. For example, nationally, organizations such as The Food Trust in Philadelphia had success in creating their own Fresh Food Financing Initiative (see Chapter 4) and received funding from the Robert Wood Johnson Foundation to support efforts to replicate the program in other states and cities across the United States. The foundation funding enabled The Food Trust to lend technical assistance to the Detroit effort. Organizers recognized that many other efforts were also underway, including urban farming initiatives, community activism, and other policy-directed efforts to improve health and well-being but emphasized the specific focal point of the work on grocery retail access. The group was formally convened three times over the span of four months and subcommittees conducted additional work between meetings. The result was several distinct reports that emphasized issues in need of attention and helped to elevate the importance of food access among industry. A summary of those findings are categorized into three main areas: (a) location of food stores; (b) buying power; and (c) health.

DFFAI Report

Location of Food Stores

Determining where food stores were located was an important goal of the DFFAI Task Force in their overarching effort to identify barriers to expanding grocery retail in Detroit. Evaluators used the industry standards of 'underserved' from the International Council of Shopping Standards, which defined underserved as areas where the grocery store space serving one person was less than 3 square feet. The number of people in Detroit was divided by the available grocery retail space and found that 62% of the city's population (580,000 people) were in underserved areas, leaving them without adequate access to food retail. And, when the calculations were performed at the local levels within Detroit, more than 50,000 residents were found to be severely underserved. The task force also reviewed data on grocery access, including the size and types of stores that residents in the city and surrounding counties had access. The evaluators used a definition of stores over 30,000 square feet for larger stores such as supermarkets, and this parameter of store size is reported by evaluators to reflect appropriate access to full grocery services. Using this metric, findings demonstrated a substantial grocery gap. Most city grocery stores had a small format, and in the region, and of the 133 larger stores in the tri-county area only 7% were in Detroit. The distance to stores also demonstrated a disparity, whereby city residents travelled, on average, a half-mile or more to reach a full-service store, and more than a quarter of residents had to travel more than 2 miles to get to a grocery store. Outside of Detroit, the average distance to a store was one mile. In 2018 the report was updated by the company StreetSense and supported these original findings.[19]

Buying Power of Underserved Communities

Equally important to the task force was assessing the underserved communities in terms of buying power to support new food retail businesses. First, the Task Force realized that the city's population was considerably larger than what had been reported in the past by the U.S. Census, both in terms of the number of people living in the city, and the density of the population. The analysis used proprietary and municipal data, such as water usage and other utilities to uncover the discrepancy. Instead of a population of 884,000 it reported an actual population of 933,043, a 5% increase, which improved the business potential. Second, the report demonstrated that prior buying power calculations were misleading. While traditional metrics rely on average household income of an area only, another important metric is the economic density of the area. The market analysis showed that by considering income in terms of population density, areas that appeared unattractive to retailers based on household income reports previously, demonstrate substantial market potential. Put simply, one person who makes $75,000 annually and lives alone on an acre of land, may have a relatively high income, but their buying power is considerably less than four renters that live in that same house, each making $27,000 annually. Authors of the report concluded:

> Higher population density in inner-city neighborhoods translates into concentrated buying power that supersedes their suburban counterparts, even in cases where average household incomes are comparatively lower.[19]

Results showed income densities of $180,000 per acre in the City of Detroit, which were three times higher than other areas in the county that were perceived to be more attractive to retailers. Third, the report called to question income levels themselves. Authors found that the income generated from the 'informal economy' within Detroit was worth more than $800 million. An informal economy is the set of economic activities that are not protected by the state, such as self-employment, unprotected jobs and other unregistered businesses, and these sources of income are not reflected in commonly relied upon U.S. Census data. Fourth, through an analysis of home buying reports and credit bureau income data, the evaluators found that income levels were 17% higher (average annual income of $48,000) than what was reported in the then seven-year-old U.S. Census, further elevating the buying potential of the area.

The cumulative effect of more buying power in the city than retailers to serve residents meant that much of the money that could be staying locally was 'leaking' into the surrounding neighborhoods. Because grocery retail was an important focus, the report provided some specific figures around the amount of the grocery leakage, including estimates based on industry standard data for retail that would be needed to serve the current population (2.8 million square feet) as compared to the actual amount of space available (2.3 million square feet). The authors concluded that the city was losing $180 million in grocery retail each year and had significant unmet grocery demand.

Food Retail and Community Health

Beyond conducting an economic analysis of the impact that a lack of food retail investment had on the city, public health impacts were also a concern to the Task Force. Therefore, in addition the leaders used existing data about grocery demand, including the layout of the food retail landscape in the city, for the task force to evaluate where supermarkets were and were not located and the relationship between store access and aggregate measures of diet-related death. From these analyses, the areas of greatest need for food retailers were determined (Figure 8.2).[20] Funded by LaSalle Bank, a consultant, Mari Gallagher Research & Consulting Group, studied Detroit's neighborhoods and examined aggregate measures of premature death to estimate the years of life lost due to poor diet. The analysis also included metrics to incorporate the abundance of fast food present in the city and the author's state: 'Fast food and other fringe food outlets are everywhere, yet there are comparatively few quality grocery stores where fresh and healthy foods can be purchased'. The authors argued that a balanced food environment was needed where residents had shorter distances to supermarkets and longer, less convenient access, to fast food. Results were compared between Metro Detroit and Detroit to reveal systematic differences in health outcomes and diet. The authors reported that for every 100 people, eleven years of life were lost due to 'out of balance food access'.

Report Conclusions

Other data important to the process included analyses of potential market needs and demand across the city of Detroit.[21] Task force members reviewed these data, and after discussions

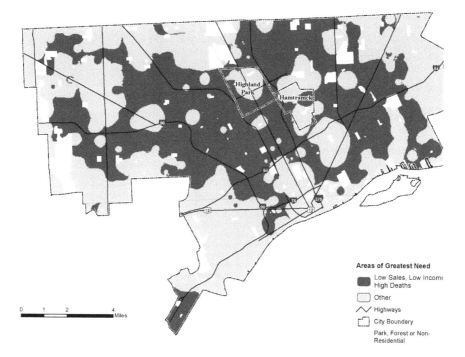

FIGURE 8.2   Map of Income and Diet-Related Deaths in Detroit, Areas with Greatest Need

(*Data:* TradeDimensions Retail Database, 2014, Michigan Department of Community Health, U.S. Census, ACS 2008–2012.)

about the implications for the report, and additional insight from local leaders contributing to the task force, established two foundational understandings among task force members: (1) neighborhoods lack full-service grocery stores where fresh foods and healthy options are available for purchase and (2) full-service stores do not always provide the selection or quality that neighborhood residents' demand.[18]

SUPERMARKET OPERATORS' BARRIERS FOR LOCATING IN UNDERSERVED AREAS OF DETROIT

The task force also entered discussions of the reasons for the challenges from the perspectives of the retailers and identified several issues, including:

- Grocery operations challenges those retailers face when serving high proportion of SNAP recipients. Because of the way that the food stamp cycle operates such that participants on SNAP receive one monthly allotment at one time, usually at the start of the month, retailers have to deal with staffing and stocking for high demand in the beginning of the month, followed by a sharp decline in purchases toward the end of the month, when stores need to continue to be stocked with produce and meats and other perishable items, despite lagging sales, thus creating waste.

- Perceived customer preferences for very large stores and wholesaler stores.

- Negative perceptions of Detroit's economy.

- Increased costs of doing business in the city.

- Challenges in processing the paperwork needed to get permits for development.

- Limited financing opportunities that meet retail needs.

- Employment or staffing challenges, such as concerns about being able to hire and retain dependable, well-trained workers.[18]

DFFAI TASK FORCE RECOMMENDATIONS

From this point, the task force further clarified its recommendations to include specifically instituting four changes that would address the retailers concerns and generate the following.[18] The solutions aimed to address barriers in underserved communities in Detroit such as: establishing resident demand for fresh food, supporting residents' need to access neighborhood stores, ensuring stores were of high quality with strong operations, ensuring that the store is compatible with the cultural norms and ethnic preferences of the surrounding community, and ensuring that financing is accessible to owners. In particular, the Task Force aimed to address the following four areas:

1. Gain improvements to the business climate, which included calls to distribute SNAP/ Food Stamps more evenly throughout the month; increase information outreach efforts to improve understanding and demand for good nutrition and healthy eating; requests to state government to reduce costs associated with item pricing and bottle deposit redemption regulations that disproportionately burden urban grocers, as well as a request to issue new state tax incentives which would encourage the development of urban grocery stores.
2. Create a new grocery store business attraction and retention program which would actively supply accurate market information, support site selection needs, establish new procedures to streamline the development and permitting process and provide financing support to grocers that qualified.
3. Build workforce development and grocer capacity, which would provide grocers with technical assistance in the operation of stores, while at the same time provide resources for current or future employees to build their skills in the industry.
4. Strengthen innovation in retailing and community relations, which include supporting efforts to partner with local community organizations, establish new transportation programs for residents, and improve the environmental impacts of stores, including addressing food waste with food rescue programs, upgrading lighting, refrigeration, and more efficient fixtures.

ESTABLISHING THE DETROIT GREEN GROCERY PROJECT

An outgrowth of the work conducted through the DFFAI was a partnership with the Detroit Economic Growth Corporation (DEGC), which created the Green Grocer Project in May of 2010.[22] This program, in response to calls from retailers, was launched with the goal of becoming a clearinghouse for grocery retailers interested in locating stores in Detroit. Experts at DEGC offered a variety of technical support to navigate the city's bureaucracy for (a) permits, (b) zoning, and (c) site selection as well as help with licensing and easements. Technical assistance was also offered to connect potential vendors to DEGC's network that included banks and vendors that could provide grants. For example, one specific type of grant offered was the Façade Improvement Program, which offered grocers matching funds to improve the exterior of grocery stores and their parking lots within Detroit city limits. Funds for the program were provided by both public and private investments including foundations like the Kresge Foundation, Lasalle Bank (now Bank of America), the Hudson Webber Foundation, Detroit Investment Fund, and the City of Detroit.

In the first several years the program supported twenty-seven retail projects with funding and technical assistance. Funding from the project has gone to address a variety of grocery retailer challenges. Sarah Fleming, the program manager at the DECG reported:

> Grants will improve everything from the type of produce in the stores, to the appearance of the stores, to the safety of the stores, to the accessibility of the stores. So, I think as these technical assistance operations, programs continue to move forward and then we're able to help the grocers fund some of these improvements through our revolving loan fund, we'll really start to see some marked improvements in access and quality and service.[23]

In the first several years of the Green Grocer Program Initiative, they provided nineteen technical assistance matching grants, provided direct assistance via the clearinghouse to more than thirty grocers, supported more than $6.3 million in funding for alternative model projects such as co-operative markets, specialty markets, and corner store conversions. The fund provided $500K in façade improvement grants which in turn were used to leverage $5.3M of other project investment. The fund is still in operation, and as recently as summer 2021 announced it was accepting proposals for funding amounts ranging from $50,000 to $300,000 intended to support pre-development, construction, renovation, and operating costs which would have verifiable, demonstrative impact on the physical, financial, or operational capacity of the store.[24] This most recent $400,000 funding pool is associated with the 2021 announcement stemming from the United States Department of Housing and Urban Development (HUD) Community Development Block Grant (CDBG). Additional support from other organizations have been seen. For example, one of the more nationally recognized food access organizations from Michigan is The Fair Food Network,[25] which has worked to collectively address the causes of inequities across many facets of the food system in both urban and rural areas by developing many, now-replicated, solutions to address the causes and consequences of discriminatory policies. With a mission to connect people to the power of food to grown community health and wealth the organization, founded by Oren Hesterman in 2009, the nonprofit has been instrumental in developing and advancing the work of nutrition incentives, which provides additional money in the form of what is called *food bucks*, to beneficiaries of the Supplemental Nutrition Assistance Program (SNAP), who in turn, can use the money to buy locally grown food.[26] The organization has also launched in 2013 an impact investing arm, called the *Fair Food Fund*.

THE MICHIGAN GOOD FOOD FUND (MGFF)

THE MICHIGAN HEALTHY FOOD ACCESS CAMPAIGN

Much like other programs across the country and in Detroit, a key to establishing the state program was forming a broad base of stakeholder support, which in part came from data demonstrating the need for food access across the state,[27] as well as an effort to convene partners to share experiences, needs, and identify solutions. The Michigan Healthy Food Access Campaign, which was like the effort conducted in Detroit, convened stakeholders statewide in October of 2015. Led by the American Heart Association, alongside partners from the Michigan Good Food Fund and Healthy Kids Healthy Michigan, the Michigan Healthy Food Access Campaign sought to create awareness of the need for more investment on the part of the state.[22] The effort used several approaches to garner additional state resources, including producing a report that highlighted areas of greatest need for healthy food retail across the state.[27] Beyond displaying need in terms of geography, the report also found that more than 300,000 Michigan children and 1.8% of Michigan residents lived in lower-income areas where supermarket access was limited. To broaden the conversation, the report also emphasized the need in areas outside of Detroit, including Grand Rapids, the largest city in West Michigan as well as rural areas across the state. Authors stated that 'Access to nutritious food is not evenly distributed in Michigan' and indicated 'this shortage of supermarkets particularly impacts lower-income residents with limited resources to maintain an adequate diet'. The authors also examined which low-income areas of Michigan were most likely to be impacted by poor diet, as evidenced by diet-related deaths (Figure 8.3).

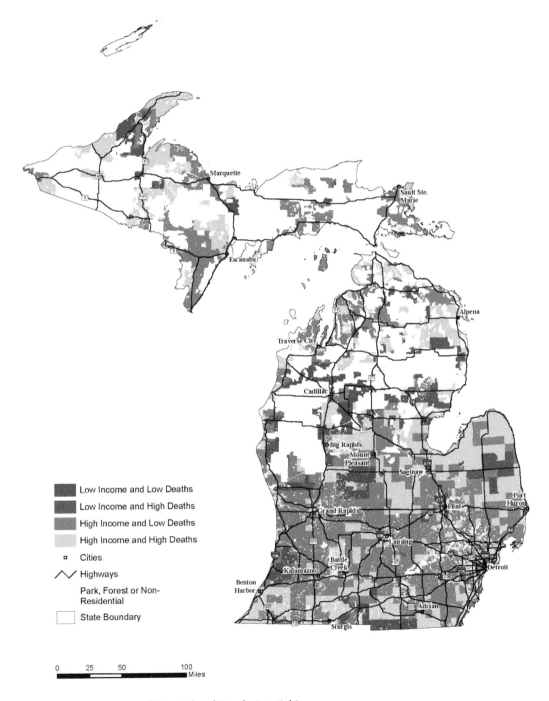

FIGURE 8.3 Income and Diet-Related Deaths in Michigan

(*Data:* TradeDimensions Retail Database, 2014, Michigan Department of Community Health, U.S. Census, ACS 2008–2012.)

MICHIGAN GOOD FOOD FUND CHARTER

Given the collective local momentum to recognize the importance of food for economic and social well-being, in June 2010 a Michigan Good Food Charter[28] was published through a multiyear collaboration with C.S. Mott Group for Sustainable Food Systems at Michigan State University, the Food Bank Council of Michigan, and the Michigan Food Policy Council, with funding from the W. K. Kellogg Foundation. Together, they sought to create a common vision for the state which would recognize the importance of the food system in promoting equity, advancing economic growth, protecting natural resources, and improving the health of residents. The goal was to establish a food system rooted in local communities and centered on, 'good food', a term first introduced by the W. K. Kellogg Foundation as part of its philanthropic work.

The reason for the charter was multifaceted, and included recognition that existing market structures, from zoning regulations which limited urban farming opportunities, to the way that public benefit programs were distributed, to how school food budgets were structured, hindered the ability for residents to get easy access to high-quality food. A key objective the charter sought to bring to the forefront of the food access movement too was to reemphasize the critical nature of working across the food system. The food system is depicted in Chapter 1 (Figure 1.1), and is characterized as the people, places, and processes involved in growing, processing, distributing, selling, preparing, and eating food, sometimes referred to as 'from farm to table' including recycling and composting food waste.[28] A term closely aligned with the food system is the food supply chain, which is described in Chapter 2. The value chain is in reference to efforts by companies to improve the efficiency of different parts of the food chain that brings a given product to market. The value chain[29] encompasses improvements to grow, produce, aggregate, process, distribute, sell and/or prepare food.

Further, Charter members recognized that the opportunities for buyers and farmers to connect were limited, and that farmers also faced barriers to maintaining good food operations, including prohibitively challenging food safety laws, limited access to capital, and limited access to farmland for growing. Adopted from the Kellogg Foundation's definition, the Charter defined 'good food' as more than local food, but rather food derived from a locally integrated food system characterized as:[28] (a) healthy – providing nourishment and enabling people to thrive; (b) green – produced in an environmentally sustainable manner; (c) fair – no one along the production line was exploited during its creation; and (d) affordable – all people have access to it.

Charter leadership envisioned that they could accomplish their goals over a ten-year span of time (2010–2020). In total they established six specific goals that could be accomplished with twenty-five policy priorities complete with accompanying strategies. Goals included:[28]

1. Michigan institutions will source 20% of their food products from Michigan growers, producers, and processors.

2. Michigan farmers will profitably supply 20% of all Michigan institutional, retailer, and consumer food purchases and be able to pay fair wages to their workers.

3. Michigan will generate new agri-food businesses at a rate that enables 20% of food purchased in Michigan to come from Michigan.

4. Eighty percent of Michigan residents (twice the current level) will have easy access to affordable, fresh, healthy food, 20% of which is from Michigan sources.

5. Michigan Nutrition Standards will be met by 100% of school meals and 75% of schools selling food outside school meal programs.

6. Michigan schools will incorporate food and agriculture into the pre-K through 12th grade curriculum for all Michigan students, and youth will have access to food and agriculture entrepreneurial opportunities.

Strategies complemented goals and included the creation of new economic opportunities for farmers and entrepreneurs, finding new ways to reduce time-consuming, or complicated regulatory processes, helping to bring good food to where people live (with an emphasis on minimally processed foods) and efforts to cultivate a mainstream culture that values the standard of food set by the Charter.

AVAILABILITY OF THE MICHIGAN GOOD FOOD FUND (MGFF)

The Michigan Good Food Fund was established because of the strong advocacy and food policy council work conducted on the part of a large group of partners and stakeholders across the state, including efforts in Detroit. Further, program visionaries looked to similar efforts in Pennsylvania and California as models. The early formal start to a Fund to support fresh food efforts came in 2013, when the Community Development Financial Institution (CDFI) called Capital Impact Partners applied for and was awarded, $3 million from the federal Healthy Food Financing Initiative.[30] With the $3 million initial investment, the initial core group of partners (Table 8.2) saw an opportunity to leverage the federal investment with other local philanthropic and community development funds to grow the overall pool of funding available for food environment projects.

At the same time, leaders had a vision for the effort to sustain a long-term approach to funding and recognized that to establish a strong, sustainable program, considerable effort was needed to establish guidelines, procedures, and partnerships that would inform the design and execution of the work. When launched in June 2015, program investors and partners had increased the fund amount from $3 million to a $13 million public-private partnership loan fund, which could provide resources to food businesses, benefiting communities across the state of Michigan. The additional $10 million investment came from the W. K. Kellogg Foundation and the Max and Marjorie Fisher Foundation.[31]

While the term *fund* is used to describe the work, there is not one set account that houses all monies available for these efforts as seen in other state and city examples in this book. Instead, the fund is comprised of a network of providers and financial intermediaries, each

TABLE 8.2
Initial Michigan Good Food Fund Core Partners

Core Partner	Responsibilities	URL Address
W. K. Kellogg Foundation	Program investors and thought leaders	Wkkf.org
Michigan State University Center for Regional Food Systems	Leads business assistance and pipeline development for agricultural production, aggregation, and distribution, as well as large processing projects	Foodsystems.msu.edu
Fair Food Network	• Provides business assistance and pipeline develop for retail grocery and small-batch processing • Leads communications and public relations for the Michigan Good Food Fund	Fairfoodnetwork.org
Northern Initiative is a Community Development Financial Institution	Lends MGFF funds from $5,000 to $25,000	Northerninitiatives.org
Capital Impact Partners	• Manages the MGFF program • Lends MGFF funds between $250,000 to $6 million	Capitalimpact.org

receiving their own funds from MGFF that they, in turn, lend (or deploy) using their own under-writing processes but based on the MGFF criteria.[29] Under the MGFF umbrella three types of financial products were provided. These include (1) technical assistance (e.g., seminars, boot camps, one-on-one meetings to help the entrepreneur understand how to secure financing, increase profitability, develop a business plan, increase sales, retain jobs, secure real estate, etc.) for those grocers or other food enterprise owners seeking loans or with outstanding loans; (2) Catalytic Investment Awards, which are comprised of grants between $10,000–$75,000 where funds are intended to grow businesses and/or prepare businesses to secure financing and are used to support renovations or as working capital, for the purchase of equipment, business planning, market research studies, or to secure real estate; and (3) loans are provided to grocers for amounts spanning between $2,500 and $6 million for retail business upgrades, expansions, inventory, equipment, and other related costs.

An effort was also made to garner state funds through the introduction of legislation that would allocate resources through the General Fund to support financing healthy food projects in the state. In December 2015, Michigan State Representative Dave Pagel introduced HB 5180[19] the Healthy Food Assistance Act which called for a $6.5 million state investment from the General Fund to: 'establish a statewide program to increase the availability of fresh and nutritious food, including fruits and vegetables, in underserved communities by providing financing for retailers to open, renovate, or expand grocery stores'. The fund would further 'provide funding for county-based programs to provide assistance to small food retailers to increase the availability and sales of fresh and nutritious food, including fresh produce, in low- and moderate-income communities'.

A year later, state Senator Geoffrey Hansen introduced a bill (SB 1110, 2016) that mirrored the bill introduced to the House a year earlier. The language of the bill delineated how the funds could be used and specified how much money could be allocated to several different loan funds. Of the $6.5 million sought, the bills indicated, for example that not more than $5 million could be used for the Healthy Food Financing grant/loan program, and not more than $1 million for the Small Food Retailer grant program, and not more than $500,000 for the Michigan Department of Agriculture and Rural Development costs of program administration.[19] While neither bill passed, both seeded momentum for future efforts across the state.

The now $30 million program is open to a variety of business applicants, including any effort that seeks to grow, process, distribute, and sell healthy food that reaches those who are in need. Applicants may include supermarkets, grocers, community markets, co-ops, food distributors, nonprofits, commercial developers, corner store owners, entrepreneurs, value-added producers, small business operators, and other innovators working to increase access to healthy food for Michigan children and families.[32] Developers sought funding parameters that would be flexible and support business ventures that might be overlooked or unable to obtain financing by traditional banks, as well as assistance to entrepreneurs to establish themselves to prepare for financing. Table 8.3 shows the program core objectives and targeted

TABLE 8.3
Good Food Fund Objectives and Outcome Criteria[29]

Fund Objective	Outcome
Healthy Food Access	Increase access to healthy food to improve the health of all Michigan residents
Economic Development	Drive economic development and job creation to grow Michigan's economy
Racial and Social Equity	Ensure equitable access to food, jobs, ownership, and flexible investment capital
Environmental Stewardship	Encourage sustainable environmental practices
Local Sourcing	Increase sourcing and supply of locally grown and regionally produced foods

outcomes for the fund.[32] The fund currently operates with partners serving in one of four roles, Program Administration (Capital Impact Partners); Technical Assistance Providers (Fair Food Network, Michigan State University Center for Regional Food Systems, Northern Initiatives); Financial Intermediaries (Capital Impact Partners, Detroit Development Fund, Grand Rapids Opportunities for Women, Michigan Women Forward, and Northern Initiatives); or as Funders (Capital Impact Partners, Max M. & Marjorie S. Fisher Foundation, Northern Trust, The Kresge Foundation, and the W.K. Kellogg Foundation).

MGFF PROGRAM OUTCOMES AND ACCOMPLISHMENTS

Since its launch in 2015, MGFF has undertaken two program evaluation efforts, including its most recent published in 2020.[31] To date the fund has invested more than $13 million into companies making or selling food. More than 280 Michigan businesses that contribute to the Michigan food system have benefited from the program, either through technical assistance or support with financing or loans (Figure 8.4). Most funds have been allocated to food processors, with only 15% for retailers. A small amount of support has been provided (14%) to operations such as farm stands, incubators, co-operatives, or aggregators such as food hubs, categorized as 'Other' on Figure 8.4. The program has created 600 jobs across the Michigan state food supply chain.

While a complete list of all projects supported is impractical, a selected number of funded ventures are provided in Table 8.4 and include support across the food system with examples that follow:[33]

- A **Full-Scale Supermarket** looking to remodel an existing site to accommodate more cases for produce, fresh meat, and dairy.

- A **Mobile Market** needing investment in vehicles and refrigeration to bring fresh, affordable product into underserved communities.

- A **Processing Facility** needing additional machinery and equipment to support expansion into new product lines or to support additional volume.

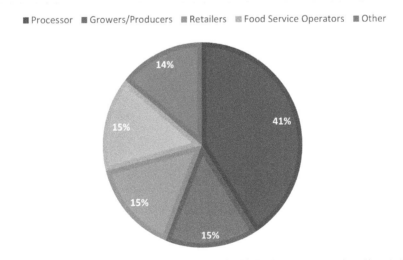

FIGURE 8.4   MGFF Program Fund Distribution within the Michigan Food System

TABLE 8.4
Selected Early MGFF-Funded Projects

Business/ Amount/Type	Description	Grant or Loan Type	Grant or Loan Use
Sofia Foods Processor-small	Producer of jarred olives and olive spread, <$25,000	N/A	Proceeds used to increase inventory
Byrne Family Farm Farm	Organic CSA farm that also sells retail to local farmers markets, <$25,000	Term Loan	Proceeds financed the construction of additional hoop houses for shoulder season production
Little Owls Organic Grocery Retail – small	Organic grocery and produce store. Offerings include a large variety of fresh organic produce, organic dry/bulk goods and environmentally friendly cleaning and beauty products, <$100,000	Term Loan	Proceeds to assist with equipment, inventory and working capital to be used for things like advertising, legal, utilities, office supplies, etc.
Flying Moose Retail small	Modern general store in downtown Marquette, Michigan that carries local and organic food lines, <$75,000	Term Loan	Proceeds used for build-out and equipment
Au Sable River Family Restaurant Restaurant	Local restaurant featuring local meat, produce, and foods, <$50,000	Term Loan	Proceeds used for renovation and expansion of dining room area
Black Pearl Processor (small)	Company sells retail and wholesale, Producer of low salt and nitrate dried meat products, <$25,000	N/A	Loan for working capital and with building inventory
PK Development – Diamond Place Retail – large	New mixed-use project with grocery store and 30 apartment units in Grand Rapids, MI. Local independent grocery operator. Apartments will include affordability component, >$3.5 million	Direct Leverage Loan as part of a potential NMTC transaction	Construction of grocery
Ken's Fruit Market Retail- small	Small food market operator in west Michigan that currently operates three locations to refinance high cost start-up debt. The first store opened in 2010, <$500,000	Refinancing	Refinance (see case study)
Park Street Market	Renovated a vacant 56,000 sq ft former grocery store in Kalamazoo, MI into a strip center anchored by a 28,000 sq ft grocery store. Kalamazoo is a blighted community on the west side of the state, and the project is in a highly distressed census tract and is surrounded by food deserts. The new store replaced a large supermarket that closed in	Direct Leverage Loan & Term Loan	Renovate a vacant 56,000 sq ft former grocery store

(Continued)

TABLE 8.4 (Continued)
Selected Early MGFF-Funded Projects

Business/ Amount/Type	Description	Grant or Loan Type	Grant or Loan Use
	2015 with a smaller store, more appropriate for the market. The site itself is not a food desert, but this is likely because the information has not been updated since the previous store closed, >$5 million		
Recovery Park Farm	Three separate but related agricultural projects: an urban farm spread out over a 2,475-acre zone on Detroit's east side, a food processing center, and an indoor fish farm. Employees will come from the community and have challenging backgrounds, >$1 million	Loan	Land reuse and employment, on farm to grow upmarket product to ship outside of community
Eastern Market Corp.	Funds to acquire >100 vacant parcels East of Eastern Market, many with structures to support local growers to sell products. Part of the plan also includes open green space and a system of storm water management, >$2 million	Line of Credit	Vacant lot to be developed for multiuse

- A **Food Incubator** in need of tenant improvements and equipment to provide commercial spaces for smaller food entrepreneurs.

- A **Food Hub** needing upgraded refrigeration space and loading platform improvements to better supply good food to corner retail and schools in under-served areas.

- An **entrepreneur** acquiring machinery to expand her business in drying, packing, and delivering dried local fruit.

- A **Producer** purchasing higher-capacity equipment that would improve yield and increase sales.

- A **Corner Store** looking to renovate store layout and acquire necessary equipment to sell fresh fruits, vegetables, and meats.

- A **Food Cooperative** seeking working capital to purchase more inventory to meet growing demand.

- A **Farmers Market** seeking financing for improvements to a permanent site, whether it be for infrastructure costs, facade upgrades, or acquisition of a leased or owned facility.

- A **Farmers Market Vendor** in need of permanent working capital to finance inventory to increase volume to be able to sell at a farmers market.

MGFF Case Studies

A detailed picture of three selected MGFF program projects are described here.

> *Imperial Fresh Market, Detroit,* is an independent grocery store and has been in operation for twenty-five years and has experienced success in a community with relatively few grocery options.[34] The 40,000-square-foot store offers local residents full-service grocery options in the heart of the community. In 2015, Sam Shina, the company's owner, decided to double the size of the store, a decision that required a $6 million investment to support the expansion. The project was in part necessary to compete with larger retailers like Meijer. Mr. Shina recalled, 'If I go back seven years, Meijer was coming into the market, and we had an older store. . . . Either you were going to get eaten up, or you were going to double down. So what we did was double down'.[34] Through the MGFF, Imperial Fresh Market was able to secure financing from Pacific Community Ventures, one of the MGFF fund administrators.

> *Ken's Fruit Market, Grand Rapids,* began as a small 7,000-square-foot produce store. The owners, Ken and Gina Courts, built a strong operation which was well-poised for growth.[34] The financing for the store however had initially been built on a complex stack of both personal and business loans, and to expand, it was most financially prudent to consolidate the debt. The project ultimately received $445,000 to refinance the store with funds that initially came to the MGFF from the Healthy Food Financing Initiative. The funds both allowed the business to reduce its financing costs and to expand its store.

> *Country Style Marketplace, Port Huron,* began with a vision to renovate a building which once housed a Woolworth operation, however it would take a while to realize their initial vision. Steve Fernandez and Michelle Jones, co-owners went to the community to learn more about local options, and what residents would like to see the old building become. Mr. Fernandez recalled,

> When we started working on cleaning up the old decals off the building, we started having people come by and asking us what was going on. And so, we started asking people walking by on the street, 'what would you want to see here?' And I'll be darned if 20 out of 20 people didn't say, 'we need a grocery store'. And so the more we started hearing that, the more we started looking into it, we started realizing, wow, that's true.[34]

At the time, the only other nearby stores selling groceries were dollar stores and a party store. However, because the space lacked a large parking lot, investors were skeptical the location would serve well as a grocery store, and the visionary partners were left without a financial mechanism to update the store infrastructure and kick-start grocery operations at the site.

So, instead, the owners identified another store about 4 miles away, outside of downtown, which offered a more traditional footprint, the Country Style Marketplace. That Marketplace in Fort Gratiot was already in operation and well-known locally for its meats. After several years of successful operations in Fort Gratiot, owners again sought to revisit their initial vision, this time as a second store. The MGFF supported the vision and helped them to secure a $3.4 million construction loan which would enable them to rehabilitate a 12,000-square-foot space for the second Country Style Marketplace to operate. They believe that the smaller store formats are well-aligned with customers visions for the revitalization of the community.

> We have numerous customers come in and tell us that they prefer to shop in a small grocery store like ours. We are always friendly, nobody's pushing or taking stuff out of your cart. And we work hard to stay that way.[34]

CONCLUSION

Efforts to improve access to healthy food in Michigan are vast and reflect a range of philosophical positions about the best ways to effectively address the long-lasting effects of discriminatory practices like redlining and blockbusting. The development of the Good Food Fund was the result of a combination of targeted advocacy efforts, commitment on the part of philanthropy, research reports describing the problem and its impacts, as well as a concerted effort on the part of the community development financing community and its affiliates to create a fund to fill gaps. As a result, more than 280 Michigan food businesses, from supermarkets to farmers markets, have benefitted from the program.

In addition to documenting the types of projects that were funded and how the funds worked to support those enterprises, lessons learned have also been gained in understanding the mechanisms by which the fund operates and how certain services have worked to support applicants. The importance of tracking data with systems intentionally developed for that purpose, with resources to initiate client outreach and management, is one such example. Other details of operations and the way that services have been used have further suggested how certain aspects of the fund may better serve some types of operations than others. For example, a recent evaluation report found that not only is technical assistance needed for retailers generally, but that growers and producers are particularly receptive to that type of support. Processors were found to account for only 16% of all loan recipients; however they represented nearly half of those that received technical assistance.[29] Another lesson learned by MGFF partners over the past few years of operations, is that in order to appeal to a broad range of types of operations, the financing options have to be diverse and flexible. Organizers have sought to address this need by relying on a network of lenders who together could enable a range of types of loans from very small to very large. A third challenge for fund administrators is to identify potential grantees. The developers of the MGFF sought to align funding efforts with the larger objectives outlined by the Good Food Charter and the term *good food* in general, which meant supporting agricultural efforts including growers and producers as well as more traditional retail operations. Leadership quickly realized however that in order to connect with potential projects across the food system, targeted and focused outreach was needed.[29]

Finally, grants made to entrepreneurs of color, and in particular Black owned businesses, under the catalytic investment award mechanism have helped owners who have experienced systematic financial discrimination.[29] In fact, a sizable proportion (69%) of the catalytic awards have gone to support entrepreneurs of color who have also received about half of all MGFF loans. Program operators find that the catalytic awards enable earlier stage businesses who may not yet be ready for larger loans and debt financing to grow their business. Overall, this support has led to improvement across the Michigan Food System that has ultimately increased 'good food' in underserved areas.

CRITICAL THINKING QUESTIONS AND EXERCISES

1. Examine the websites of one or more advocacy organizations noted as being influential in Detroit. Reflect on their likely stance regarding the work of the MGFF.
2. Examine the data reported in the MGFF 2015–2019 Evaluation with particular consideration toward its ability to effectively address racial discrimination. Has the fund done so? Why or why not?
3. Compare the process undertaken in Michigan to that of New Orleans or Colorado. In so doing, consider how the role of philanthropy has contributed to the establishment of the fund.
4. To get an interactive look at redlining across America, scholars across America, including the University of Richmond's Digital Scholarship Lab team created a

website, *Mapping Inequality*. Go to the website and examine the differences between Redlining in New Deal America 1935–1940 (https://dsl.richmond.edu/panorama/redlining/#loc=5/39.1/-94.58) and the way that Family Displacements occurred through Urban Renewal 1950–1966 (https://dsl.richmond.edu/panorama/renewal/#view=0/0/1&viz=cartogram).

5. Understand key terms in this chapter including a food system, a food value chain, and food apartheid. How are these terms relevant to Detroit in particular?

6. Describe the process for developing the MGFF and contrast the program to one other state initiative described in this book.

7. Review the types of projects resulting from the MGFF at all levels of the food system. Do you think the program is effective at improving food access for underserved areas? Connect the program objectives listed on Table 8.3 with the projects funded on Table 8.4.

8. Articulate how the MGFF has impacted low- and moderate-income communities across the state and within Detroit.

REFERENCES

1. Thomas R. *Life for Us Is What We Make It: Building Black Community in Detroit 1915–1945*. Bloomington, IN: Indiana University Press; 1992.
2. Hill A. Detroitography: Detroit Redlining Map 1939. https://detroitography.com/2014/12/10/detroit-redlining-map-1939/. Accessed July 11, 2021.
3. Brown E, Barganier G. *Race and Crime: Geographies of Injustice*. Oakland: University of California Press; 2018.
4. Rothstein R. *The Color of Law: A Forgotten History of How Our Government Segregated America*. New York: Liveright Publishing Corp/W. W. Norton; 2017.
5. Appel I, Nickerson J. Pockets of Poverty: The Long-Term Effects of Redlining. 2016; Available at SSRN: https://ssrncom/abstract=2852856 or http://dxdoiorg/102139/ssrn2852856.
6. Krysan M, Farley R, Couper M. In the eye of the beholder: Racial beliefs and residential segregation. *Du Bois Review 5*. 2008;1:5–26; https://igpa.uillinois.edu/system/files/cas/media/pubs/Krysan_Farley_Couper_2008.pdf.
7. Quick K, Kahlenberg R. Attacking the Black-White opportunity gap that comes from racial segregation. *Race & Inequality*. 2019; https://tcf.org/content/report/attacking-black-white-opportunity-gap-comes-residential-segregation/?session=1. Accessed July 11, 2021.
8. Sadler RC, Bilal U, Furr-Holden CD. Linking historical discriminatory housing patterns to the contemporary food environment in Baltimore. *Spatial and Spatio-Temporal Epidemiology*. 2021;36:100387.
9. Editors of the Encyclopedia of Chicago. Blockbusting. 2021; www.encyclopedia.chicagohistory.org/pages/147.html. Accessed July 14, 2021.
10. Posner G. Motown: Chapter 1. *The New York Times*. 2003; www.nytimes.com/2003/2001/2012/books/chapters/motown.html.
11. Perkins T. Why Are There No Black-owned Grocery Stores in Detroit? 2017; https://fairfoodnetwork.org/news/why-are-there-no-black-owned-grocery-stores-in-detroit/. Accessed July 11, 2021.
12. Detroitblogger John. City's sole African-American grocer becomes an icon. In: Times DM, ed. *The Black Market*. Vol. 2021; www.metrotimes.com/detroit/the-black-market/Content?oid=21491212012.
13. Sorge M. Fair Food Network Fights for Detroiters. https://fairfoodnetwork.org/news/fair-food-network-fights-for-detroiters/. Accessed July 11, 2021.
14. Hill AB. The History and Conflict of Food Access in Detroit. 2012; https://alexbhill.org/2012/05/02/the-history-and-conflict-of-food-access-in-detroit/. Accessed July 14, 2021.
15. Detroit Black Food Security Network. Who We Are. https://detroitblackfoodsecurity.org/. Accessed July 11, 2021.
16. Lu I. Food Apartheid: What Does Food Access Mean In America? 2020; https://nutritionstudies.org/food-apartheid-what-does-food-access-mean-in-america/. Accessed July 11, 2021.

17. Reed J, Yates B, Houfek J, et al. A review of barriers to healthy eating in rural and urban adults. *Online J Rural Nurs Health Care*. 2016;16(1):122–153.

18. Detroit Economic Growth Corporation. *Detroit Fresh Food Access Initiative: Report of Taskforce Findings*. August 2008.

19. Michigan House Fiscal Agency. Legislative Analysis: Healthy Food Assistance Act House Bill 5180. 2016; www.legislature.mi.gov/documents/2015-2016/billanalysis/House/pdf/2015-HLA-5180-E803B30B.pdf. Accessed July 14, 2021.

20. Gallagher M. *Examining the Impact of Food Deserts on Public Health in Detroit*. Chicago, IL: Mari Gallagher Research & Consulting Group; 2007.

21. Social Compact Inc. *Detroit Grocery Initiative: Catalyzing Grocery Retail Investment in Inner-City Neighborhoods*. 2008.

22. Healthy Food Access Org Editors. Policy Efforts to Watch: Michigan Healthy Food Access Campaign. 2016; www.healthyfoodaccess.org/michigan. Accessed July 12, 2021.

23. Michigan Radio: What's Working. Trying to Improve Detroit's Grocery Stores. 2011; www.michiganradio.org/post/trying-improve-detroits-grocery-stores. Accessed July 12, 2021.

24. Economic Development Corporation of the City of Detroit. Green Grocer Project Notice of Funding Availability and Notice of Request for Proposals. In: June 25, 2021:5.

25. Fair Food Network. Who We Are. https://fairfoodnetwork.org/. Accessed July 11, 2021.

26. Mann J, Miller S, O'Hara J, Goddeeris L, Pirog R, Trumbull E. Healthy food incentive impacts on direct-to-consumer sales: A Michigan example. *Journal of Agriculture, Food Systems, and Community Development*. 2018;8(1):97–112.

27. Manon M, Church D, Treering D. *Food for Every Child: The Need for Healthy Food Financing in Michigan*. Philadelphia, PA: The Food Trust; 2015.

28. Colasanti K, Cantrell P, Cocciarelli S, et al. *Michigan Good Food Charter*. East Lansing, MI: C.S. Mott Group for Sustainable Food Systems at Michigan State University, Food Bank Council of Michigan, Michigan Food Policy Council; 2010.

29. Pacific Community Ventures. *Growing Michigan's Good Food Future: An Evaluation of the Michigan Good Food Fund 2015–2019*. 2021.

30. Fund MGF. What Is the Michigan Good Food Fund? In:2018.

31. Capital Impact Partners. Michigan Good Food Fund Launches to Grow Michigan's Good Food Future. June 9, 2015. www.capitalimpact.org/michigan-good-food-fund-launches-to-grow-michigans-good-food-future/. Accessed July 12, 2021.

32. Michigan Good Food Fund. Michigan Good Food Fund Brochure: Growing Michigan's Good Food Future. In: Fund MGF, ed2016.

33. Northern Initiatives. Michigan Good Food Fund. 2021. https://northerninitiatives.org/apply-for-a-michigan-small-business-loan/michigan-good-food-fund/. Accessed July 13, 2021.

34. Donnell M. In the Midst of the COVID-19 Pandemic, Local Independent Grocers Double Down to Feed Their Communities. In: Vol. 2021; www.capitalimpact.org/capital-impact-independent-grocers-healthy-food-access-covid-pandemic/; Capital Impact Partners, Michigan Good Food Fund; October 23, 2020.

Section III

Food Store Implementation
and Evaluation

This section of the book is intended to describe the formative research that has been conducted on local food environments as well as introduce readers to approaches for program evaluation targeting the influence of new foods stores (or other food environment modification) on the economic and health benefits for underserved communities. Chapter 9 describes the formative research that has documented food retail disparities in the United States as well as the associations with diet and obesity, which have been used to support the HFFI legislation and the state initiatives. Chapters 10–12 provide methods for formative and summative program evaluation beginning with the development of public-private partnerships and conducting needs assessments within specific underserved areas of the United States. Chapter 11 portrays the program planning, implementation, and process evaluation necessary for monitoring program fidelity, with an emphasis on logic models and behavioral theories to support the expected outcomes and impacts of the planned food environment change. Also in Chapter 11, the National Academy of Medicine's Translational Pipeline is introduced to readers as a framework for adopting implementation and dissemination science for evaluating the influence of HFFI and other food environment projects. Finally, Chapter 12 introduces readers to methods for evaluating the short-term outcomes and longer-term impacts of the changes in food retail among underserved communities by utilizing a mixed methods approach.

DOI: 10.1201/9781003029151-11

9 Food Environments
Formative Evaluation

CONTENTS

INTRODUCTION

This is the first of four chapters in Section III and focuses on program planning and evaluation in relation to local food environments. The purpose of this chapter is to provide the reader with a description of the formative research that has been used to justify state and federal funding to support new supermarkets and food retailers in underserved areas of the United States. The chapter describes the research that documents disparities in access to supermarkets as well as the potential impact supermarket accessibility has on diet and diet-related behaviors for Americans. In addition, because these formative studies are based on secondary data analyses, this chapter presents readers with factors to consider in the interpretation of statistics from these studies. Overall, the chapter describes the formative research up to when the Healthy Food Financing Initiative was presented to Congress and explains why program planning to utilize capital that is now available to food retailers is the most pressing next step in rectifying disparities in access to supermarkets in low-income, predominately Black, and other communities.

DOI: 10.1201/9781003029151-12

The state initiatives described in Chapters 4–8 and elsewhere in this volume garnered the momentum for the United States Congress to adopt the Healthy Food Financing Initiative with support through three departments of the U.S. government. This federal initiative (and the state programs that have preceded the HFFI) are justified with formative research that aimed to answer the following questions.

- Are there disparities in access to supermarkets in the United States, and who is affected by the disparities?

- Do disparities in access to supermarkets have any impact on attaining U.S. dietary recommendations?

- Do disparities in access to supermarkets affect rates of diet-related health conditions such as obesity?

Formative research and evaluation is the first step taken in program planning[1] and is conducted to document the problem, identify the group or groups of people that are most affected by the problem, and pinpoint potential programs to resolve the problem. Formative research is needed to garner funding for program planning and implementation of specific programs. The next stage of formative evaluation will involve assessing the feasibility and appropriateness of a particular program as a solution and the acceptability of that program by the community.

To understand the impact that the presence of a supermarket has on the behavior of eating, one must first appreciate the complexity of dietary intake. Dietary intake is a unique health behavior because, unlike other behaviors, we must eat every day and usually multiple times per day. There are very few mandatory behaviors for humans. It has been estimated an individual makes an average of 200 food-related decisions each day,[2] and one of these decisions is purchasing food. The way in which food is purchased for home preparation and consumption is thought to be different from eating away from home. Grocery shopping is one specific behavior where individuals purchase foods from grocery stores or supermarkets with the intention of cooking at home and eating the foods with family members. The behavior of purchasing foods at convenience stores or corner markets has also gained attention; however those food purchases are believed to support a more immediate hunger or food craving. This is distinguishable from the meal planning and typical grocery list that may accompany a person to a grocery store with the aim to purchase foods for many meals to nourish a family for several days, a week, or longer. Also, because the act of grocery shopping involves the purchasing of foods for multiple days, those foods purchases contribute to a greater proportion of meals consumed. This is the conceptual reasoning researchers have used to hypothesize that the presence of supermarkets are significant contributors to healthy food consumption.

DISPARITIES IN THE PLACEMENT OF SUPERMARKETS

As discussed in previous chapters, over time there has been a disinvestment in neighborhoods across the United States due to real estate and banking practices that have failed to support predominately Black, low-income, and other segregated areas (see Chapter 3–8). This disinvestment has left these neighborhoods without commercial resources such as banks, affordable housing, and supermarkets. The disparities in the presence of supermarkets are associated with both wealth and the racial makeup of areas. For example, in a study conducted by Morland et al., where the presence of supermarkets were evaluated within four states, most supermarkets were located in predominately White wealthy areas (Figure 9.1).[3] There were 68 supermarkets located in predominately White areas, providing service to 259,500 people; whereas only five supermarkets were in predominately Black areas aiming to serve 118,000 people. The racial disparities observed were independent of the wealth of the neighborhoods.

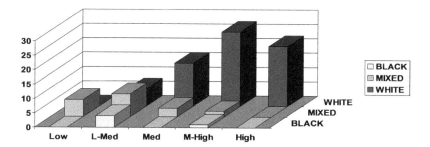

FIGURE 9.1   The Number of Supermarkets Present by Racial Segregation and Wealth of Neighborhoods

Although the measurement of local food environments and their impact on health began in the late 1990s, consumer advocate groups such as the Consumers Union had conducted studies to measure disparities in retail environments between neighborhoods prior to this time.[4] Others have also documented the influence of economic decline and the decrease of low-cost retailers within American inner cities during the 1960s and 1970s.[5] The urban grocery gap during the late 1980s and early 1990s was captured by the Food Marketing Policy Center of the Department of Agriculture and Resources Economics of the University of Connecticut, where Cotterill and Franklin published a report on 21 American cities and the associations between low-income areas and the presence of supermarkets.[6] The authors report that there were serious distribution problems in some U.S. cities in terms of food delivery, and stated that: 'Given the recent cuts at the Federal level in food programs and the clear-cut need to improve the efficiency of distribution of federal food program dollars, the focus on the ability of the supermarket food distribution system to deliver food in an efficient, i.e., reasonably priced fashion, to low-income urban neighborhoods is extremely timely'. These findings were supported by the work conducted by the U.S. House of Representatives Select Committee on Hunger where the migration of supermarkets to the suburbs and lack of transportation was determined to contribute to the malnutrition among low-income Americans.[7,8] Other economic experts have investigated issues related to attracting supermarkets to inner cities, noting that citywide grocery initiatives are rare within the 32 U.S. cities investigated.[9]

This earlier work guided the development of new investigations to evaluate if these disparities in food retail continue within the same communities. The following summarizes 25 studies that were published prior to the initiation of the Healthy Food Financing Initiative and have been used as formative research to support the federal and state funding initiatives that aim to place supermarkets and other healthy food retailers in underserved communities.

Overall, investigators have consistently documented disparities in the placement of large-scale food stores, such as supermarkets, by either the wealth of areas investigated or the racial composition of area residents.[3,10–18] Some have shown that the lack of availability of healthy food options is also associated with inequality in the presence of supermarkets within urban centers.[12–14,19–21] Others have documented disparities in the availability of selected healthy food options independent of supermarket presence[22–26] and those differences have been associated with demographic and urbanization factors. Only one study documented lower prices of foods within supermarkets,[27] although other studies that have measured price difference report price not being a significant factor between local food environments.[13,20,28,29]

There is a remarkable consistency of findings across these studies. Most investigators have found disparities in access to healthy foods by racial and economic characteristics of areas, which supports earlier investigations. The consistency of findings has led to a report to Congress from the USDA called *Access to Affordable and Nutritious Foods: Measuring and Understanding Food Deserts and Their Consequences*.[30] The USDA reported that (1) 11.5 million low-income Americans live more than a mile away from a supermarket; (2) food costs are lower within supermarkets; and (3) low-income households are more likely to utilize super-centers, when possible, because of lower prices. These conclusions were drawn from the studies conducted by the ERS and from many of the studies summarized in the previous paragraphs. Findings between studies are rather consistent, even though investigators have utilized different methods. The size of the studies varies greatly, with some representing smaller geographic areas and others measuring all areas of the United States. Variations between studies may be due to difference across the country but can also be due to the selection of comparison groups, sampling, and methods for determining food stores, food types to study, and measurement methods for the cost of foods.

Few studies have measured the changes in local food environments over time. This is an important component of understanding disparities between local food environments and how residents' exposure may be constant over time. One study measured the fluctuation of supermarket presence in Brooklyn from 2007 to 2011 and found that there was an increase in the number of supermarkets during that period; in fact, the greatest proportion of new supermarket locations was found in the lowest income areas. The higher wealth areas had the greatest supermarket stability, meaning the greatest proportion of stores remained open during the 5-year period of investigation.[18] A better understanding of the types of fluctuations within local food environments may aid in understanding how motivations for behavior change are influenced by the stability of local food environments. For instance, within a community-based participatory project to address poor access to healthy foods, a community group opened a new community-owned-and-operated food store in East New York. Comments from store patrons as to why they were not using the new food store with any regularity reflected their familiarity with a volatile retail environment; stating they were hesitant to rely on a new food store because they expected it would shut down within a year or two.[31] These comments were despite the recognition by the community that the store was needed and contained foods that were desired and served the community.[32] Unfortunately, residents were correct and the store was not able to sustain itself for more than two years.[33]

In summary, there is strong formative research that specific groups of Americans live in areas with poor access to supermarkets and that these disparities appear to tract in communities with higher concentrations of people of color and low income. Some believe that these disparities are the result of a food system that has increasingly evolved toward factory farming and mass merchandising requiring large spaces for these corporations to conduct their businesses. Others believe that disparities are due to the business principal of 'supply and demand', placing the onus of supermarket disparities on lack of desire for the foods sold by local residents. Still others argue that businesses that operate on a 2%–3% margin, like supermarkets, cannot make a profit in areas where the consumer base lacks resources. Regardless of the reason, the result is the same. Even with the progress made by cities and states described in Chapters 4–8 many low-income, Black American and other racial minority groups in the United States do not have convenient access to supermarkets.

MEASUREMENTS OF THE GEOGRAPHIC BOUNDARIES DEFINING SUPERMARKETS ACCESSIBILITY

One of the main issues that arose while conducting formative research on supermarket disparities was how to conceptualize poor neighborhood accessibility to supermarkets, called *underserved areas,* in this text. Because this work began before the state initiatives and before the Healthy Food Financing Initiative, it was an important issue for formative evaluators because these definitions were expected to be used in future program planning in order to place supermarkets within underserved communities. However, this issue played an unusually complicated role with investigators measuring supermarket densities in regions as small as block groups to others who have used boundaries as large as zip codes. There has been little behavioral theory to support the boundaries. The different geographic areas that have been used in these formative studies are described in the sections that follow.

CENSUS-DEFINED BOUNDARIES

The U.S. Census Bureau conducts an enumeration of the American population every decade, whereby trends in population density, demographics of Americans, and other information can be used publicly.[34] The U.S. Census Bureau presents data within several different geographic boundaries that fall within a standard hierarchy, beginning with the nation. The nation is subdivided into regions (e.g., the Southeast), then subdivided into divisions, and then further subdivided into states. Within states, there are counties, which contain census tracts, block groups, and blocks. Importantly, the geographic boundaries of each one of these entities do not cross the hierarchy of borders. In other words, there are a certain number of census tracts within a specific county and those tracts do not cross county lines. One attractive feature of U.S. Census–defined borders from a formative researcher's perspective is that the racial distribution and income of the populations residing within those borders has already been collected. Therefore, for the formative research studies that are aiming to look for racial and economic disparities between local food environments, these census-defined borders are extremely useful. In addition, using this type of secondary data is how research is conducted when looking for geographic differences in disease rates, hence validating the method.[35] However, there are exceptionally large differences in the sizes of the census geographic boundaries; and it is therefore important to remember that local food environment disparities are conceptualized to take place at the neighborhood level. Also noteworthy is the fact that U.S. Census–defined boundaries can change at each new decennial of investigation.

Counties

Counties are the first level of geographic unit smaller than states. County borders do not cross state lines. Second, the size of counties varies within states and across the nation, as does the population size within counties. The sizes of counties vary quite considerably. For instance, Brooklyn is one of the five boroughs of New York City, and the entire borough is one county, Kings County. In 2010, Kings County contained 2,504,700 people within a landmass of 71 square miles. Comparatively, during the same census, Fresno County, California, contained far fewer people (930,450 people) within a much greater landmass (5,958 square miles). Difference in landmass and population characteristics of counties can be viewed interactively through the U.S. Census Bureau's website.

Census Tracts

Census tracts are the next unit of measurement smaller than counties that are measured by the U.S. Census Bureau. Tracts are smaller geographic units of measurement containing roughly 3,000–5,000 people. Census tracts also vary in size, and although they do not cross county borders, they do sometimes cross neighborhood boundaries, limiting the use of census tracts as direct measurements of actual neighborhoods. As an example, in Figure 9.2, the neighborhood of Bay Ridge in Brooklyn, New York, is presented overlaid with over twenty census tracts, demonstrating the comparative size of the census tracts to the New York City defined neighborhood. Also, census tracts vary in size and shape.

Blocks and Block Groups

The census blocks are located within census tracts and are noted in Figure 9.2 with light gray lines within each tract. These geographic boundaries generally represent city blocks and hence also vary in size and shape. Block groups are another census geographic boundary, in

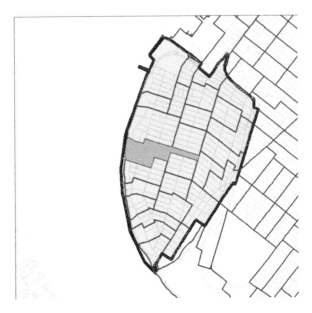

FIGURE 9.2   Bay Ridge, Brooklyn, New York Neighborhood, Census Tracts and Blocks

size, between blocks and tracts where several blocks within a tract are grouped (not shown in Figure 9.2).

Zip Code Tabulation Areas/U.S. Postal Service–Defined Boundaries

Zip codes are geographic boundaries defined by the U.S. Postal Service for the purpose of delivering mail. Unlike the census-defined boundaries, the intention of these boundaries was not to enumerate Americans. However, zip code tabulation areas are created by the U.S. Census Bureau, which marries the U.S. Postal Service zip code boundaries with U.S. Census data. These areas also vary in size and may cross county and state lines. They are also a largest geographic area often containing over 100,000 people.

GEOGRAPHIC INFORMATION SYSTEMS–DEFINED BOUNDARIES

In addition to the census-defined boundaries, formative evaluation researchers have also utilized geographic information systems (GIS) defined boundaries. GIS is software (e.g., ArcGIS) that has been used by geographers, urban planners, and other professionals to develop maps. Some GIS base maps showing the streets of areas are publicly available and information (such as locations of supermarkets) can be layered onto these maps. For instance, the New York City Department of City Planning provides several maps of the city that can be used with GIS software. The DCPLION is a base map of New York City streets and includes other geographic features such as shorelines, surface rail lines, and boardwalks. Because this type of data is publicly available for most of the United States, there has been an increase in secondary data analyses using these types of techniques within food environment research. Once the base maps are in place, many types of data can be layered onto the maps by geocoding the latitude and longitude of an address for placement on the map. The geocoding of addresses is commonly used by researchers to place individuals and/or the locations of food retailers onto maps. If addresses are not complete or not known, geographic positioning system devices can be used to collect that information. These handheld devices record the latitude and longitude of a specific place when standing in front of the business or place of residence. Finally, because the usefulness of GIS has expanded, agencies are providing more prepared maps that may be useful in formative research. For instance, NYC provides the geographic boundaries for the FRESH program, where zoning and discretionary tax incentives are available for the development, expansion, and renovation of full-line grocery stores and supermarkets. This is a geographic file created by the New York City Department of City Planning, showing eligible areas for the zoning incentives adopted May 11, 2009, through the New York City Industrial Development Agency.

Buffer Zones

Buffer zones of many sizes have been used to characterize the geographic space surrounding a specific address, such as a home address. In Figure 9.3, a 300-meter radius buffer zone, or circle, has been drawn around a residential address using ArcGIS. Instead of a census tract or block group, this buffer zone would be used by researchers to characterize the boundary for which a supermarket is accessible to the resident. These types of measurements have the advantage of placing an individual in the middle of the geographic area, eliminating some of the concern with the census-defined boundaries where exposure is assigned to an individual regardless of where they may be located within that geographic area.

Distance Measurements

In addition to buffer zones, instead of using geographic boundaries, distance have also been used as a measurement of accessibility. Distance measurements are calculated using GIS tools as a straight line between two points, a Euclidian distance, sometimes called a *crow flies distance* is depicted in Figure 9.3. This type of measurement does not take the roadways, sidewalks, or other street features such as dead ends or traffic volume into account in terms of how a person would walk or drive from one location to the other. Users of the crow flies distance recognize street features would affect residents' access to supermarkets; however it is justified as a simple and direct proxy measurement of distance. Nevertheless, GIS software also offer applications for more complicated network distances that take street features into account. With network distances the fastest distance, the shortest route, or a path described by a study participant can be measured.

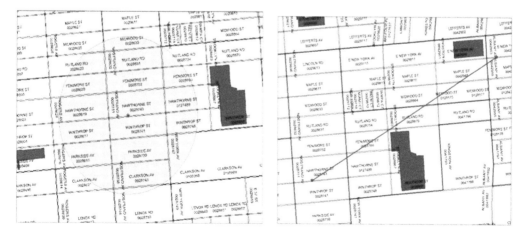

FIGURE 9.3 GIS-Derived Measurements of Local Food Environments: (1) 300-Meter Buffer Zone around Residential Address; and (2) Straight Line (Euclidian) Distance between Two Addresses

Neighborhoods

Finally, although uncommonly used in local food environment research, it is possible to utilize the geographic boundaries of neighborhoods as boundaries of local food environments. The geographic boundary of the neighborhood Bay Ridge is shown in Figure 9.2. These types of geographic boundaries may be available from city agencies and may or may not be available with demographic data.

Summary of Limitations for Each Type of Boundary

Again, formative studies that have used these different types of boundaries preceded the work from the Obama administration that decided to group poor access to supermarkets within an existing term used by the federal government called *underserved areas*. For the federal government, these areas of the United States are underserved by retailers in general and other capital that would bring private businesses to the communities. However, at the time and now existing in the formative local food environment literature, studies have used the boundaries described previously, and not without criticism. For example, census-defined borders have been criticized primarily because an individual may live anywhere within that boundary, perhaps even on the perimeter of two adjacent boundaries, thus introducing potential misclassification of access to a supermarket. Moreover, because the size and shape of these boundaries vary, there is inconsistency in the definition of local food environments within and between studies. Further, any given census-defined boundary may be a moderate-to-poor proxy of actual neighborhood availability of food with some boundaries possibly being too small (e.g., blocks) and others being too large (e.g., counties). Although the GIS-defined borders have addressed some of these concerns, these boundaries have also been criticized because the GIS boundaries are an individual-level measurement, which conflicts with the concept of the shared environments inherent to neighborhoods. Moreover, the size and shape of the GIS-defined boundaries are not based on any empirical evidence or validated with any behavioral research. The presentation of multiple sizes of buffer zones, which is commonly done with buffer zone studies, demonstrate the authors do not have a hypothesis or behavioral theory to support one size over the other. Often these studies are not powered to make distinctions between different size geographic boundaries making findings difficult to interpret. The buffer zones also change the research question from availability to utilization by centering the geographic boundary around the individual. This is a conceptual flaw that is incongruent with the policies and business practice described in Chapters 1–3, which have been shown to give rise to the disinvestment in Black, low-income, and other underserved neighborhoods. Finally, distance measures are limited by the need to determine distance to what specific establishment is of interest. Is the distance to the primary food store reported by the study participant the best definition of healthy food availability? If so, this store may be far away from a person's home and would more accurately be describing utilization rather than the effects of the restricted nature of the food environment that is closer to home.[36] Also, this type of measurement focuses on a single food retailer and therefore does not account for the interdependencies between area retailers.

MEASUREMENT OF SUPERMARKETS

In addition to defining the geographic boundary of supermarket accessibility, investigators have also used secondary data sources to gain the placement of supermarkets and other food stores for formative research. The location of food stores, as a density measure or a distance between two points, is accomplished with the use of GIS. The latitude and longitude of a store address can be determined by geocoding its address; hence the location of that establishment can be placed on a map. Once addresses have been geocoded, density measurements (number of stores within the geographic boundary) or distance measurement, as described previously, can be calculated. These variables are then used in statistical models as predictors of health behaviors and health outcomes, as well as outcome variables in studies aimed to determine disparities in access to healthy foods. These formative studies have been an important foundation of data for Congress and other state legislators to move public policy forward and gain funding for food retailers seeking to locate in underserved areas.

There are several ways by which investigators have determined the location and types of food stores, but the three main avenues include (1) government sources, (2) private companies that compile lists, and (3) primary data collection. All the sources have strengths and limitations. The first two are convenient and used in most studies as secondary sources of information. Food store addresses can be easily obtained through government sources. The disadvantage is that government data is usually cross-sectional with no historical data kept by these agencies limiting the ability for retrospective longitudinal studies. Also, the type of store is not usually coded (e.g., supermarket, convenience store). A second option is private firms, such as InfoUSA, that track all types of businesses, and their lists can be used to obtain the name and addresses of food retailers, usually for a fee. These agencies often provide additional information about the businesses, such as the type of retailer. However, businesses sometimes need to register to be listed, and therefore information regarding some of the smaller, independent stores may not be captured. Third, because of the limitations of the secondary datasets, some investigators have conducted primary data collection to determine the locations and types of food stores within geographic areas. Several studies have enumerated the placement of food stores by conducting walking or driving audits of specified areas. For instance, in the National Institute of Health–funded study called the *Cardiovascular Health of Seniors and the Built Environments*, all streets within a 300-meter radius buffer zone of each participant have been studied repeatedly, resulting in the longitudinal evaluation of 23,667 streets located in all areas of Brooklyn.

Quantifying types of food stores has also been a challenge. Often, secondary datasets will not contain detailed classification information about food stores, so investigators will have to make assumptions about the type of venue. The rationale for coding the type relates to the concept that different types of food stores sell different amounts and varieties of healthy food options at different prices. For instance, price differences between large-scale supermarkets that can benefit from mass merchandising versus smaller food stores have been documented prior to the genesis of local food environment research.[37] Nevertheless, many studies using secondary data to evaluate the placement of food stores rely on name recognition to determine the types of food stores and restaurants. These methods can provide relatively good specificity for determining supermarkets and fast-food establishments, such as Kroger or McDonald's, because most chains are well recognized. However, misclassification is a concern for smaller types of retailers where the content of the stores cannot be determined from the name. Therefore, some investigators have utilized other information provided about the business, such as the amount of retail space, the number of cash registers, or sales to distinguish the larger stores from the smaller stores. In the end, the aim has been to distinguish the types of food sold and the pricing of those goods.

Studies that focus solely on the placement of different types of food stores rely on the inherent fact that mass marketing requires a large volume of goods to be available for sale to sell goods at lower prices. With the larger volume of goods sold, these retailers can provide a greater proportion of healthy food items, particularly perishable items compared to smaller stores. The U.S. government has the North America Industry Classification System (NAICS), whereby the definitions of each type of industry conducting business in the country has been defined and is monitored by the U.S. Census. The definitions for the U.S.-based supermarkets and grocery stores are described in Chapter 2 (Table 2.1).

SUPERMARKET DISPARITIES AND FRUIT AND VEGETABLE INTAKE

Even with the variety of ways neighborhood accessibility to supermarkets have been measured, supermarket disparities have been well-documented by researchers and the U.S. government. Therefore, the second research question that was pertinent to the formative evaluation that preceded the HFFI was, do people living in areas without supermarkets have a more difficult time meeting dietary recommendations? Because the implementation of any program is both expensive and time consuming, we rely on formative evaluation prior to the implementation of a program to gain information on not only who would benefit most from the new program but also estimate the potential impact of the proposed intervention. Opening a new supermarket is a multimillion-dollar project. Therefore it is reasonable to question if the investment is likely to have an impact on the local community. One potential impact is on diet. This formative research is needed because the funding for a new supermarket is costly, and the project requires a public-private partnership which can be challenging to arrange. Therefore, quantifying the potential improvements to diet can aid in the investment of such a project from parties in both the private and public sectors.

As with studies that have measured the disparities in supermarket availability, most formative evaluation studies that evaluate the placement of supermarkets and residents' diets also rely on secondary datasets. The use of secondary datasets is an efficient and low-cost method for gaining this necessary information to guide program planning. Prior to when the Healthy Food Financing Initiative (HFFI) bill was discussed by Congress in 2013, seven cross-sectional studies had been published that aimed to measure the association between the availability of supermarkets on the one hand and fruit and vegetable intake among adults on the other. Investigators chose fruits and vegetables as a dietary outcome for this formative research because fruits and vegetables are a recommended food group by the USDA.[38] There is now considerable evidence linking various health benefits to fruit and vegetable consumption, which is fueling increased focus from the scientific and policy communities on factors related to intake. The dietary guidelines have emphasized fruits and vegetables as separate food groups since the 1980s and continues to recommend a plant-based diet high in fruits and vegetables to reduce the risk of chronic disease and maintain a healthy weight.[39] Healthy People 2020, the report of health goals for the nation that is reviewed every ten years, also outlines targets for increases in fruit and vegetable consumption for all populations over two years of age. Despite the array of health evidence underlying the promotion of fruits and vegetables, and advice from the scientific community, it is estimated that fewer than 20% of adults in the United States consume the recommended five daily servings.[40] In low-income populations, the consumption patterns appear to be worse, with even fewer servings of fruits and vegetables consumed.[41]

Several studies have hypothesized that the presence of supermarkets would be associated with a higher intake of foods recommended for health, such as fresh fruits and vegetables. As presented in Chapters 2–3, perishable foods such as fruits and vegetables are more prevalent in larger supermarkets. Therefore, in addition to being a measure of healthy eating, this food group is also a marker of a food that is more readily available within supermarkets compared to other types of food vendors, which adds specificity to the formative research conducted that use fruits and vegetables as the dependent variable. By contrast, fat is ubiquitous in many food items sold by many types of food vendors; therefore a hypothesis that lower-fat diets are associated with the presence of supermarkets lacks specificity. For example, investigators have evaluated the effect of ubiquitous food groups such as whole grains, meats, and dairy.[42–45] Similarly, diet quality scores, such as the healthy eating index, are also a measure that contains ubiquitous food items in the score and therefore lacks specificity as a dependent dietary variable for these secondary data analyses.[46–48]

All the studies that measured the effect of supermarkets on consumption of fruits and vegetables were conducted before the HFFI was reviewed by Congress and were secondary data

TABLE 9.1

Supermarkets and Fruit and/or Vegetable Consumption: Adults and Children

| Author (Year) | Effect Size | | Statistical Significance | |
	Risk Ratio	Mean Difference (in grams* or servings)	95% CI	p-value
Morland (2002)	RR = 1.54		1.11–2.12	
Rose (2004)		72		0.061
Bodor (2008)		−0.09		0.93
Zenk (2009)		0.69		0.002
Sharkey (2010)		0.012		0.004
Caspi (2012)*		0.23		0.21
Gustafson (2013)	OR = 3.04		1.13–8.17	
Hattori (2013)*		−0.010		0.025

analyses. In other words, none of the studies were designed specifically to look at the relationship between diet and food environments. Instead, secondary sources of dietary data (e.g., existing food frequency questionnaires collected from a population aimed to address a different hypothesis) and food environment data (e.g., names and locations of food stores from private companies) were used. The effect size and statistical significance of findings from these seven studies are shown on Table 9.1. For example, Morland et al. found a 54% increase in meeting recommendations for fruit and vegetable intake among Black Americans living in areas with a supermarket compared to Black Americans living in areas without supermarkets.[49] Similarly, Zenk et al. found Black Americans living in areas with large grocery stores increased their daily serving of fruits and vegetables by 0.69 servings compared to Black Americans living in areas without larger grocery stores.[50] Bodor et al. measured residential distance to the nearest supermarket and found a 0.09 daily serving decrease in fruit intake for each additional kilometer a supermarkets was located away from a person's home.[51] Rose et al. found that when supermarket access was made easy, there was a 72 gram greater daily intake of fruit compared to people who lived in areas where there was no supermarket access.[52] Gustafson et al. found that people living within 0.5 miles of a supermarket had a three times greater odds of consuming at least one serving of vegetables per day compared to people that lived further away from supermarkets.[42] Finally, Sharkey et al. found a 0.012 daily serving decrease in fruit intake per mile between urban older adults' residences and the nearest supermarket.[53] Most of these findings were statistically significant at an alpha level of 0.05, with some studies such as Bodor et al. lacking statistical power with small study samples.

Finally, other investigators measured the effect of supermarkets and intake of fruits and vegetables among children and adolescents. Like Gustafson, Caspi et al. also measured the association between distance to the nearest supermarket. These investigators found that for every kilometer a supermarket is located further away from an adult's home, there is a 0.23 daily serving increase in servings of fruits and vegetables.[54] This finding is counter to the hypothesis that having access to supermarkets near will improve intake of fruits and vegetables. Caspi used the HIC study as their secondary data source where information about cancer was collected among 743 study participants living in twenty housing projects. Distance to supermarkets was measured from the housing projects and therefore there were only twenty different distance measures for the 743 people. This lack of variation in distance for individuals in the study is likely to limit the power of the study to detect an effect. Finally, Hattori measured the difference in fruit and vegetable intake among two cross-sectional samples of the California Health Interview Survey (CHIS) and found a small inverse effect for intake of fruit for people living within one mile from a supermarket.[43] This study was well powered to detect an effect with a sample size of 97,678 people. However, the authors did not target the low-income population or specific minority groups hypothesized by other investigators to be the groups at risk in their analyses. This secondary data analysis includes mostly White adults (48.8%) with a low prevalence of Black Americans (5.9%) who have a median household income of $69,127. Overall, most of the studies produced measures of effect in the direction expected to support the hypothesis that supermarket availability is likely to affect fruit and/or vegetable intake.

Multiple Dietary Outcomes

It can be confusing when an author presents effect estimates for a number of dietary outcomes within the same study, and there are discrepancies in the direction and/or magnitude of the effects of supermarkets between the dietary outcomes. For example, Gustafson presented a strong effect between living within 0.5 miles of a supermarket and consumption of vegetables; however an effect in the opposite direction was observed for fruit intake (OR = 0.83, 95% CI [0.51,1.34]). When evaluating the literature that is conducted for the purpose of formative evaluation, readers are reminded that these studies are intended to detect patterns of associations only. Because formative evaluation relies on existing data (secondary datasets), these studies are not rigorous, because the size of the study populations, the characteristics of the study populations, and methods used to measure diet are all dependent on whatever methods were intended to address the hypothesis for the parent study, not the formative evaluation study. Because of this, we aim to use these studies to detect patterns of association instead of causal relationships. For example, in the Gustafson study, diet was measured using one twenty-four-hour recall, which may be sufficient to rank participants in the Healthy Eating Index and was the intention of the parent study. However, a single twenty-four-hour recall is likely to underestimate the intake of most foods and nutrients.[55] The underestimates reduces the validity of the dietary outcomes as a measurement of usual diet and hence hampers the ability to detect effects. For the Gustafson study, there is evidence of an underestimate of both fruit and vegetable intake among the population with an average intake of less than one serving of fruit and one serving of vegetables per day reported, which is significantly lower than the national average.

Because of the reliance on existing data in formative evaluation studies such as these, an inconsistency of effect across all hypothesized dietary outcomes should not be interpreted as lack of evidence of a relationship between supermarkets and diet. Rather, the inconsistencies are an expected result of the study design and methods used in the parent studies that collected the data to investigate an entirely different hypothesis. Because the methods used in parent studies may make the ability to detect an effect between supermarkets and produce intake more difficult, a reliance on the statistical significance of findings only limits what can be learned from these existing datasets. Rather, consistency in the direction and strength of associations between studies are indicators of patterns we aim to detect with these formative studies.

Statistical Inference

In addition to the ability to detect an effect using secondary data sources, when interpreting the meaning of statistical significance in formative research readers need to be reminded that the secondary data analyses may not be powered to detect an effect. Similarly, readers should be wary of large studies with sufficient power to detect effects, but researchers fail to stratify data to detect these effects among populations found to be at risk in other studies. In addition, many authors focus on statistical testing (p-values) to determine if there is an association between supermarkets and a dietary outcome, largely ignoring the size and direction of the effect measure. So, for instance in the Bodor study, although the authors found a 0.09 daily serving decrease in fruit intake for each additional kilometer a supermarket was located away from a person's home; because the associated p-value was 0.93, the authors concluded that there is no association between supermarket access and fruit intake. A p-value is the result of a statistical test that allows the investigators (and readers) to reject, or fail to reject, the null hypothesis.[56] In the Bodor analysis, the null hypothesis was that there is no association between distance to supermarkets and intake of fruit among study participants. The p-value of 0.93 is greater than 0.05 and therefore warrants the reader to fail to reject the null hypothesis. However, a failure to reject the null hypothesis is not the same as accepting the null hypothesis. A p-value greater than 0.05 is not to be interpreted that the null hypothesis is true, particularly in observational studies.[57] We may fail to reject the null hypothesis for a variety of reasons: (a) the study is not powered to detect an effect; (b) the measure of diet is underestimated; and/or (c) the measure of supermarkets is imprecise. The interpretation of the p-value of 0.93 in conjunction with the measure of effect tells a reader that there is a 0.09 daily serving decrease in fruit intake for each additional kilometer a supermarket was located away from a person's home, however we cannot rule out the possibility that there is no association. The interpretation of the p-value in these formative studies is particularly susceptible to not reaching statistical significance because the secondary datasets were not powered to detect an effect for these formative hypotheses.

In addition to measuring the association between supermarkets and the diets of adults, two studies used large secondary datasets to measure the association between supermarket access and fruit and vegetable consumption among children and adolescents. Like Hattori, An et al. used the CHIS 2005–2007 data to measure the impact of a large supermarket being located within a 0.5-mile buffer zone of a child or adolescent's residence on the intake of fruit.[44] For example, small differences in fruit intake were observed for children living near supermarkets (mean difference =1.02, p = 0.016). Small differences were also observed by Powell et al., who measured the presence of supermarkets within zip codes of residence, and fruit (mean difference = 0.0010, p = 0.0125) and vegetables (mean difference = 0.0146, p = 0.0112) among teens.[58] These studies contribute to the formative evaluation of the potential effect of supermarket availability and fruit and vegetable intake in relation to who the target population for the program should be, specifically the targeted age group. The authors of the An and Powell studies did not provide a conceptual framework to support the focus on children and teens. For adults, supermarkets are used to purchase groceries for home cooking to support the nutritional intake for the shopper and their family members. For children and adolescents, a supermarket is not used to purchase groceries for a family. Behavior theory to support the contextual assumption in these statistical models that a child or adolescent would purchase fruit in a supermarket would give the findings meaning. For example, Powell used zip codes as areas a child would use to purchase fruits from a supermarket and this assumption in their statistical analysis requires justification to be a helpful formative evaluation study. Secondly, both studies utilize large existing datasets where statistically significant results are almost assured of any association measured and therefore like the adult studies, the direction and magnitude of the effects need to be assessed in addition to the p-value to draw conclusions for the formative evaluation.

MEASUREMENT OF DIET

Among studies that hypothesize that supermarket availability will be associated with a higher level of fruit and vegetable intake, understanding how fruit and vegetable intake is measured introduces the reader to potential information bias (e.g., misclassification) that may affect the ability to detect effects in these secondary data analyses. The most common and validated types of dietary assessments are described that follow.[59]

Twenty-Four-Hour Recall

The twenty-four-hour recall is often considered the gold standard for measuring dietary intake in an individual because it provides the highest validity, least biased dietary information relative to other methods of diet data collection.[55] In the twenty-four-hour recall, the respondent is asked to report everything eaten and drunk during the previous 24 hours and to provide details regarding every item consumed (when, where, how, how much, with what). The 20–40-minute interview is usually conducted in person or over the phone by trained interviewers who are taught to probe for all foods and beverages consumed including preparation. It is recommended that two or more recalls are collected from individuals within the same seven-day period, including both weekday and weekend intake, to approximate an individual's usual intake.[55]

Collecting dietary data using the twenty-four-hour recall approach necessitates dietary software that contains an extensive food and nutrient database. Once foods and beverages are reported by study participants, those foods and beverages are converted to nutrients based on a USDA database of foods and nutrients or using a proprietary database such as the Nutrition Data System for Research (NDSR) at the Nutrition Coordinating Center at the University of Minnesota. Because the conversion of nutrients from reported food items are based on a standardized database, some ethnic foods and other foods eaten by fewer people may not be in the database and require interviewers to enter ingredients for the recipe in the serving proportion reported by the study participants. In addition to the NDRS, the National Cancer Institute has developed a computer-assisted self-report recall system, called the *Automated Self-Administered 24-Hour Recall* (ASA24), which is free to use.

The benefit of the twenty-four-hour recall is that it does not require a high level of literacy (if being administered by an interviewer), and because of the immediacy of the recall period, respondents are generally able to remember their intake. Further, it is the most accurate tool to determine usual intake of specific foods and nutrients if two or more twenty-four-hour recalls are collected. The downsides of this method of data collection are that it tends to be impractical for large-scale research due to its expense and reliance on trained interviewers and the fact that multiple days are needed to estimate the usual intakes of individuals. Estimating the usual intake, is important because dietary recommendations are intended to be met over time, and diet-health hypotheses are based on dietary intakes over the long term. Also, for foods such as fruits and vegetables, unless multiple twenty-four-hour recalls are assessed over a long period, there is a concern that seasonality is not captured, and these food groups may be underestimated. Despite this and other limitations, the twenty-four-hour recall approach is the most accurate and comprehensive and, if used to capture a group mean intake, is the best approach for measuring usual intake of nutrients.

Food Frequency Questionnaires

The Food Frequency Questionnaires (FFQ) ask respondents to report the frequency of consumption of foods over a specified period. The FFQ is most often used to obtain a crude estimate of total diet intake over a specified time, such as the past month, six months or, year. A list of foods is provided to the respondent, and details on frequency of consumption are asked. Some FFQs will incorporate questions on portion sizes but little detail regarding other food characteristics (such as method of cooking) is collected. For example, FFQs often group similar items into a single question (e.g., pork, beef, lamb), which could be considered cognitively challenging to someone who frequently eats beef, but only occasionally eats pork, lamb, or other similar meats.

The challenge with an FFQ is creating an appropriate list of foods that captures the breadth of the target population's diet, is culturally appropriate, and is the least cognitively challenging. Compared to the twenty-four-hour recall, the FFQ is less expensive as it is often self-administered.

However, measurement error, especially underreporting of caloric intake, is common due to many details of diet intake not being measured and inaccuracies due to incomplete listings of foods. Research has suggested that longer FFQ lists may overestimate intake of fruits and vegetables, whereas shorter lists may underestimate intake.[60] Like the twenty-four-hour recalls, the FFQ responses are transferred to the USDA or another nutrient database to sum daily nutrients across foods and beverages reported. There are many versions of the FFQ, which attests to its easy adaptability for specific populations and purposes. Most FFQ have between 120 and 160 food items or groups and take forty-five minutes to an hour to complete. A few of the most common versions that have been validated include the Block Questionnaire, the Willett Questionnaires and the NCI's Diet History Questionnaire.[61]

Brief Dietary Screeners

Finally, short dietary assessment instruments, often called *screeners*, can be useful in situations that do not require assessment of total caloric intake, the total diet, or quantitative accuracy in dietary estimates. Although estimates of intake from short dietary assessment instruments are not as accurate as those from more detailed methods, such as twenty-four-hour dietary recalls, screeners are often used to characterize a population's average intakes, distinguishing between individuals or populations with regard to higher versus lower intakes, examining interrelationships between diet and other variables, and comparing findings from a smaller study to a larger population study. It is common for screeners to be developed if a specific component of diet is of interest, as is the case with fruit and vegetable screeners used in the BRFSS and the CHIS studies.

The obvious advantage to using a short screener to assess intake is the shorter amount of time burden on the study participant. Also, fewer resources are required to administer the questionnaire because the screeners are usually self-reported. In addition, instead of relying on an extensive food and nutrient database, a score based on the frequency with which the foods are consumed can be tallied. However, despite this advantage, short screeners do have some limitations. Most significantly, they do not capture information about the entire diet and therefore caloric intake cannot be calculated, which is a standard adjustment in nutritional research.

SUPERMARKET DISPARITIES AND RISK FOR OBESITY

In addition to the effect a supermarket might have on the intake of fruits and vegetables, investigators conducted formative research to examine the effect of supermarkets availability and diet-related diseases. The most commonly measured diet-related disease in these formative studies has been obesity. These analyses hypothesize that the lack of supermarkets in an area effect obesity because in order to avoid the experience of hunger when resources are limited, individual's choices are restricted to cheaper foods that often have less nutritional density.[62] The effect of different types of food retailers on the prevalence of obesity has been measured by Morland et al.[63] Figure 9.4 shows the increased risk of obesity given the presence of different combinations of food retailers within neighborhoods. All comparisons use people living in areas with only a supermarket as the reference. These findings show that in areas where there is at least one supermarket and there is also at least one convenience store, a 35% increase in the prevalence of obesity is observed compared to areas where there is at least one supermarket only. However, the greatest risk of obesity is shown in areas without supermarkets and instead have other types of food retailers such as small grocery stores only (relative risk (RR) = 1.48, 95% confidence interval (CI) [1.12,1.94]); convenience stores only (RR = 1.45, 95% CI [1.16, 1.82]) or small grocery stores and convenience stores (RR = 1.60, 95% CI [1.28, 2.00]). Although causation cannot be determined from this cross-sectional analysis, the pattern of associations suggest supermarkets may be an important environmental factor in the prevention of obesity.

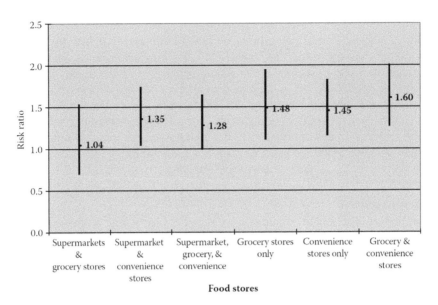

FIGURE 9.4 Relative Risks and 95% Confidence Intervals of the Associations between Different Combinations of Neighborhood Food Retailers and Obesity Prevalence

In addition to this study, others have investigated the relationship between the presence of supermarkets and obesity with results summarized in Table 9.2. Most investigators have found a protective effect between the presence of supermarkets and risk for obesity, albeit the size of the effect varies. Although, causality cannot be determined with these secondary data analyses, the consistency of point estimates under 1.0 suggest the placement of supermarkets in underserved areas may benefit residents in the prevention of obesity.

OBESOGENIC FOOD ENVIRONMENTS

Because investigators began to consider the composition of food environments instead of a single food retailer such a supermarket as potential risk factors for obesity, investigators considered the availability of 'unhealthy' retailers as well. For instance, fast-food outlet availability has been theorized to influence consumption of unhealthy food items – either as cheaper food options when food environments are limited or because the food item is seen as a complement (i.e., soda, high-fat vegetables). One study found that fast-food outlet density was positively associated with fried potato consumption and soda consumption.[43] In a sample of Boy Scouts (10–14 years) from Houston, Texas, greater residential distance to the nearest fast-food restaurant predicted lower fruit and juice intake and lower high-fat vegetable intake.[64] Boone-Heinonen et al. (2011) conducted a secondary data analysis using longitudinal data from the CARDIA study and found[65] that although a higher number of fast-food outlets close to respondents' homes (<1 km compared with 1–2.99 km) predicted greater fast-food consumption among low-income men, among women, and men in higher income groups, over the fifteen years the associations between fast-food exposure and fast-food consumption were not significant. However, additional studies found no association between fast-food outlet availability and foods characterized as unhealthy.[44,66]

The investigation of unhealthy food environments was driven in part by socioeconomic trends that Americans work more hours and food consumption away from home is on the rise. Between 1970 and 2006, foods purchased and eaten away from home have increased from 26.1% to 41.7%.[67] Specifically, 37.4% of sales of meals and snacks outside of the home are at limited service eating establishments such as fast-food restaurants. Fast food is estimated to account for 15% of daily energy intake, and in children the percent of energy consumed at these locations now surpasses the amount consumed in schools.[68] This trend is alarming due to the associations with fast-food consumption and diet quality[69–71] and poor diet-related health outcomes.[72,73]

TABLE 9.2
Association between Supermarket Presence and Obesity Prevalence

Author (Year)	Risk Ratio	95% Confidence Interval
Hutchinson (2012)	1.33	(0.79, 2.23)
Drewnowski (2012)	1.01	(0.97, 1.05)
Dubowitz (2012)	0.86	(0.79, 0.92)*
Block (2011)	0.98	(0.94, 1.01)
Ford (2011)	0.97	(0.79, 1.18)
Gibson (2011)	1.00	(0.98, 1.01)
Gustafson (2011)	0.77	(0.23, 2.59)
Black (2010)	0.90	(0.86, 0.95)*
Black (2010)	0.90	(0.86, 0.95)*
Bodor (2010)	0.93	(0.88, 0.99)*
Ford (2010)	2.53	(2.36, 2.74)*
Janevic (2010)	0.88	(0.81, 0.94)*
Ford (2009)	0.93	(0.86, 1.01)
Morland (2009)	0.78	(0.63, 0.95)*
Rundle (2009)	0.87	(0.78, 0.97)*
Brown (2008)	0.28	(0.08, 1.04)
Wang (2006)	0.74	(0.57, 0.96)*
Morland (2006)	0.94	(0.90, 0.98)*

* Indicates statistically significant at alpha = 0.05.

While these trends may be a cause for concern, the increase in foods eaten away from home do not outweigh the proportion of meals consumed at home by Americans. And these home cooked meals are made with ingredients from foods purchased at grocery stores and supermarkets for most Americans. A high density of restaurants may create a synergistic effect in raising obesity rates in areas without supermarkets. As seen in Figure 9.4, in the absence of supermarkets, all types of food vendors are associated with an increase in obesity. So, an obesogenic food environment is not characterized by the presence of fast-food restaurants or convenience stores per se; rather, an obesogenic food environment stems from the absence of supermarkets.

CONCLUSION

In 2004, Ralphs closed fifteen supermarkets in southern California noting low sales and a small customer base, which has limited their profitability.[74] More recently in 2021, two North Long Beach supermarkets, a Ralphs located at Los Coyotes and Diagonal and a Food For Less located on South Street near Cherry Avenue also closed,[75] causing a food desert according to a neighborhood resident.[76] These supermarket closures are not unique to California, as Fairway in the neighborhood of Red Hook in Brooklyn New York, also closed in 2020, leaving residents at the time with no grocery store.[77] These examples demonstrate that, in addition to supermarket disparities prior to the initiation of the Healthy Food Financing Initiative (HFFI), these inequalities continue to intensify with supermarket closures in poorly served areas today. These formative studies, albeit based on secondary data analyses, provide a consistency of associations across studies suggesting potential dietary and health benefits from supermarket accessibility.

These formative studies are not rigorous. They are based on secondary data, mostly cross-sectional, and have unspecific measurements of dependent and independent variables.

However, formative research, by its definition, relies on inexpensive research to show patterns of associations, not causal effects. This is because formative research is just that, the early stage of program planning where funding has yet to be identified. Nevertheless, this body of formative research, along with the advocacy efforts of The Food Trust and other organizations, has resulted in state and federal programs specifically designed to correct the disparities in the placement of supermarkets in the United States. The Fresh Food Financing Initiative in Pennsylvania, the HFHC Program in New York, and other state initiatives described in Chapters 4–8 have recognized the necessity of public-private partnerships to remedy these disparities. The dedication of state and federal funds aimed to entice supermarket and grocery store retailers to underserved areas is seen in the forms of grants, tax incentives, and low interest loans as described in previous chapters.

Typically, formative research would be applied during the program development of one specific intervention. However, by design, the leadership of The Food Trust recognized that the disparities in access to supermarkets could not be solved with the intervention of just one new store. Rather, The Food Trust aimed to use these formative studies, not to justify one intervention, but rather to support their arguments to persuade state legislators to earmark funds for supermarket developers to open multiple stores in underserved areas throughout Pennsylvania. These leaders understood that one new supermarket in an underserved area will have little influence over the larger systemic problem of poor supermarket access within multiple neighborhoods, cities, and states. Funds are needed to provide venture capital for many multimillion-dollar projects. These interventions cannot be funded with National Institute of Health grants or other funds that would typically be used to support a new nutrition program. Also, building a new supermarket, running the store, and sustaining its growth is far beyond researchers' capacity of nutrition interventions; it is necessary to partner with supermarket retailers who have the expertise to successfully run a food store. These formative studies have been used to persuade state and federal legislators to allocate capital investment to food retailers through CDFIs as described in Chapter 3.

Because of The Food Trust's success with their assistance in promoting similar programs in other states and championing the HFFI, the need for the type of formative research described in this chapter has now waned. It is well-accepted that disparities in the location of supermarkets exists in the United States. It is also well accepted that supermarkets are an important component of the U.S. food system and communities' benefit by their presence, both nutritionally and economically. Although easy and inexpensive to conduct, these secondary analyses are no longer useful in understanding local food environments. New studies do not add to the knowledge gap that was present twenty years ago when the questions at the beginning of this chapter were first being examined. Instead, program planning for community projects that will utilize the state and federal funding now available to food retailers is the next step in continuing to decrease the disparities in access to healthy and affordable food in the United States. Additional methods for program planning and evaluation are described in the following chapters.

CRITICAL THINKING QUESTIONS AND EXERCISES

1. Draw a diagram of how the absence of supermarkets might affect the intake of fruits and vegetables by some Americans. How does this diagram help you to understand the causal pathway by which supermarket accessibility effects diet for some people?

2. Oprah Winfrey lives on a 42-acre estate in Montecito, California, placing her far away from a supermarket. Would you expect her to consume fewer vegetables and fruits because she is far away from a supermarket? Why or why not? What other groups of people may not benefit from supermarkets being in proximity? How does

this help identify a target population that might benefit from a supermarket in their neighborhood?

3. Supermarkets offer benefits beyond nutrition to community members. List and discuss the economic benefits of a conveniently located supermarket for underserved communities.

4. Describe resources for secondary dietary information. Go to these resources and describe how the dietary information has been collected and the limitation of its use in a causal analysis.

REFERENCES

1. Centers for Disease Control and Prevention. Types of Evaluation. 2020; www.cdc.gov/std/Program/pupestd/Types%20of%20Evaluation.pdf. Accessed February 18, 2021.
2. Wansink B, Sobal J. Mindless eating: The 200 daily food decisions we overlook. *Environmental Behavior.* 2007;39:106–123.
3. Morland K, Wing S, Diez Roux A, Poole C. Neighborhood characteristics associated with the location of food stores and food service places. *Am J Prev Med.* 2002;22(1):23–29.
4. Troutt D. The Thin Red Line: How the Poor Still Pay More. In: Consumers Union West Coast Regional Office, ed. San Francisco, CA; 1993.
5. Anderson A. The Ghetto marketing life cycle: A case of the underachievement. *Journal of Marketing Research.* 1978;15:20–28.
6. Cotterill RW, Franklin AW. *The Urban Grocery Store Gap.* Mansfield, CT: Food Marketing Policy Center; 1995.
7. U.S. House of Representatives Select Committee on Hunger. Obtaining Food: Shopping Constraints of the Poor. In: Washington, DC: Government Printing Office; 1987.
8. U.S. House of Representatives Select Committee on Hunger. Urban Grocery Gap. In: Washington, DC: Government Printing Office; 1992.
9. Pothukuchi K. Attracting supermarkets to inner city neighborhoods: Economic development outside of the box. *Economic Development Quarterly.* 2005;19:232–244.
10. Alwitt LF, Donley TD. Retail stores in poor urban neighborhoods. *Journal of Consumer Affairs.* 1997;31:139–164.
11. Zenk SN, Scultz AJ, Hollis-Neely T, et al. Fruit and vegetable intake in African Americans and income and store characteristics. *American Journal of Preventive Medicine.* 2005;29:1–9.
12. Baker EA, Schootman M, Barnidge E, Kelly C. The role of race and poverty in access to foods that enable individuals to adhere to dietary guidelines. *Prev Chronic Dis.* 2006;3(3):A76.
13. Block D, Kouba J. A comparison of the availability and affordability of a market basket in two communities in the Chicago area. *Public Health Nutr.* 2006;9(7):837–845.
14. Moore LV, Diez Roux AV. Associations of neighborhood characteristics with the location and type of food stores. *Am J Public Health.* 2006;96(2):325–331.
15. Morland K, Filomena S. Disparities in the availability of fruits and vegetables between racially segregated urban neighbourhoods. *Public Health Nutr.* 2007;10(12):1481–1489.
16. Powell LM, Slater S, Mirtcheva D, Bao Y, Chaloupka FJ. Food store availability and neighborhood characteristics in the United States. *Prev Med.* 2007;44(3):189–195.
17. Sharkey JR, Horel S. Neighborhood socioeconomic deprivation and minority composition are associated with better potential spatial access to the ground-truthed food environment in a large rural area. *J Nutr.* 2008;138(3):620–627.
18. Filomena S, Scanlin K, Morland KB. Brooklyn, New York foodscape 2007–2011: A five-year analysis of stability in food retail environments. *Int J Behav Nutr Phys Act.* 2013;10:46.
19. Sloane DC, Diamant AL, Lewis LB, et al. Improving the nutritional resource environment for healthy living through community-based participatory research. *J Gen Intern Med.* 2003;18(7):568–575.
20. Jetter KM, Cassady DL. The availability and cost of healthier food alternatives. *Am J Prev Med.* 2006;30(1):38–44.
21. Leise AD, Weiss K, Pluto D, Smith E, Lawson A. Food store type, availability and cost of foods in a rural environment. *Journal of the American Dietetic Association.* 2007;107:1916–1923.

22. Fisher BD, Strogatz DS. Community measures of low-fat milk consumption: Comparing store shelves with households. *American Journal of Public Health.* 1999;89:235–237.

23. Lewis LB, Sloane DC, Nascimento LM, et al. African Americans' access to healthy food options in South Los Angeles restaurants. *Am J Public Health.* 2005;95(4):668–673.

24. Horowitz CR, Colson KA, Hebert PL, Lancaster K. Barriers to buying healthy foods for people with diabetes: Evidence of environmental disparities. *Am J Public Health.* 2004;94(9):1549–1554.

25. Algert SJ, Agrawal A, Lewis DS. Disparities in access to fresh produce in low-income neighborhoods in Los Angeles. *Am J Prev Med.* 2006;30(5):365–370.

26. Hosler AS, Varadarajulu D, Ronsani AE, Fredrick BL, Fisher BD. Low-fat milk and high-fiber bread availability in food stores in urban and rural communities. *J Public Health Manag Pract.* 2006;12(6):556–562.

27. Chung C, Myers SL. Do the poor pay more for food? An analysis of grocery store availability and food price disparities. *Journal of Consumer Affairs.* 1999;33:276–296.

28. Hayes RA. Are prices higher for the poor in New York City? *Journal of Consumer Policy.* 2000;23:127–152.

29. Cole S, Filomena S, Morland K. Analysis of fruit and vegetable cost and quality among racially segregated neighborhoods in Brooklyn, New York. *Journal of Hunger and Environmental Nutrition.* 2010;5:202–215.

30. ver Ploeg M, Breneman V, Ferrigan T, et al. *Access to Affordable and Nutritious Foods: Measuring and Understanding Food Deserts and Their Consequences.* Washington, DC: United States Department of Agriculture; 2009. AP-036.

31. Morland K. Communication with ENY Food Co-Op Customer. In: 2006.

32. Munoz-Plaza CE, Filomena S, Morland K. Disparities in food access: Inner-city residents describe their local food environments. *Journal of Hunger and Environmental Nutrition.* 2008;2:51–64.

33. Morland K. An evaluation of a neighborhood-level intervention to a local food environment. *American Journal of Preventive Medicine.* 2010;39:e31–e38.

34. U.S. Census Bureau. U.S. Census Bureau Website. www.census.gov/. Accessed March 5, 2021.

35. Meade M, Florin J, Gesler W. *Medical Geography.* New York: The Guilford Press; 1988.

36. Morland KB, Filomena S. The utilization of local food environments by urban seniors. *Preventive Medicine.* 2008;47:289–293.

37. Cotterill RW, Franklin AW. *The Urban Grocery Gap.* Connecticut: University of Connecticut; 1995.

38. United States Department of Agriculture. Dietary Guidelines for Americans: 2020–2025. 2020; www.dietaryguidelines.gov/sites/default/files/2020-12/Dietary_Guidelines_for_Americans_2020-2025.pdf. Accessed February 7, 2021.

39. United States Department of Agriculture. Dietary Guidelines for Americans, 2020–2025. In: United States Department of Agriculture, ed. Washington, DC; 2020.

40. Blanck HM, Gillespie C, Kimmons JE, Seymour JE, Serdula MK. Trends in fruit and vegetable consumption among U.S. men and women, 1994–2005. *Prevention of Chronic Diseases.* 2008;5:A35.

41. Kirkpatrick SI, Dodd KW, Reedy J, Kreb-Smith SM. Income and race/ethnicity are associated with adherence to food-based dietary guidance among U.S. adults and children. *Journal of the American Dietetic Association.* 2012;112:624–635.

42. Gustafson A, Lewis S, Perkins S, Wilson C, Buckner E, Vail A. Neighborhood and consumer food environment is associated with dietary intake among Supplemental Nutrition Assistance Program (SNAP) participants in Fayette County, Kentucky. *Public Health Nutrition.* 2013;16:1229–1237.

43. Hattori A, An R, Sturm R. Neighborhood food outlets, diet and obesity among California adults 2007–2009. *Preventing Chronic Diseases.* 2013;10:1–11.

44. An R, Sturm R. School and residential neighborhood food environments and dietary intake among California children and adolescents. *American Journal of Preventive Medicine.* 2012;42:129–135.

45. Christian W. Using geospatial technologies to explore activity-based retail food environments. *Spatial Spatiotemporal Epidemiology.* 2012;3:287–295.

46. Moore L, Diez-Roux AV, Nettleton JA, Jacobs DR. Associations of the local food environment with diet quality: A comparison of assessments based on surveys and geographic

information systems: The Multi-Ethnic Study of Atherosclerosis. *American Journal of Epidemiology*. 2008;167:917–924.

47. Laraia BA, Siega-Riz AM, Kaufman JS, Jones SJ. Proximity of supermarkets is positively associated with diet quality index for pregnancy. *Preventive Medicine*. 2004;39:869–875.

48. Franco MA, Diez-Roux AV, Nettleton JA, et al. Availability of healthy foods and dietary patterns: The multi-ethnic study of Atherosclerosis. *American Journal of Clinical Nutrition*. 2009;89:897–904.

49. Morland K, Wing S, Diez-Roux AV. The contextual effect of local food environments on residents' diets: The Atherosclerosis risk in communities study. *American Journal of Public Health*. 2002;92:1761–1767.

50. Zenk SN, Schultz AJ, Kannan S, Lachance LL, Mentz G, Ridella W. Neighborhood retail food environment and fruit and vegetable intake in multi-ethnic urban population. *American Journal of Health Promotion*. 2009;23:255–264.

51. Bodor J, Rose D, Farley JA, Swalm C, Scott SK. Neighborhood fruit and vegetable consumption and the role of small food stores in an urban environment. *Public Health Nutrition*. 2007;11:413–420.

52. Rose D, Richards R. Food store access and household food and vegetable use among participants in the U.S. food stamp program. *Public Health Nutrition*. 2004;7:1081–1088.

53. Sharkey JR, Johnson CM, Dean WR. Food access and perceptions of the community and household food environment as correlates of fruit and vegetable intake among rural seniors. *BMC Geriatrics*. 2010;10:1–12.

54. Caspi CE, Kawachi I, Subramanian SV, Adamkiewicz G, Sorensen G. The relationship between diet and perceived and objective access to supermarkets among low-income housing residents. *Social Science and Medicine*. 2012;75:1254–1262.

55. Baranowski T. 24-hour recall and diet record methods. In: Willett WC, ed. *Nutritional Epidemiology*. New York: Oxford University Press; 2013:49–69.

56. Rosner B. Hypothesis testing. In: *Fundamentals of Biostatistics*. 4th ed. New York: Duxbury Press; 1995:193.

57. Rothman KJ. Random error and the role of statistics. In: *Epidemiology: An Introduction*. New York: Oxford University Press; 2012:151–152.

58. Powell LM, Han E. The cost of food away at home and away from home and consumption patterns among adolescents. *Journal of Adolescent Health*. 2010;48:20–26.

59. Willett WC. *Nutritional Epidemiology*. New York, NY: Oxford University Press; 2013.

60. Kreb-Smith SM, Heimendinger J, Subar AF, Patterson B, Pivonka E. Estimating fruit and vegetable intake using food frequency questionnaires: A comparison of instruments. *American Journal of Clinical Nutrition*. 1994;59:238S.

61. Subar AF, Thompson FE, Kiphis V, et al. Comparative validation of the block, Willett and National Cancer Institute food frequency questionnaires: The eating at America's table study. *American Journal of Epidemiology*. 2001;154:1089–1099.

62. Brown JL. Nutrition. In: Levy BS, Sidel VW, eds. *Social Justice and Public Health*. New York: Oxford University Press; 2006.

63. Morland K, Diez Roux A, Wing S. Supermarkets, other food stores and obesity: The Atherosclerosis risk in communities study. *American Journal of Preventive Medicine*. 2006;30:333–339.

64. Jago R, Baranowski T, Baranowski JC, Cullen K, Thompson D. Distance to food stores & adolescent male fruit and vegetable consumption. *International Journal of Behavioral Nutrition and Physical Activity*. 2007;4:35.

65. Boone-Heinonen J, Gordon-Larsen P, Keiefe CI, Shikany JM, Lewis CE, Popkin BM. Fast food restaurants and food stores: Longitudinal associations with diet in young to middle aged adults: The CARDIA study. *Archives of Internal Medicine*. 2011;171:1162–1170.

66. Powell LM, Han E. The cost of food at home and away from home and consumption patterns among U.S. adolescents. *Journal of Adolescent Health*. 2011;48:20–26.

67. McGuire S, Todd JE, Mancino L, Lin BH. The Impact of Food Away from Home on Adult Diet Quality. In: United States Department of Agriculture, ed. Washington, DC; 2011.

68. Poti JM, Popkins BM. Trends in energy intake among U.S. children by eating location and food source, 1977–2006. *Journal of the American Dietetic Association*. 2011;111:1156–1164.

69. Bowman SA, Vinyard BT. Fast food consumption of U.S. adults: Impact on energy and nutrient intakes and overweight status. *Journal of the American College of Nutrition.* 2004;23:163–168.

70. Bowman SA, Gortmaker SL, Ebbeling CB, Pereira MA, Ludwig DS. Effects of fast food consumption on energy intake and diet quality among children in a national household survey. *Pediatrics.* 2004;113:112–118.

71. Sebastian RS, Wilkinson C, Goldman JD. U.S. adolescents and MyPyramid: Associations between fast food consumption and lower likelihood of meeting recommendations. *Journal of the American Dietetic Association.* 2009;109:226–235.

72. Duffy KJ, Gordon-Larsen P, Jacobs DR, Williams OD, Popkin BM. Differential associations of fast food and restaurant food consumption with 3-y change in body mass index: The Coronary Artery Risk Development in young adults study. *American Journal of Clinical Nutrition.* 2007;85:201–208.

73. Pereira MA, Kartashov AI, Ebbeling CB, et al. Fast food habits, weight gain, and insulin resistance (the CARDIA study): 15-year prospective analysis. *Lancet.* 2005;365:36–42.

74. Writer S. Ralphs to close 15 stores. *The Progressive Grocer.* 2004; www.theprogressivegrocer.com/ralphs-closes-15-stores. Accessed March 5, 2021.

75. Holmes M. World's Largest Company Closes Two Long Beach Stores to Avoid Paying Workers More. In: *Eater.* 2021.

76. Niebla C. Customers urged to boycott Long Beach's highest performing Ralphs, demonstrators say. *Long Beach Post News.* February 21, 2021.

77. Zagare L. Fairway Red Hook expected to close permanently by July 17. *Bklyner.* June 26, 2020.

10 Food Store Needs Assessment

CONTENTS

INTRODUCTION

As stated at the end of Chapter 9, in terms of improving access to healthy and affordable foods, much has been accomplished over the past twenty years. Most importantly, policymakers have recognized the importance for supermarkets and other healthy food vendors to be located within underserved areas in America. The Healthy Food Financing Initiative (HFFI) was supported with funding from federal departments in 2014, and state initiatives supported healthy food retailers prior to the HFFI as described in Chapters 4–8. These programs have received bipartisan support, and the HFFI has had continued aid through the Obama, Trump, and Biden administrations. Other programs, such as opportunity zones, which aim to bring venture capital to areas that lack investment, are also promising avenues of support for healthy food retailers. The next step in diminishing disparities in access to healthy foods in America is for community groups, academics, food store owners, and others to work together to identify strategies to utilize the available federal and state resources to build new food stores in underserved areas, making food more accessible.[1]

As described in Chapters 4–8, state and federal funding has supported the building of new food stores or the improvement of existing ones to carry recommended healthy foods. The process by which these projects have been selected vary. For example, in Pennsylvania, The Food Trust (see Chapter 4) took the responsibility of identifying projects to be funded with

DOI: 10.1201/9781003029151-13

FFFI. The state projects originated with funding from the state legislature and/or foundations that required an organizational structure to select viable projects. Once federal funds became available through the Healthy Food Financing Initiative, any business that meets the criteria set by the Reinvestment Fund is eligible to receive HFFI financing. Additional federal financing opportunities for food environment projects continue to be available through the Treasury Department such as the New Markets Tax Credit and selection of Opportunity Zones for the project (see Chapter 3). Therefore, any community that has poor access to grocery stores can organize to gain access to these federal funding opportunities.[2]

First, the community or geographic area in need of grocery stores needs to be identified. As mentioned, the state projects had existing organization structures that identified these areas. Described here are methods to conduct a needs assessment. Simply put, a needs assessment is a gathering of information that will inform the identification of a needy area as well as the program planning and implementation of a community intervention.[3,4] This type of assessment is the earliest phase of program development and aims to provide information to support the decisions made by the steering committee of the project. With evidence-based decision-making, the quality of decisions are improved, and thus the overall project will benefit.[5] Personal biases and assumptions prevent most people from making the best decisions. For example, a community group may believe they know best where to locate a supermarket in their neighborhood, or a nutritionist might believe they know best what to stock in stores. These prior assumptions by decision-makers may lead to quick decisions without exploring all options, which may impact the success of the project. A needs assessment is intended to explore options, to determine the parameters of the project that solves the disparity of supermarket availability best for the community, and mitigates factors that may impede the long-term success of the project. The needs assessment begins with questions, questions that may challenge the inherent assumptions of project leaders. The aim of the needs assessment is to gain information to answer these questions to characterize the scope and feasibility of the food environment intervention and inform the second phase of the project, implementation, which will be discussed in Chapter 11.

There are general guidelines for needs assessments, and here we present a guide for a needs assessment specifically related to making environmental changes to food environments.[6,7] By environment, we mean structural changes to residential-built environments focused specifically on food retailers. This guide is intended to be project specific, meaning that for each underserved area, the process described in this chapter, beginning with the development of a steering committee, must take place. It would be a poor decision to assume that a single approach to solve supermarket disparities in one underserved community would have the same effect in all underserved communities. This chapter presents a guide for community groups, researchers, food policy councils, or other people who have identified an underserved area, to conduct a needs assessment to identify the best intervention to solve the food environment disparity for a specific community.

ESTABLISHING THE STEERING COMMITTEE AND WORKING GROUPS

STEERING COMMITTEE

A needs assessment begins with people who are vested in the problem of low access to supermarkets for a particular community. These people may be community members, academics from a local college or university, local government personnel, and others. These people are sometimes called *key stakeholders*. A steering committee may be initiated by any of these groups of people but ideally needs to have representation by all these groups and possibly more. A steering committee generally consists of approximately ten people, and these members function as the decision-makers for the needs assessment.[6] Some of these members may continue onto the steering committees for the implementation and evaluations stages of the project. Ideally, participation from representatives of the following groups of people would serve as members of the steering committee for a residential food retail environment modification. These groups include:

- *Community Groups.* Community groups are represented by community leaders that are aware of the supermarket disparity in their residential neighborhood. Depending on the neighborhood, several representatives may be needed that characterize differences in age, race/ethnicity, or socio-economic status within the neighborhood. These leaders may be reached from local social service agencies within the community, churches, or advocacy groups.

- *Community Development Financial Institution (CDFI) Bankers.* CDFIs are the financial institutions that will be familiar with the funding opportunities provided by the HFFI and other federal and state resources that would support the retail project proposed by the committee. CDFI's are described in Chapter 3, and the identification of a local one to support the region where the food environment modification will take place is described in this chapter.

- *Supermarket and Food Store Owners.* Owners of regional supermarket chains and family-run independent supermarkets as well as smaller grocers as described on Table 2.1 in Chapter 2 should be identified and asked to participate on the steering committee. The group has the expertise to offer questions to be answered that pertain to the feasibility of the project as well is its sustainability.

- *Academic Faculty and Students.* Academics from local universities or colleges in departments of public health, city planning, nutrition, and others will benefit the needs assessment in a number of ways. First, faculty members bring their expertise and training from these disciplines that can be used for data collection and analysis. Second, faculty members have students who can collect information. Third, faculty have the support of the university and/or college resources including software (e.g., GIS mapping capabilities, statistical software such as SAS); libraries (e.g., access to journals and reports); and potential funding (e.g., small grants that might be applied for costs incurred by the needs assessment).

- *City Government Officials.* City government officials in city planning that are aware of zoning restrictions, and/or city government officials in health and human services that are aware of local program for nutrition assistance may be helpful in identifying the neediest areas within the region. City government officials may also have existing food policy councils, be aware of the neediest communities, and have resources that may benefit the needs assessment.

- *Realtors.* As stated by Mr. Green, the former Vice President of Operations at Kroger in Chapter 2, the initial assessment of a location for a new supermarket involves information from realtors. Therefore, including a realtor that is familiar with the demographic and commercial trends in the local area can provide resources to help the committee with questions of location and sustainability of the food store.

The steering committee will be in place for the duration of the needs assessment which may take six to twelve months to complete. The committee will determine a chair or co-chairs during the first meeting; agree upon a schedule for regular meetings; and determine a timeline for the completion of the needs assessment.

WORKING GROUPS

The working groups are spearheaded by members of the steering committee. As questions are identified by the steering committee, the appropriate member of the committee will take responsibility for gaining information for that question and utilize their working group. For instance, the steering committee may need information on where a targeted community is currently shopping for food. A working group of academics and students may take the lead on this question by developing a survey and sampling a group of local residents or perhaps conducting focus groups.

STATEMENT OF OBJECTIVE

One of the primary tasks for the steering committee is to be clear about the objective of the needs assessments. Needs assessments are used for many purposes, and the objective can influence the questions and research as well as the composition of the steering committee. For example, the steering committees that oversaw the development of the Fresh Food Financing Initiative had an objective to influence policy by making state funds available to businesses that provide healthy foods to underserved communities in Pennsylvania. This objective is different than an intention to place one new food store in one underserved area.

DEVELOPMENT GOALS AND QUESTIONS

The steering committee will develop guidelines that allow for a nonconfrontational discussion in order to document questions and concerns regarding the project. The questions may be derived as an iterative process whereby the answers brought back to the committee by the working groups may lead to additional questions before the committee can reach a decision on each issue. The questions will fall under a series of development goals. For example, one development goal might be: determine the type of food stores that should be targeted for the area. Under this goal there may be a series of questions that will inform that decision by the steering committee. Examples of development goals and questions can be found on Table 10.1.

TABLE 10.1
Development Goals and Questions

Area Targeted for the Food Store Intervention
- Where is the underserved area?
- How large is the area and how many people reside in the area?
- What are the economic and demographic characteristics of the area?
- What are the economic and demographic characteristics of adjacent areas?
- Does the area qualify as an opportunity zone?

Type of Food Store
- What types of food vendors currently serve the area?
- Are there any supermarkets currently serving the area or in the recent past?
  - Why is the supermarket not successful?
  - What does the current supermarket look like inside?
  - Where is the supermarket located?
  - Can the store be refurbished?
  - Is the store owner willing to sell to another vendor?
  - Is another vendor willing to purchase the current supermarket?
- What size of a grocery store is needed to meet the needs of the area?

Food Shopping Habits of the Targeted Community Residents
- Where do residents shop for food?
- What is the estimated retail food leakage for the area?
- What are residents' perceptions of barriers to obtaining groceries?
- What types of transportation are utilized for grocery shopping?

Feasibility of the Development
- Who are the potential grocery store chains or family-owned businesses that would be a good fit for the development and how can they be reached?
- What are the potential funding sources for the development?
- What is the timeline for the development?

Leadership for the Implementation of the Project
- What type of public and private leadership will be needed to implement the project?
- Who are the specific people that will fill these roles and provide the time commitment?
- What are the specific tasks that will be needed from leadership to implement the project?
- Who are additional stakeholders that would be assets to the project?

RESOURCES AND METHODS FOR COLLECTING NEEDS ASSESSMENT INFORMATION

Once the questions of the steering committee have been documented, the working groups can get started to collect information that will resolve concerns raised and be in a better position to make informed decisions. Described in this section are several methods working groups may choose to use to gain information.

SECONDARY DATA

As described in Chapter 9, secondary data can be useful for the purpose of gaining formative information about the scope of the problem for a newly investigated area of public health. Whereas the secondary data analyses described in Chapter 9 have been used to support the effort to gain state and federal funds for food retailers, secondary data can also be useful when conducting a needs assessment for a single program project. There are several publicly available resources of information that may be useful in characterizing the targeted area for the intervention. While some of the studies presented in the previous chapter aimed to answer questions about disparities in access to healthy food in other area using similar resources, the focus of a needs assessment is to gain information about the specific area the steering committee is looking to make a modification. The Centers for Disease Control and Prevention (CDC) lists a number of public resources related to the placement of food stores.[6] However, because it is important to be gaining information about one specific geographic area targeted for the intervention, information at the county, zip code, city, or larger geographic areas is not helpful for the needs assessment. The next section discusses two resources where information is available within census-defined borders.

Reinvestment Fund and Policy Map

The Reinvestment Fund is a CDFI located in Philadelphia that administered the Pennsylvania Fresh Food Financing Initiative (FFFI) projects and has also been designated by the U.S. Department of Agriculture to administer discretionary funds allocated in the current Farm Bill to provide capital investment to food retailers who locate in underserved areas. Because of the Reinvestment Fund's partnership with The Food Trust, this CDFI has been a leader in modifications to local food environments. As part of their work, the Reinvestment Fund developed the Limited Supermarket Access (LSA) analysis, which is a tool to help investors and policymakers identify areas that have inadequate access to healthy food and also a sufficient market demand for new or expanded food retail operations.[8] This tool was originally developed to support the Reinvestment Fund's role to attract supermarkets to distressed communities or assist small stores to expand or upgrade their facilities through the FFFI. The tool aims to distinguish areas that are well-served with supermarkets from limited-access areas. For this tool, the Reinvestment Fund defines supermarkets, access to supermarkets, and limited supermarkets access (LSA) areas in the following ways.

- *Supermarkets*. A supermarket is a grocery store with at least $2 million in annual sales. The Reinvestment fund rationalizes this definition because supermarkets, compared to smaller stores (e.g., corner stores), most consistently offer the greatest variety of healthy foods at the lowest prices (see Chapter 2). In addition, stores under 5,000 square feet are excluded as well as wholesale clubs and military commissaries.

- *Access to supermarkets*. Access to supermarkets is based on a comparison to areas that are well-served by supermarkets. Well-served areas are defined within six classes based on levels of population density and car ownership. Using these reference groups, the typical distance traveled to the nearest supermarket by residents of these well-served block groups were measured. These reference areas will generally contain commercial resources such as banks and supermarkets because incomes are above average. Each block group is then assigned a Low Access Score (LAS) based on the percentage by which a block group's distance to the nearest supermarket would need to be reduced to equal the distance for well-served block groups. The Reinvestment fund defined block groups with a LAS greater than or equal to 0.45 as limited access. In those limited-access block groups, residents must travel almost twice as far to a supermarket as residents in well-served block groups with similar population density and car ownership.

- *Limited supermarket access (LSA)*. Finally, contiguous limited access block groups with a collective population of at least 5,000 people are combined to form LSA Areas. These areas have limited access to supermarkets and potentially enough market demand to support new or expanded supermarket operations.

The Reinvestment Fund has used these matrices as a surveillance tool for assessing changes in local food environments across large regions of the United States. For instance between 2010 and 2016, within the Philadelphia metropolitan area there was a 2% increase in LSA areas.[8] Theses matrices are used to both define an area's need for supermarkets and qualify areas for venture capital through the HFFI and therefore an important component of a needs assessment aiming to bring healthy food retailers to underserved communities.

The Policy Map is an interactive map that is available to assess the supermarket needs of a community. The Policy Map has been created by the Reinvestment Fund and therefore allows users to overlay contents on maps including characteristics of the LSA (www.policymap.com/maps). Within this tool, a user can select the option called *Quality of Life* from the top bar and within that pull-down menu select Reinvestment Fund Limited Supermarket Access (LSA) Areas under Food and Grocery Store Access. This results in an added layer onto the map with points indicating LSA Areas across the United States. By zooming into the State and City you are interested in, specific LSA areas can be seen in detail on the map in blue. Each LSA Area point provides the following information about the areas: the low access score; estimated retail food demand in dollars; estimated retail food supply in dollars; estimated retail food leakage in dollars, percent of food demand, population size, and number of households within the LSA area. As described in previous chapters, retail food leakage is the amount of money that is being spent by residents on food outside of their residential area. For example, a LSA area has been noted by the Reinvestment Fund in East Los Angeles, including a cluster of block groups by the cities of Commerce and Montebello. Table 10.2 describes the information provided for that LSA area and provides important formative information for the needs assessment. For example, the residents in the area are estimated to be spending over $18 million per year on

TABLE 10.2
Area Measurements of an LSA Area in Los Angeles County, California

Low Access Score	62
Estimated Retail Food Demand ($)	$ 18,170,000
Estimated Retail Food Supply ($)	$ 961,000
Estimated Retail Food Leakage ($)	$ 17,209,000
Estimated Retail Food Leakage (%)	95%
Population (N)	16,006
Households (N)	4593

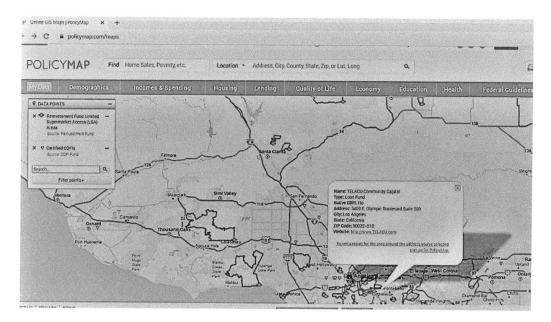

FIGURE 10.1   Policy Map of Los Angeles, California with a Pop-up of a Certified CDFI

groceries, and most of this money is spent outside of the community, supporting the economic growth of adjacent communities. For a retailer who might consider locating in this area, this is potential revenue for his store with little to no competition for those food dollars.

In addition to characterizing the LSA areas, the Policy Map also contains other important information that the needs assessment team will use for assessing the feasibility and potential funding to bring food retailers to underserved areas. For example, in addition to plotting the location of LSA areas, the Reinvestment Fund has also plotted all the certified CDFIs across the nation. In Figure 10.1, the map of Los Angeles is seen with the LSA areas indicated in orange figures and CDFI in green triangles. The pop-up window of the CDFI closest to the LSA area described in Table 10.1 indicates the name and location of the CDFI.

United States Department of Agriculture Food Access Research Atlas

In addition to the Policy Map, the United States Department of Agriculture (USDA) has created a resource where census tracts across the nation have been characterized as low income and/or low access to supermarkets or large grocery stores. This resource can be accessed at: www.ers.usda.gov/data-products/food-access-research-atlas/go-to-the-atlas/.

As part of the recognition of the importance of expanding the availability of nutritious food as a driver of the Healthy Food Financing Initiative, the USDA aimed to characterize food deserts across the United States. The Food Access Research Atlas describes food access at the census tract level based on definitions related to distance to a supermarket, wealth of the census tract, and car ownership. The definitions for access are stratified by urban and rural areas, allowing users to use the half-mile or 1-mile distance for urban areas and the 10-mile or 20-mile distance for rural areas. This information is based on census data available in 2010 and 2015. Other data available include poverty rates, median family income, race and Hispanic ethnicity, and number of households enrolled in the SNAP program. The 2015 and 2010 list of supermarkets is from the 2010 Decennial Census and the American Community Survey (2010–2014 and 2006–2010).[9]

United States Census Bureau Data

In addition to the two sources previously stated that allow a user to find information about food store placement, other data may be useful to gain information about economy or demographics of an area. However, this type of data is usually only available in geographic units larger than census tracts. Nevertheless, this information can be useful to document the economic stability of a targeted area and surrounding vicinity to support the potential placement of a food store. For this type of information, the United States Bureau of the Census can be helpful. For example, the zip code where Progress Plaza is located in Philadelphia can be seen in Figure 10.2. The economic variables: median income, number of occupied housing units, median home value with a mortgage, proportion of homes with a mortgage less than $100,000, and median real estate taxes are described by year as indicators of economic stability for the area surrounding Progress Plaza between 2011–2016 (Table 10.3). The information presented on Table 10.3 shows an upward trend in economic growth for this area during the six-year period. Census variables, such as home values and real estate taxes, were chosen as proxies for area wealth, as opposed to personal wealth (e.g., income) because area wealth signifies the economic

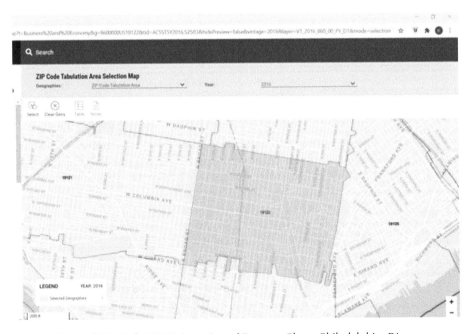

FIGURE 10.2   Map of Zip Code 19122: Location of Progress Plaza, Philadelphia, PA

TABLE 10.3
Area Economic Trends for Zip Code 19122: 2011–2016

Year	# Occupied Housing Units	Median Income ($)	# Owner-Occupied Housing Units with a Mortgage	Median Home Value for Homes with Mortgage ($)	Proportion of Homes with Mortgages Worth Less Than $100,000 (%)	Median Real Estate Taxes ($)
2011	6186	20697	1103	153,200	35.4	703
2012	6150	21929	1180	157,900	30.8	746
2013	6108	23509	1124	159,300	23.9	731
2014	5948	29442	1201	158,600	23.1	759
2015	5906	29815	1291	166,500	19.8	863
2016	6087	33448	1350	173,100	19.4	969

vitality of the neighborhoods. By presenting a series of years, the upward economic mobility of the area can be documented. These and other types of information can be accessed using the United States Census Bureau website (www.data.census.gov).

To access this type of secondary data, a user can reach the U.S. Census Bureau's website and select 'advanced search' below the search box. A new screen will appear allowing the user to browse topics by geographic size and year. The topics include business and economy; families and living arrangement; housing; income and poverty; population and people; and race ethnicity. A user can choose the geographic area that they would like to see the information prior to choosing the topic. Not all information is available at every level of census-defined borders. The census-defined areas are discussed in detail in Chapter 9. In addition to the topics just described, the website also allows users to select codes from the advanced search menu, which include NAICS codes (as described in Chapter 2), where the number of food stores with additional information about the industry can be assessed at the county level.

PRIMARY DATA COLLECTION

Some of the questions posed by the steering committee can be answered with secondary data using the resources described in the previous paragraphs. However other types of information that pertains specifically to the residents of the targeted community who will be the 'end-users' of the new food store, may require primary data collection. Primary data collection is information collected by the working group and includes quantitative data collections (e.g., surveys); qualitative data collection (e.g., focus groups) and direct observation (e.g., windshield tours). The choice of the method used among those described in the next section can be determined by the working groups and will depend on the questions being asked.

Quantitative Measures and Methods

This type of data collection involves assessing the frequency of responses and/or the average response. These measures allow the working groups to document a number of qualities that may be useful to the steering committee such as: the attitudes and beliefs of the targeted community regarding the need for a new food store; the current food shopping patterns of the residents around a proposed site; the dietary patterns of local residents. In addition, information may be necessary from key informants, such as city officials knowledgeable of zoning laws or public transportation, or current food store owners who have knowledge about patrons, purchasing power, and retail leakage.

Surveys

Questionnaires are useful tools for collecting many types of information. This method of data collection can be interviewer-administered or self-administered, depending on the questions being asked and the amount of probing that will be necessary to gain the required information. In addition, surveys are a flexible tool where information can be completed on paper copies and mailed or completed electronically through existing platforms such as SurveyMonkey. Although the development of survey questions may seem straightforward, the consideration of the type of responses offered to respondents (e.g., multiple choices, open-ended, true or false) do influence the quality of the information gained from surveys. The methods for making these decisions are beyond the scope of this chapter but would be useful when developing these instruments.

In addition to developing new surveys, depending on the questions posed by the steering committee existing validated questionnaires may be appropriate. For example, as discussed in Chapter 9, there are a number of validated methods for measuring dietary intake that may be appropriate for the needs assessment if the committee is interested in documenting the nutritional needs of a targeted population. Access to existing software for data collection and nutrient analysis for this type of information is described in Chapter 9.

Direct Observation

In addition to surveys, measures of direct observation may be useful for answering some questions posed by the steering committee, particularly as those questions relate to the physical environment. For example, counting food stores can be accomplished on foot or by car and may be another method for documenting the disparity in access for specific communities. In addition, direct observation of store content can clarify the types of foods as well as the quality and costs that are available in targeted areas. Many tools are available for this type of assessment, including market basket surveys, audits, and the Nutrition Environment Measures Survey (NEMS) tool.

Qualitative Measures and Methods

In addition to the collection of quantitative data, needs assessment may benefit by integrating ethnographic and other qualitative research approaches that will serve to complement the quantitative data collection. Such an approach will result in richly detailed representations of questions asked, including why and how the answers are meaningful in the context of participants' complex, multifaceted everyday lives. Such information is unlikely to surface with only a quantitative data collection approach. Thus, the qualitative methodology proposed for a needs assessment includes: (a) individual interviews; (b) focus groups; and (c) ethnographic participant observation. Interviews should be guided by unstructured and semi-structured protocols, and focus groups should be conducted using open-ended moderators' guides. Research activities may occur at various venues, including homes, libraries, churches, and other public or private locales. Interviews should ideally be audiotaped with the consent of the participants. The qualitative interviewer should document important aspects of interviews, interactions, and field observations in detailed notes. The goal of the needs assessment may require gaining information from people who are in the social networks of the end users of the proposed food stores such as: family members, current food store owners, and other social service agencies involving food distribution to the community, who may all take part in successive qualitative components. This approach offers a critical contribution to the project's success, namely, a deep understanding and interpretation of residents' daily experiences around access to and participation in food acquisition.

Focus Groups

Focus groups might be used to gain information from residents regarding issues such as: (a) food they would like to see available; (b) perceptions about obtaining food in their neighborhood; and/or (c) attitudes and suggestions for food retailers. The number of focus groups will be determined by the working group but usually requires two to four groups before reaching saturation. Each focus group should have no more than twelve participants, giving everyone enough time to contribute. Focus groups generally take an hour to an hour and a half to complete and should be facilitated with a trained interviewer and note taker. Participants may need to be paid to attend and offered refreshments. All focus groups and other qualitative interviews should ideally be taped and transcribed verbatim and analyzed for themes using qualitative software such as ATLASti. Results should be prepared for presentation to the steering committee, which can then use the information to make decisions about the scope and implementation of the project.

Individual Qualitative Interviews

In certain cases, a focus group is not the best method to gain qualitative information. For example, if prospective interviewees are busy, it may not be feasible to have everyone in one place at one time to conduct a focus group. Also, focus groups are intended to gain information within a dynamic environment where people are responding to comments from others. Sometimes, the qualitative information that the working groups may be aiming to gain is simply a single person's perspective. In these instances, an individual qualitative interview is more appropriate where there is a one-on-one interview between the participant and interviewer using an unstructured or more directed semi-structured interview guide. An example of this type of qualitative interview may be key stakeholder interviews. Key stakeholders are people identified by the steering committee (or during the needs assessment) as individuals with valuable knowledge that would benefit the project. For instance, a key stakeholder may be a person who owns a small chain grocery store and therefore understands the grocery store business. Another example may be an executive director of an area program that provides food service to the targeted community. In other words, a key stakeholder is any person that can provide 'insider knowledge' that will allow the steering committee awareness into the specific needs of the community. These types of interviews can take place as surveys, but typically a key stakeholder may play a larger role in the development and implementation of the project; therefore qualitative interviewing is a method where information can be gained while also building a relationship with a person in this group.

Ethnographic Participant Observation

In addition to the individual and group interviews, another qualitative research method is ethnographic observation. This type of observation might be conducted for general populations, such as observing characteristics of shoppers in a particular grocery store. Alternatively, this method might be used to evaluate the patterns of food shopping for selected participants by accompanying participants on food shopping trips in order to observe the decision-making processes for determining both location of the food store and selection of foods.[10]

IDENTIFYING THE INTERVENTION

DISSEMINATION OF NEEDS ASSESSMENT AND STAKEHOLDER BUY-IN

After the needs assessment has been completed, the next step before implementation is to disseminate the findings to the broader community. This outreach may be to other community members, local government officials, funders, and/or other people that would be interested in the new food market. This dissemination may take place as one large meeting as described in the next section on the East New York Food Cooperative. More likely, the presentation of the needs assessment and scope of the project will require a series of smaller meetings that may take place at churches, schools, community social services, board rooms of funders, and other locations. The purpose of these meetings is to raise awareness of the new food store and provide the community and funders a timeline on when they can expect the stages of implementation to begin and end. These bidirectional meetings are opportunities to gain additional insight from a broader community into facets that may promote the success of the project and/or gain additional stakeholders. For instance, during outreach Jeff Brown found that some residents that would become patrons of his new ShopRite in Philadelphia would like to be involved in sourcing some culturally specific foods to be sold at his store.[11]

SCOPE OF THE PROJECT

The scope of the project is determined by the steering committee once the working groups have completed their collection of information and all questions have been answered. The scope of the project may range from acknowledging that the group does not have all the key stakeholders necessary to open a new store and the scope is to gain technical assistance. Alternatively, a food retailer may be a member of the steering committee and ready to renovate or open a new store, and therefore the scope of the project may be larger and more expensive. It is also possible that the steering committee has decided that a smaller store, such as a food co-op that can be run by the community, is the best fit for addressing the needs of the underserved community. Ultimately, the scope of the project is evidence based on findings from the needs assessment.

FUNDING FOR THE PROJECT

Funding for the project is dependent on the scope of the project. Depending on the size of the project, it may require grants, loans, and/or private investment; therefore the steering committee should be in contact with a local CDFI to gain information on potential revenue for what is being proposed. The CDFI will be able to inform the committee members about opportunities available through the Healthy Food Financing Initiative, New Markets Tax Credit, state funding, private investment through opportunity zoning, and other resources. In addition to funding through USDA, funds are available through the U.S. Treasury and Health and Human Services as described in Chapter 3.

CASE STUDY: THE EAST NEW YORK FOOD COOPERATIVE

East New York (ENY) is a residential neighborhood in the borough of Brooklyn in New York City. It is located in the east side of Brooklyn within Community Board 5 and contains approximately 175,000 residents who are predominately Black and Latino. A walking tour of the residential area and main commercial corridors can be viewed in the following video called, *NYC's Roughest Neighborhood? Walking in East New York Brooklyn*, (January 22, 2021): (www.youtube.com/watch?v=HarqoSWaeRU)

ENY is part of the East Brooklyn Improvement District, which was incorporated in 1983. Business leaders and area residents aimed to work with the City of New York to advance real estate and structural improvements under the New York City Industrial Business Zone Program. This program focuses on a specific forty-block area of Brooklyn, part of what is seen in the video above, with the primary objective to strengthen economic activity.[12] As part of this effort, the Local Development Corporation of ENY, a nonprofit organization, is located in the neighborhood and promotes the mission of economic stability by empowering low-income people of color and women to build commerce, create jobs, and improve the economic vitality of the neighborhood.[13] It is within the Local Development Corporation of ENY that the ENY Food Policy Council arose. The ENY Food Policy Council had a specific mission within the strategy of building economic growth, which was to bring retail to the area that would provide healthy and affordable foods to ENY residents.

A COMMUNITY'S NEEDS ASSESSMENT

The Local Development Corporation of East New York (LDCENY) approached Hunter College's Urban Development Department in search of collaborators to conduct a community needs assessment in ENY.[14] The steering committee of the ENY Food Policy Council was focused on addressing the food environment disparities in ENY with a community owned-and-operated food store. The steering committee was interested to document the disparities in access to healthy foods within this predominately Black and Hispanic area of Brooklyn and assess whether a food co-op would be a viable solution to make high-quality perishable foods more accessible and affordable to residents of ENY. Community leaders gained the following information as part of their needs assessment.

- *Observation of the Food Environment.* The names and addresses of food stores in ENY were collected. There were 321 food stores located in ENY, with only 4% chain supermarkets. The area also has a fair number of convenience stores (6%) and specialty food stores (8%). There are on average five food stores per census tract although some tracts have as few as none and some have as many as thirteen. The fourteen chain supermarkets are located in ten tracts, where one census tract contains three supermarkets, and two others contain two supermarkets each. Five (36%) of the supermarkets are in predominately White Hispanic census tracts, and these supermarkets are located primarily in the northern region of ENY. The remaining supermarkets are clustered toward the southern part of ENY, leaving many residents living in the center portion of ENY without access to supermarkets. In addition, no supermarkets are in census tracts defined as predominately Black (80% or greater proportion of the residents are Black Americans).

- In addition, fifty-six food stores were surveyed for the presence of fresh produce in predominantly Black and White areas of Brooklyn. This included: forty-one bodegas, seven small grocery, four supermarkets, two delis, and two other stores. A handheld computer was used to collect information about the availability, variety, price, and quality of fresh, canned, and frozen produce. Only 64% of the stores carried fresh vegetables, 66% carried fresh fruit, 29% carried frozen produce, and 94% carried canned produce. Figure 10.3 presents the proportion of stores that carry the most commonly found fresh produce: bananas, apples, tomatoes, lemons, oranges, limes, mangoes, potatoes, pears, and grapefruit. Over 40% of all stores carry bananas. For the predominately White areas, all these types of fresh produce can be found in roughly 30–40% of food stores. However, for the predominately Black neighborhoods, with the exception of bananas, potatoes, and lemons, fresh produce is found in less than 20% of food stores.[15]

- A survey consisting of eighteen questions was administered to 100 residents. Responses from the survey revealed the community's perception and acceptance of a food co-op for improving the local food environment. Although 73% had not heard of a food co-op prior to taking the survey, 97% reported they would consider

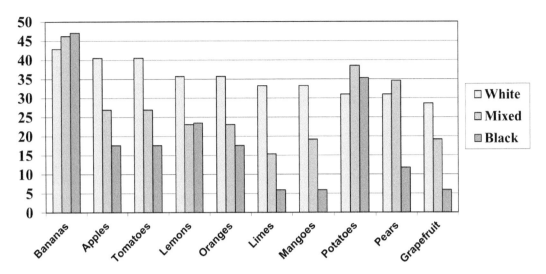

FIGURE 10.3 Percent of Stores That Carry the Ten Most Commonly Found Types of Fresh Produce in Brooklyn by Racial Segregation of Neighborhoods

shopping at a food co-op if one were located in ENY. Interestingly, they preferred a location for the food co-op that was somewhere along Pennsylvania Avenue. About 50% of respondents said Pennsylvania Avenue would be the most convenient location for them to access the food co-op. Many residents (87%) were willing to pay a fee and volunteer their time (71%) at the food co-op. About 40% reported they would be comfortable paying $25 to $50 a year for a membership fee. Some of the residents surveyed were willing to pay more for the membership fee in exchange for not volunteering at the food co-op because their schedules did not afford them the time to volunteer.

- A ENY farmers market survey was also administered to shoppers aiming to understand the food needs of the community. The Farmers Market provides fresh fruits and vegetables from local growers every Saturday between June and November. The products customers would like to see sold at the farmers market or within the community included: (a) a larger variety of fruits and vegetables; and (b) more variety of fresh foods, specifically dairy and eggs. Other food items mentioned included: baked goods, fish, meat, and ethnic food choices. What customers reported liking most about the farmers market was the fresh fruits and vegetables and believed the market could be improved with more vendors. Customers mostly walked (42%) or drove (38%) to the market. The most common types of other food stores utilized included primarily supermarkets: Pathmark, Key Food, and Associated.

- Focus groups were conducted to gain information from community residents regarding their food preferences, shopping patterns and perceptions of the SNAP Program. When asked what kinds of food participants normally eat, produce included: sweet potatoes, yams, green beans, peas, okra, potatoes, tomatoes, onions, garlic, corn, broccoli, spinach, greens, Brussel sprouts and carrots; bananas, kiwi, apples, grapes, strawberries, gineya and plantains; and sources of protein included chicken, pork chops, beef patties, sausage, eggs, seafood, and beans. A youth group described food normally eaten as 'ghetto foods' (chicken wings, onion rings, fried rice, Chinese food, McDonald's) and soul food, particularly on Sundays (shrimp, string beans, cabbage, and tomatoes) however they don't eat regular meals with their families. When asked where foods are normally purchased and why, community members reported the convenience of obtaining foods; the freshness of the food; and costs were the biggest issues. Some people said they bought what was on sale and were willing to travel further for a better price. Residents reported having to stop at several stores to complete their food shopping; for instance they may go to CTown (a supermarket) for a sale on bread but would not purchase produce there because of the poor quality. Others reported doing one large shopping once a month, and in between large shopping trips, then buying from the bodegas intermittently. Participants also report difficulty finding selections of food within their community that met their cultural needs. For instance, a Jamaican woman remarked, 'I have trouble finding yellow yams and heartier bread, which we are used to at home'. Still others reported that when they do buy fresh fruit, they or their children eat it right away, so it is 'gone too quick'. Regarding the quality of the foods available in ENY, most community members felt the quality of foods in general was lower than in other areas. Some reported that there were too many bodegas that go unchecked by the health department and expressed a belief that often dairy products in ENY, especially ice cream, had been through several supermarkets before reaching them. One participant said, 'there isn't much selection, and you have to take what you can get'. Another woman said she goes out and buys unhealthy take-out food because it's difficult to find good food in grocery stores (in the area), saying, 'If you had the good stuff at home, you probably wouldn't want the junk'. Most people who participated in the focus groups either used or had used food stamps or the Women Infants and Children (WIC) programs to supplement their food budgets. The reviews were mixed about these federal programs. Some felt 'discouraged, they treat you with no respect'. Another community member responded that she 'left government programs because of how they treat you' and others said they 'avoid government programs because [they] don't like to feel small'. More negative comments included one person who said. 'Food stamps were not worth the hassle'. Other participants' comments suggested that 'the hassle' included multiple appointments, long waits, being treated rudely, and being forced to answer personal questions. Spanish speakers in particular expressed frustration with food stamps saying, 'If you don't speak English, they discriminate and don't want to help you', and reported being told that a passport was not a valid ID. However, some in the group depended on food stamps; one participant said, 'I feel if I had to buy food with my income, we'd be close to the starving line'.

- Multiple Key Informant Interviews were conducted with community residents and professionals to get expert opinion on the feasibility of the proposed food co-op. These key informant interviews provided the opportunity to speak with residents and professionals, who were vested in the ENY community and wanted to see an improvement in the quality and price of food that is currently available. Five people were interviewed, and each expressed support for the proposed food co-op. Walter Campbell, district manager of Community Board 5, encapsulated the sentiments of the community regarding the proposed establishment of a food co-op in ENY when he said, the ENY food co-op will be a success if the Local Development Corporation of East New York does two things: 'Make it affordable, and make it accessible!'

IDENTIFYING THE INTERVENTION

- *Dissemination of the Needs Assessment Finding and Stakeholder Buy-in*. The East New York Food Policy Council hosted a conference called *the Food, Justice and Healthy Families Conference* at the Roberto Clemente Public School in East New York. The focus of the conference was presented as 'Strengthening Community Networks to Promote Equal Access to Food and Nutrition'. Attendees included community members (adults and youth); academics; local government officials and members of nutrition related community-based organizations in New York City. The sessions were dedicated to the topic of food justice in the ENY community and included the presentation of findings from the needs assessment. The conference engaged attendees with a series of workshops focused on topics such as building purchasing power, stretching food dollars, and improving wellness. The last session included an ENY-FPC committee session where community members were asked to direct the next steps to address issues of food injustice in their community. Community members overwhelmingly wanted a locally owned, locally governed, food cooperative.

- *Scope of the Project*. The scope of the project was determined to be a locally owned-and-operated food cooperative, located conveniently near public transportation, ideally near Pennsylvania Avenue. The store was planned to function as a small grocery store providing both fresh and shelf-stable foods to members of the Co-op. The store was to be opened and managed by the Local Development Corporation of East New York.

- *Funding for the Project*. The Local Development Corporation of East New York collaborated with Mount Sinai School of Medicine after the community conference to prepare a grant to the National Institute of Environmental Health Sciences (NIEHS) for funding. Through the Environmental Justice Program at NIEHS, this project called *Building Food Justice in East New York*, was funded with $971,081 to support the costs of rent, food, cooking classes, and other elements needed for the infrastructure and community outreach and evaluation of the new food store. The funding was available for four years, after which time the ENY Food Co-op was planned to be self-sufficient. A description of the implementation of the ENY Food Co-op is summarized in the following ten-minute documentary film called *Building Food Justice in East New York* (https://vimeo.com/rainlake/review/538866567/715ad6bcfb).[16]

CONCLUSION

A needs assessment is a critical first step in the implementation of an environmental change that will address disparities in access to healthy and affordable foods. It is necessary because with information gained, the intervention can be targeted to the needs of the community the food store plans to serve. With this information, the store is more likely to succeed. The second and equally important function of the needs assessment is to gain stakeholder buy-in. These projects require public/private collaboration and will not be successful without the buy-in of food store owners who understand the food retail trade. Jeff Brown, owner of seven profitable supermarkets in food deserts, states the following, when responding to why so many food stores located in underserved areas fail, 'A lot of the time it is inexperienced entrepreneurs; so, they aren't accustomed to running a food business at all. They are just trying to do something good'.[11] Finally, the needs assessment will allow the steering committee to scale the project depending on their findings. For example, although the community may recognize the lack of healthy foods within the community, once a needs assessment is conducted, the steering committee may recognize additional technical assistance is necessary, a larger sum of funds is required; or additional leadership is necessary before embarking on adding a new store to the neighborhood or renovating an existing one.

CRITICAL THINKING QUESTIONS AND EXERCISES

1. Using a phone or other device, take a thirty-minute walking tour video in your neighborhood documenting the major residential and commercial corridors. Compare and contrast the video to other students' videos and the video of East New York.
2. Watch the Rainlake documentary, *Building Food Justice in East New York,* https://vimeo.com/rainlake/review/538866567/715ad6bcfb. Discuss aspects of the needs assessment that could be improved that might have helped the food co-op stay open for more than two years.
3. Use the Policy Map to identify an underserved area near your residence and describe characteristics of the LSA. Compare to other students' LSA.

REFERENCES

1. Healthy Eating Research. *A National Research Agenda to Support Healthy Eating through Retail Strategies.* 2020.
2. The Reinvestment Fund. America's Healthy Food Financing Initiative. www.investinginfood.com/who-we-are/. Accessed April 4, 2021.
3. Watkins R, Meiers MW, Visser YL. *A Guide to Assessing Needs.* Washington, DC: The World Bank; 2012.
4. Center for Community Health and Development. The Community Tool Box. 2021; https://ctb.ku.edu/en. Accessed March 21, 2021.
5. Egan BD. A Guide for Making High-Quality Decisions. 2016; https://d1w1nui6miy8.cloudfront.net/media/965911/wp-a-guide-for-making-high-quality-decisions.pdf. Accessed March 22, 2021.
6. Centers for Disease Control and Prevention. *Healthier Food Retail: Beginning the Assessment Process in Your State or Community.* Atlanta, GA; 2014.
7. Heath Care Without Harm. Engaging the Community to Understand Food Needs: Healthy Food Playbook. https://foodcommunitybenefit.noharm.org/resources/community-health-needs-assessment/engaging-community-understand-food-needs. Accessed March 22, 2021.
8. The Reinvestment Fund. Assessing Place-Based Access to Healthy Foods: The Limited Supermarket Access (LSA) Analysis. July 2018; www.reinvestment.com/wp-content/uploads/2018/08/LSA_2018_Report_web.pdf. Accessed March 9, 2021.
9. Economic Research Services (ERS), United States Department of Agriculture. Food Access Research Atlas. 2020; www.ers.usda.gov/data-products/food-access-research-atlas/about-the-atlas/. Accessed March 23, 2021.
10. Munoz-Plaza CE, Morland KB, Pierre JA, Spark A, Filomena SE, Noyes P. Navigating the urban food environment: Challenges and resilience of community-dwelling older adults. *J Nutr Educ Behav.* 2013;45(4):322–331.
11. PBS News Hour. Building an Oasis in a Philadelphia Food Desert. August 7, 2015; www.pbs.org/newshour/show/building-oasis-philadelphia-food-desert. Accessed April 20, 2021.
12. East Brooklyn Business Improvement District. East Brooklyn Business Improvement District. www.eastbrooklynbid.org/. Accessed April 13, 2021.
13. Local Development Corporation of East New York. Local Development Corporation of East New York–Home Page. www.ldceny.org/. Accessed April 14, 2021.
14. Dugan C, George T, Knox R, Owusu S. *A Food Co-Op Grows in Brooklyn: A Community Needs Assessment of the Potential Growth and Support for a Food Cooperative in East New York, Brooklyn.* New York: Hunter College; December 2004.
15. Morland KB, Filomena S. Disparities in the availability of fruits and vegetables between racially segregated urban neighborhoods. *Public Health Nutrition.* 2007;10:1481–1489.
16. Rainlake Production. Building Food Justice in East New York. 2009; https://vimeo.com/rainlake/review/538866567/715ad6bcfb. Accessed April 19, 2021.

11 Program Planning, Implementation, and Process Evaluation

CONTENTS

INTRODUCTION

This chapter is a continuation of the program planning and implementation that takes place after the needs assessment described in Chapter 10 has been completed, and the purpose for the program can be stated. We can use the work of The Food Trust, The Reinvestment Fund, and the Pennsylvania Department of Community and Economic Development as an example of how groups worked together to implement a program such as the Fresh Food Financing Initiative (FFFI).[1] The mission of the FFFI was to improve access to healthy foods across the state of Pennsylvania. This exceptionally large program project identified that barriers to supermarket operators locating in underserved urban centers included lack of sufficient capital, costly site assembly, higher development costs, and workforce development needs. The program aimed to find solutions to these barriers. Don Hinkle-Brown, previous president and CEO of The Reinvestment Fund said,

> In underserved areas, you typically don't have nice, big, clean sites that are ready to go. You have brownfields, odd-shaped lots, small lots, historic buildings, all of which can make supermarket development more expensive. If we can take care of those front-end costs, it can be enough to encourage developers and operators to build in these areas.[1]

The details of the development and implementation of the FFFI is described in Chapter 4 and includes the eighty-eight food retailers that were supported by this program and remained open in 2020, demonstrating the sustainability of the program's outcome.

The FFFI is an outstanding example of a program that has impacted both state level policy change and local level food retailers. In some ways, the FFFI can be viewed as two program projects. The first program project for the stakeholders was to raise capital. The FFFI stakeholders accomplished program planning and implementation that led to the earmarking of $300 million of state funds allocated to the program.[1] These funds were then matched with $48.7 million in federal New Markets Tax Credits; $32.4 million in bank syndicated loans; $26.5 million in funds contributed by retail operators/developers; $8.4 million in federal, local and foundation grants; and $1.4 million from the Reinvestment Fund core loan fund. The stakeholders then developed a second program plan for the administration of the funds to qualified merchants that would fulfill the goal of the program by locating and/or modifying foods offered in underserved areas. The program plan for this second project is described in Figure 11.1. Examples of program aims for this project were to increase the number of supermarkets operating in underserved areas of Pennsylvania and increase job opportunities.

Whereas the FFFI is an exceptional example of a program project to change local food environments statewide and has been implemented successfully by other states in the United States (Chapters 4–8), the FFFI program plan is not applicable to the implementation and evaluation of individual local food environment (LFE) programs. For example, the mission of the FFFI was to increase the number of supermarkets across Pennsylvania; but the mission of Kennie's Market in Gettysburg, PA, was to expand the food store to offer customers more fresh produce. These program projects are related because Kennie's Market received FFFI funding, but they are two separate program projects that have different inputs and outcomes and hence would be evaluated with different measures. For example, the former may measure the number of businesses awarded FFFI funding as an outcome, whereas the latter may measure sales of fresh produce at Kennie's Market. This chapter aims to describe the steps in planning, implementing, and evaluating individual food environment programs, such as the effects Kennie's Market might have, on improvements in economic and dietary factors of the underserved community.

PROGRAM PLANNING

Program planning is the process stakeholders take to determine the most effective solution to the problem identified during the needs assessment, whereby a series of action items and expected outcomes are developed as well as an evaluation plan to measure the efficacy of the program.[2] The purpose of program planning is for the stakeholders to focus their priorities and formalize a unified objective before moving forward. The program plan contains timelines and a set of expected outcomes throughout the implementation of the program. The program planning also allows stakeholders the opportunity to define roles and responsibilities as well as describe outcome and impact measurement tools and methods. A program plan is a written document that delineates how the program will be implemented and evaluated. Effective program plans begin with a brief description of the program and describes the following components of the plan in detail.[2]

- *Who or What Is the Target of the Program?* This question makes clear to program planners where they expect to see the effect of the program. For example, the initial target for the FFFI program was state and city lawmakers. The intention was to educate lawmakers of the need for food stores in underserved areas of Pennsylvania in order to change policies that would mediate barriers for supermarket development, such as gaining capital and reducing regulatory obstacles. This is a different target than for Kennie's Market. For this program project, the target is the local underserved community where Kennie's market is located. The target for the program is important for stakeholders to identify early in the program planning process because the determination of the target influences all other program planning decisions. Note also that the target of a program plan does not have to be people. The target can be the environ-ment, such as a program aiming to increase the number of food stores in an area.

- *What Do the Stakeholders Expect the Targeted Population to Do?* This is an important question because it forces stakeholders to consider the reasonableness of their expecta-tions. For example, if the program project aims to increase fruit and vegetable intake by residents living near a new food store, the stakeholders must be concerned about the process by which dietary changes occur. Also, stakeholders would consider the neces-sary assessment tool to detect the behavior and assess the validity of those instruments.

- *How Much Change in the Environment or Individual's Behavior or Health Is Expected?* This is another important component of program planning, which is to be realistic about how much change is likely to occur due to the implementation of the program. Using diet again as an example, is it expected that the program will generate an increase as large as an average of one increased serving of fresh fruit per day? The rec-ommendation for fruit intake is two servings (two cups) per day and most Americans consume an average of 0.9 cups per day.[3] The average intake of 0.9 cups includes fresh, frozen, and canned fruit. Therefore, the estimated effect of a one serving per day increase would be a considered large effect because program planners are expecting the community to double their intake of fruit based on the availability of fresh fruit from one food store. An environmental change such as new food produces in a new or existing food store may produce more modest changes (e.g., a half of a serving per day), which are still clinically significant because any increase in recommended foods is beneficial. Program planners need to be realistic about the amount of change expected in the time allowed for follow-up and properly determine the study size sample based on these expectations.

- *When Will the Change Occur?* All programs are time-limited and typically determined by the funding mechanism. Therefore, what can be accomplished within the time period needs to be a realistic assessment of the time necessary to implement the program and outcomes and impacts within the community to occur. Expectations for individual change need to be sensible estimates based on behavioral and/or biological models. Individual changes can also be influenced by a number of other program fac-tors such as: financial resources for the program that may influence it's fidelity; exter-nal factors such as policies or environmental influences that support or do not support the intended change; and components of the program plan such as incentives.[2]

LOGIC MODELS

A logic model is a chronological series of activities and expected outcomes set by stakehold-ers during program development and is typically accompanied by a written program plan. The activities, called *inputs* are followed by the expected short-term and long-term goals of the project, called *outputs*. A logic model is typically portrayed in a visual diagram, such as the one developed by The Food Trust in Figure 11.1. For example, after legislation was passed in Pennsylvania to fund the FFFI, the input into administering the FFFI program (referred to ear-lier as the second program project of the FFFI stakeholders) consisted of: (a) the development of public-private partnerships; (b) funding specific food store projects; and (c) the identifica-tion of communities in need of food retailer as detailed in the first box on the logic model under financing legislation passed. These inputs were planned to be supported by activities described in the second box, which are called the implementation of the program. The Food Trust lists: (a) technical assistance; (b) program outreach; (c) identifying eligible operators and locations; and (d) matching underserved communities to eligible operators as the main

Problem statement: A healthy diet contributes to obesity prevention. Limited access to healthier food choices in terms of availability and/or quality is a major barrier to maintaining a healthier diet among children in families with low incomes.

Pre-Program Inputs

Community need

Political will and leadership (program champion)

Establishment of evidence with background data collection

- Educating decision makers on findings

Task force representing a diversity of interests and committed to process

- Health interests
  - University researchers
  - Dept. of Public Health (to offer evidence)
- Industry operators
- Dept. of Planning

- Non-profit civic groups

Advocate at state and local levels for funding, building relationships among community sectors

Financing and selective grant-making to reduce structural barriers

Community buy-in

Tax credits for economic development

Financing Legislation Passed

Inputs

Community need

Political will and leadership

Public-private partnerships

- The Reinvestment Fund
- The Food Trust

- The Greater Philadelphia Urban Affairs Coalition
- Commonweath of Pennsylvania

Process for funding grants and loans

- Funding leveraged (New Market Tax Credits)

Financing or distribution mechanism to help establish or assist supermarkets in underserved areas

- Grants
- Debt financing

Activities/Process

Ongoing response to constituent need

Provision of technical assistance and human resources assistance to qualifying grantees and borrowers

- The Food Trust
- The Reinvestment Fund
- Others

Outreach to promote programs to communities and operators/locations

Determine eligible operators/locations

Match communities to willing operators

Land assembly (obtain space for construction of new supermarkets)

Community commitment to deal with hurdles

Outputs

Amount of funding to resource program

Number of applications for grants or loans

Number of grants and loans made

Number of stores constructed or renovated

Number of operators matched to communities

Number of new options for produce/ healthier food

Number of jobs created

Short-Term Outcomes

Increase in number of supermarkets opening and operating in underserved areas

Revitalization of old stores and construction of new stores

Increased access to (and increased variety

of) affordable fresh produce and/or healthier food options

Cost savings for community members

- Lower food prices
- Reduced transportation costs

Jobs for community members

Supermarkets both meeting needs of consumers and meeting probability objectives

Greater food diversity

Intermediate Outcomes

Increased purchase and consumption of fresh produce and/or healthier food options

Increased selection of fresh produce at markets in underserved areas

Increased workforce capacity

Increased safety due to improved lighting, access, and security

Increased development of other small enterprises

- Supermarkets anchor developments for other retail

Bundled health and social services in supermarkets

- Other positive community outcomes/spinoffs

Increased knowledge of new healthy foods

Long-Term Outcomes

Increased consumption of healthier food options

Ongoing construction of markets in underserved areas and maintenance of existing markets

Create jobs, revitalize commercial real estate, leverage private sector capital, and increase tax ratables

Provide lower cost, nutritious foods and savings on transportation

Promote a nutritionally balanced diet which leads to reduced rates of diet-related disease

Goals

Contribute to improving the access of fresh foods

Economic development

Improved health outcomes due to:

- Reduction in diet-related disease
- Increased social capital
- Improved well-being

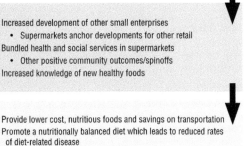

FIGURE 11.1   Logic Model Used for the FFFI Program

components of implementation of the program. These activities are typically measurable and are part of the process evaluation used to evaluate the fidelity of program implementation. The short-term outcomes are products of the program that are expected to happen quickly after program implementation has been completed. For example, The Food Trust expected the following to occur in each neighborhood that had an FFFI implementation project: (a) an increase in the number of supermarkets in underserved areas; (b) revitalization of old food stores or construction of new food stores; (c) increased availability and variety of affordable fresh produce and other healthy foods; (d) lower food prices; (e) lower transportation costs; and (f) an increase in jobs. The intermediate and long-term outcomes are called the impact of the program implementation. These are typically behavioral factors, changes in health, or long-term economic indices as described in the final boxes in Figure 11.1. The logic model is an important part of program planning because it presses program planners to clearly delineate the program goals (long and short term) as well as the steps that are needed to achieve those goals. The logic model is also useful in program evaluation, whereby investigators apply the inputs to identify measurable factors that are used in process, outcome, and impact evaluation.

BEHAVIORAL THEORIES

Food environment program plans need to be embedded in grounded behavioral theories because the programs aim to change the behaviors of food shopping and eating. Many traditional health behavior theories do not explicitly consider how our environment, such as opening a new food store, might influence our health behaviors. For example, the Knowledge-Attitude-Behavior Model postulates that as a person accumulates knowledge, attitudes change, and hence behaviors change.[4] The Health Belief Model adds to this principal by stating that people must use their knowledge of perceive risk or benefit before a behavior change will occur. Both models focus on individuals' knowledge and have been the cornerstones of health education campaigns to change behaviors, such as reducing sodium intake to prevent hypertension. Social Cognitive Theory (SCT) builds on these individual level behavioral theories by adding the concept of self-efficacy and the availability of environmental resources to support a behavior change. Self-efficacy is the degree to which an individual believes that they have the ability to execute a behavior.[5,6] In terms of dietary behaviors, this theory postulates that an individual needs a high level of self-efficacy regarding the dietary change, which typically includes knowledge, and an environment that supports the behavior change, before the behavior change will occur. The 'environment' referenced in this theory has typically been conceptualized as a social environment, such as a home environment that would support the change in diet.[7] For example, using SCT, the success of a teenager becoming a vegan is based on their self-confidence in abstaining from eating animal products, but the teenager's success is equally dependent on their home environment, which includes the food shopping and cooking patterns of their parents. A fourth theory or model, the Socio-Ecological Model, postulates that human behaviors happen in the context of many interrelated environments (e.g., social, physical, political).[8,9] For example, this theory has been used to hypothesize that a behavioral change to increase consumption of fresh produce is dependent on the convenient availability of fresh produce. Whereas this behavioral theory asserts that a modification of a food environment will lead to improvements in diet, the implementation of food environment programs using this theory is problematic. This is primarily because the physical availability, in terms of the placement of a food store or the content of foods sold within a store, is corporate controlled in the United States. Consequently, nutritionists, public health professionals, activists, government agencies, and others cannot control, which is required in traditional randomized controlled trials, without the involvement of food store owners. In other words, it might be possible for a city to include more green space to promote physical activity and measure the effect of this environmental change, but cities have little control over where food stores are located other than perhaps zoning laws. Therefore, evaluators must rely on usage of food stores as they exist. This limits minor modifications during the implementation stage that may lead to a successful adoption of the store by residents. A public-private partnership during evaluation of these projects would minimize this limitation; however, these types of partnerships are not currently common in program evaluations of local food environments. The second challenge with the Socio-Ecological Model as a basis for developing programs to improve food environments in underserved areas is that the behavioral model describes the interdependent environments that influence human behavior but falls short of postulating how these environments are expected to produce a behavioral change. Users of this theory are left with a 'build it and they will come' framework, which does not consider the series of cognitive and behavioral responses individuals have when encountering a new environmental stimulus. The fifth and final behavioral model that is pertinent to dietary change is the Transtheoretical Model (also called *Stages of Change*), which proposes that a person moves through a series of five stages before a new behavior is fully adopted.[7] These stages are pre-contemplative, contemplative, planning, action, and maintenance. As an example, for a person to use a new food store, the theory postulates it would involve: (a) the pre-contemplative acknowledgment of the new store and what the store has to offer; (b) a contemplative consideration of switching from the person's current grocery store to a new one; and (c) planning the transportation and other logistics involved in using the new store as opposed to the existing one. These three stages happen before the action of shopping at the new store takes place, which precedes the adoption of the new store as the person's primary grocery store (maintenance). Although these stages are postulated to happen sequentially, the timing between the stages and/or the total time it would take to complete the five stages of change is dependent on the specific behavior and the type of intervention. Although the 'build it and they will come' ecological theory sets a stage for the necessity for a change to the physical environment in an underserved area, the stages of change may take residents weeks, months, or even years to fully adopt the new store as their primary grocery store. Equally important, some residents may not complete the five stages of change and therefore never adopt the new store as their primary grocery store. As we aim to evaluate the impact of building a new food store (or modifying the content of an existing one) on dietary changes or diet-related health outcomes of an underserved community, these behavioral theories are essential for mitigating expectations of program impact, developing realistic hypotheses, and conducting rigorous implementation research.

IMPLEMENTATION

Public health program projects have traditionally been implemented and evaluated using methods from program evaluation. The Centers for Disease Control and Prevention has many helpful documents that describe the process whereby a program project is implemented and evaluated with the aim to improve a health behavior or health outcome.[10–12] For example, public health program projects might focus on the implementation of health education,[13,14] a change in the availability of foods in a school,[15] or providing cash incentives[16,17] to increase the consumption of fresh produce among a targeted population. These programs aim to measure the efficacy of the intervention on a changed behavior and consumption of fresh produce with an overarching aim to utilize effective interventions in other populations, schools, and locations. Conceptually, for these studies it is believed, for instance, that if a cash incentive will work in one area, there is a high likelihood it will work in another similar area. And for some interventions, this may be a reasonable assumption. Converting evidence-based programs into other real-world environments is known as translational research.

Recently, the urgent need for rapid implementation of evidence-base practices within clinical care has been recognized.[18] It has been reported that efficacious clinical procedures measured in lab settings can take nearly two decades to make their way into best practices within health care settings.[19] This acknowledgment has led some to consider the barriers within the U.S. health care system that prevent the early adoption of effective treatments. Implementation and dissemination science is a relatively new area in clinical care that aims to utilize knowledge gained in efficacy trials to observe how the new health care protocol works within specific health care systems, using effectiveness trials.[20] Implementation and dissemination science focuses on the health care system, with objectives that aim to identify facilitators and barriers involved in the uptake of efficacious procedures by doctors, nurses, patients, and administrators within real-life dynamic health care delivery locations. The health care system in the United States is a complex structure consisting of places such as hospitals and pharmacies; providers such as doctors, nurses, and administrators; and users such as patients. The health care system is further complicated by access factors for the users such as medical insurance; convenient proximity of health care facility to home or work; and medical literacy. Therefore, translating a new medical procedure from bench science into a specific health care facility requires an understanding of the hospital and patients being served. The National Academy of Medicine has described the pipeline of translational research in Figure 11.2. Shown is a stepwise progression from 'could a program work' (efficacy lab studies) to 'does a program work' (within a specific community – effectiveness studies). Researchers conducting effectiveness studies recognize that the efficacious procedures may need minor adjustments to tailor the intervention to the needs of the specific community being served. Hence, part of the stepwise process described in Figure 11.2 includes systematic modifications to implementation protocols in the final stage of translational research, called *making a program work*.

Effectiveness studies are site specific and consist of four stages: exploration, preparation, implementation, and sustainment (Figure 11.2). Exploration is the needs assessment described in Chapter 10. Adoption/preparation is the program planning, such as the identification of the site selection, defining leadership roles and development of the logic model, and a written program plan. The implementation phase entails the whole implementation strategy, including the specific intervention being adopted as well as the support structures and evaluation

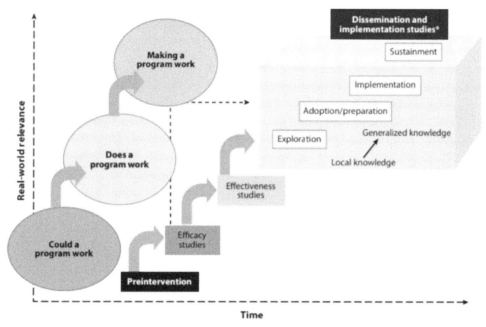

FIGURE 11.2 National Academy of Medicine 2009 Translational Pipeline

components necessary to measure its success. Implementation is the process whereby the intervention is delivered and includes monitoring the planned activities. Part of implementation is also collecting the necessary information for process and summative evaluation. This may involve recruiting study participants, administering study instruments, training researchers, and gaining fidelity measures, in addition to opening the new store or stocking an existing one with new food products. Sustainment is the final phase and refers to how the program is maintained long-term (e.g., after funding has ended).

Because the translational model described in Figure 11.2 focuses on how a system change (e.g., a new hospital procedure) affects a targeted community, it can be useful for understanding how other system changes might affect residents, such as a modification to a food environment. The U.S. food system, like the health care system, is a complex structure consisting of places (e.g., supermarkets and small grocers); providers (e.g., food store and supply chain owners); and users (e.g., customers). The food system also has access factors similar to the health care system including the affordability of products, convenient location of food stores, and nutritional literacy. However, unlike medicine, where researchers can discover 'could a program work' in a lab setting, local food environment implementation (by definition of being a change to a neighborhood) requires that the efficacy studies are conducted within places. In other words, medical studies can transfer knowledge gained in labs to real life medical clinics to answer 'does a program work'; local food environment research can only answer 'does a program work' because there are no controlled lab environments to measure the efficacy of a new food store on the diets or health outcomes of individuals. Therefore, food environment research projects are always site-specific and therefore cannot be interpreted as efficacy trials where findings can be easily translated to other underserved areas. These site-specific program evaluations are effectiveness trials.

There is a plus and a minus for building a body of evidence-based interventions about food retailing and its effect on underserved communities using effectiveness trials. The advantage is effectiveness trial researchers recognize that all communities, even if they share the description of underserved, are not the same. Site specific interventions allow evaluators, food providers and the community to tailor food store interventions to the needs of the community and incorporate those changes as a dynamic feature of the implementation process. This bidirectional relationship between the stakeholders creates a win-win for the food store owner who learns what food products are desired by the community while also meeting the nutritional needs of the underserved community as witnessed in Jeff Brown's ShopRite store in Philadelphia.[3] The site-specific need for tailored food environment interventions is also shown by the variety of programs proposed and funded by the HFFI in 2019 and 2020. The disadvantage is because effectiveness trials place a greater emphasis on the external validity of the intervention (by 'making the program work'), the internal validity compromises the ability to translate the specific intervention to other communities,[21] which means each underserved community needs a unique implementation and evaluation plan. This model is contrary to standard public health promotion that aims to identify an intervention that can be delivered to many people at once. The reason the public health model does not apply here is because it is expected with an effectiveness trial that modification of the program protocol will be necessary for the adoption of the implementation by a specific community. In an efficacy trial, this would compromise the internal validity of the study because the original implementation protocol is intended to be rolled out to other underserved areas. Once modified, evaluators have changed assumptions and expectations for the intervention implemented that may no longer produce similar results in other communities. Therefore, general lessons learned can be gained with effectiveness trials, but implementation of the specific LFE intervention in multiple sites is not the intention of effectiveness trial evaluation. The implementation strategies and process evaluation are described in this chapter, and the methods for the outcome and impact measures will be described in Chapter 12.

PROCESS EVALUATION

Process evaluation is a means whereby evaluators can understand the mechanisms behind the success and failures of a food environment intervention.[22,23] These methods have been developed to measure the fidelity and quality of the implementation, allowing investigators to identify contextual factors that might mitigate outcome and impact effects of the intervention. Because food environment effectiveness trials are embedded in both a food system and an economic system, which perpetuates the poor delivery of other resources within underserved communities, the application of process evaluation using a systems approach empowers program planners to understand proximal and distal factors that may influence the success of their intervention. A systems approach orients evaluators to consider the real world in which the intervention will be received by the targeted community, instead of a reductionist approach that focuses on the intervention only,[24] and calls for evaluators to be sensitive to the interaction of multiple systems, which may results in nonlinear responses to changes in food environments.

Process evaluation from a systems perspective allows evaluators to not only measure the mechanisms of the intervention that produced a desired impact but also to consider the dynamic nature of an intervention and its impact on multiple systems. For example, a new supermarket may affect the food system with a greater variety of healthy food options and also effect the economic system with an increase in jobs. These impact factors may work in tandem to improve the health of the community. It is important to distinguish between a systems approach from a complex intervention. Whereas the former is a viewpoint from which program planners postulate how other systems will effect one intervention, complex interventions contain multiple interventions and the measurable interdependencies between the interventions are hypothesized to effect the outcomes and impacts.[25] The challenges of complex interventions in food environment effectiveness trials are discussed in Chapter 12.

Process evaluation requires planning and the input of multiple stakeholders who are knowledgeable of the multiple systems that are affecting the targeted community.[26] With this knowledge and behavioral theories, the process evaluation planners will develop an understanding of how they expect the program to work. This understanding will guide the development of the process evaluation plan whereby the mechanisms thought to be part of the success of the program (e.g., measures of changes), can be measured along with factors that may reduce the use of the new food store (e.g., because there are no jobs in the area, residents spend working hours in other neighborhoods where food is purchased). Having a well-planned process evaluation allows stakeholders to understand at what point the intervention is not on course to be successful, identify the factors causing the problem, and resolve the issue with changes to the implementation protocol. Therefore, the process evaluation for effectiveness trials is an iterative process whereby the questions for the process evaluation may change after protocol modifications have been made and methods for gaining information may also vary.

Once planned, process evaluation begins at the start of the intervention and ends when all expected outcomes and impact of the intervention have occurred,[26] and requires the collection of information from many sources and various times during the implementation phase. Many studies have utilized qualitative methods to answer process evaluation questions, but recently value is has been in a mixed-methods approach.[27,28] Suggested components of a food environment intervention are described in Table 11.1 along with potential questions and mixed methods sources for gaining the information to answer the process evaluation questions. For example, qualitative interviews can also be used in key stakeholder interviews. These interviews aim to gain information from people involved in the planning and implementation of the food environment intervention to gain perspectives on factors leading to the successes and failures of the implementation project. Other types of information needed for process evaluation may require other types of data collection by the program planners. This type of information may be in the form of market basket surveys at the food

TABLE 11.1
Components of the Food Environment Intervention for Process Evaluation

Component	Questions	Measurement Sources
Costs	Is the project on budget? What have been the unexpected expenses and why have they occurred? How have unexpected expenses been addressed? Are the costs for rent, employees, product costs, and marketing on budget? Is additional capital necessary? Where can the capital be gained? Is the cash flow amendable to the spending for the project?	Accounting
Customers	Is the store drawing in customers? Are the customers residents of the underserved community? Has the store operator engaged with the community and in what ways? How are limitation with drawing customers being resolved?	Marketing; community engagement; community focus groups
Dose	Are the store hours consistent with the program planning? Are the key food products consistently available at affordable prices? If not, what will be done to correct this?	Observation/tracking
Incentives	Has the program utilized incentives to encourage shopping at the store and/or the purchase of items? What are the incentives, and have they been utilized by patrons? If the incentives are not being used, what at the reasons? How will the use of incentives be corrected?	Accounting; community focus groups
Leadership	Have program planning leaders taken responsibility in their roles for the project? Have leaders left the project? What has caused departures? What have been the resolutions for program leader's underperformance or departures?	Observations/ key stakeholder Interviews
Stocking	Does the store stock the planned food items? If not, what are the reasons? Are the items of good quality? What are the factors influencing quality for the store? How can they be corrected? Are the prices of the food items affordable and as planned? If not, what is causing the higher prices? How can the prices be offset to remain affordable by customers?	Market basket surveys
Sustainability	Are the sales from the store meeting benchmarks for sustainability? What are the reasons the store is not meeting benchmarks of profitability? What is being done to improve the profitability of the store?	Store sales and cost records
Timing	Did the store open on time? What caused the delays? How are the delays being corrected?	Observation/tracking
Other Systems	Is the community economically distressed? Do community members have a high burden of disease? Are there public and private transportation issues within the community? Does the store take food stamps?	City records of unemployment and disease rates; City records of the location of bus stops; U.S. Census information on car ownership rates

Note the implementation strategy includes collecting information for the formative and summative evaluation as well as the implementation. Therefore, additional components, questions and data sources for the evaluation are needed to complete the process evaluation for the whole implementation strategy.

store, where a selected number of food items are collected repeatedly (e.g., quarterly) and evaluated for their availability, quality, and cost. Other information may be collected by observation such as the store hours, the timing of when the store opened, or the number of customers on a given day. However, these findings will likely need to be followed with qualitative interviews to illicit reasons when components are not meeting the benchmarks set in the program plan.

Finally, process evaluation is also critical for understanding the outcomes and impact of the program. For instance, if a store is not sustainable, then any impact hypothesized becomes unrealistic because not enough residents will have the opportunity to adopt the store as their primary food store. As an example, the East New York Food Co-op had low sales during the entire project,[29] suggesting sustainability of the store might be difficult. Community members voiced a skepticism that the store would stay in business because of their experience that most businesses failed in East New York.[30] Understanding the mechanisms that led to the business failure after opening is an important part of process evaluation. The majority of HFFI funds have been awarded to noncorporate food retailers. For these new food retailers to successfully transform the food system, it will require evidence-based evaluations of successes and failures. Because of their smaller sizes and nature of the businesses funded, the corporate business models described in Chapter 2 may not be suitable. It is therefore vital that program planners of these innovative projects have the ability to learn from each other through published lessons learned using process evaluation.

PROGRAM FIDELITY

Program fidelity is a measure of how well the implementation of a program matched the intended program as written by program planners.[31] For efficacy studies, program fidelity is important because the aim is to utilize the same protocol in many different sites. It is therefore important to be sure that the program was implemented as planned so that the same effect can be achieved when rolled out to other communities. For effectiveness trials, fidelity plays a different role. Even though evaluators using effectiveness trials do not aim to roll out the exact protocol to other underserved communities, evaluators need to know what was implemented to understand the effect of the implementation on outcomes and impacts. When program plans require modifications to fit the needs of a community, these changes need to be implemented systematically. First, the stakeholders need to meet and address the benchmark not being met with suggested solutions. The group needs to agree on the change from the protocol and document the: (a) modification to the protocol; (b) timing for the implementation for the modification; and (c) person responsible for implementing the change. This information should be recorded in meeting minutes as well as the program plan. Evaluators can then use either of these resource for documenting the type and timing of the protocol change.

CASE STUDY: THE EAST NEW YORK FOOD CO-OP

PROGRAM PLANNING

As an example of the program planning and process evaluation, we turn again to the Building Food Justice Program introduced in Chapter 10. Upon receiving funding, the program planners used the logic model shown in Figure 11.3 to implement and evaluate the food environment program.[29] As shown in the logic model, the aim of the East New York Food Justice program planners was to increase food justice in East New York. The specific outputs were to create a sustainable food co-op, expand the community's capacity around food justice in East New York, and produce products for dissemination to other underserved communities, local government agencies, and national conferences. The program planners saw the inputs for the program as the community outreach activities, such as advertising the food co-op, cooking classes, and health screenings. These community outreach activities were expected to result in intermediate factors that would assist in opening and sustaining the new community owned-and-operated food store. For instance, galvanizing the local community to shop at the store was planned to be influenced by building community capacity around the food store with participation on the community advisory board and volunteer hours at the store. The program

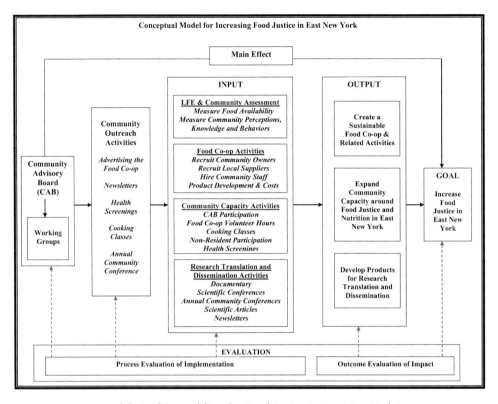

FIGURE 11.3 Logic Model Used for Building the Food Justice in East New York Program

planners also viewed the additional inputs, such as recruiting community owners and hiring staff from the community, as necessary for sustaining the food co-op. The logic model also describes the plan for program evaluation, which includes process evaluation of the input measures and evaluation of the expected output, such as sustaining the community owned-and-operated food cooperative.

PROCESS EVALUATION

The goal of the project was to place a sustainable food store that provided healthy food options to ENY residents in this underserved area. Goals of the program were not to measure the impact of the store on the local residents with endpoints such as changes in diet or incidence of obesity because this was a four-year project, determined largely by the funding mechanism. The program planners recognized that it would take time, once funding was received, to find a location, prepare the location as a food store, recruit volunteers, and identify food suppliers. The program planners also believed there would be low statistical power for impact evaluation. For example, planners recognized that it would take time for East New York residents to shop at the East New York Food Co-op and eventually adopt it as their primary food store. Also, the business plan was projecting for a relatively small customer base each year of regular shoppers, e.g., 100 during year 1, which would be a sample size too small to detect realistic dietary changes.

Because the main goal was to implement and sustain a community owned-and-operated food store, ENY program planners developed a business plan for this purpose. The process evaluation aimed to compare benchmarks from the business plan to those achieved and understand successes and failures from the perspectives of the community. For example, barriers to the cost of the planned program protocol included comparing the budgeted cost for the East New York Food Co-op project and the implemented expenses, which were evaluated by stakeholders using process evaluation. The estimated costs projected in the business plan were compared to itemized quarterly spending. Program planners identified that: (a) excess spending on perishable items at the start of the project limited funds for food products in future months, resulting in the stocking of more shelf-stable foods; (b) cost projections for staffing the food store included five personnel, a full-time general manager and sales assistant, and three part-time positions for community organizing and coordination with urban agriculture; program planners found that only one sales assistant managed the store when open four days a week; (c) the revenue plan stated the pricing of all food products would be based on a flat 20% (over wholesale and shipping & handling) markup but did not account for the higher cost of perishable items; therefore stakeholders adopted a tiered markup plan after year 1; and (d) estimated revenue for the store for year 1 was based on the assumption that 100 members would join the co-op and spend $20 per week. The stakeholders met the membership goal at the first year, but half of the members were not from the ENY community, and the expected weekly spending was not met. All of this information was gained with accounting records, and the information can impact the fidelity of the project. In addition, personal interviews with key stakeholders identified other limitation with cash flow. Because the project was funded with a grant from the National Institutes of Environmental Health Sciences, funds are dispersed to institutions after purchases were made. This type of cash flow assumes the institution has the capital to make purchases and then be reimbursed. This was also identified as a barrier to stocking the store.

As stated previously, program planners were interested in gaining information from community members about their experience with a community owned-and-operated food cooperative as a solution to poor food access as part of the process evaluation for opening and sustaining the store. Part of the process evaluation was a thematic analysis from community members who had joined the East New York Food Co-op. Evaluators aimed to understand factors that contributed to the poor sustainability of the food store from the perspective of the membership. The opinions of ENY community members and the major themes identified during the qualitative analysis are presented here.[32] Using qualitative methods, process evaluators identified themes related to: (a) motivation to join the ENY Food Co-op; (b) how the store met expectations; (c) opinions about the store structure, pricing of items, and shopping habits; (d) the communities perspective of the store; and (e) recommendations. A summary of these findings follows.

Motivation to Join

To start the interviews, members were asked, 'Please tell me why you originally decided to become a member-owner of the ENY Food Co-op?' In response, all the members noted that they were previously familiar with the concept of a food cooperative, due to their exposure and/or awareness of the Park Slope Brooklyn food cooperative. One member said:

> [my first impression of the store was that] . . . it had potential. . . . They didn't carry a lot of things, so that I could understand how people didn't want to jump right in and join because it didn't carry a lot of products and it looked kinda bare. But I saw the potential because I had heard of the other food co-op.

While members agreed that they joined the co-op, in part, because they would personally benefit from more convenient access to fresh food, they suggested that they were also driven by a desire to support a social justice effort in their community; a community they perceive as lacking access to fresh produce:

> [S]o, I saw that this co-op started with the same mentality and initiative to provide good foods and low prices to people that can't really access it. And I do live in East New York myself and I saw this as a way for myself to help out the community . . . spread the word . . . that was my thinking behind joining the co-op. Not necessarily to get the access to the foods, because I had that through the other co-op as well. But just to help the community get more educated and have better choices.

> Being a part of something in my community to help build [it up] . . . being a part of helping people with their health challenges and eating the foods that we need to eat to stay healthy.

Meeting Expectations

When asked about what expectations they had for the food cooperative when they joined, the primary expectation identified was the desire for fresh fruits and vegetables, with less emphasis on packaged goods:

> I wanted the store to have the things that I need for everyday purposes. . . . The food that I like, I like to buy a lot of vegetables, I like to buy beans and things like that. Lettuce. Tomatoes. Cucumbers. Mangos. And all those different things.

> I expected to find an emphasis on fresh produce and bulk items. Like grains and what have you, and less in terms of canned or packaged food. I also expected a nice variety of organic dairy and soy products.

However, each of the members conceded that the food cooperative was unable to meet this primary expectation – to consistently provide a wide array of fresh fruits and vegetables. All the members noted that the store had problems with the refrigeration system:

> Because in the beginning when I joined the refrigeration wasn't good at ALL [her emphasis]. I think they had second hand equipment and they had to clean it, it didn't smell good, it was very few vegetables.

When asked if the co-op met her expectations, another member responded, 'I was a little put off by the canned goods and sort of the more run-of-the-mill items. I mean, things like ketchup that actually sort of seemed odd to me'. Still another member elaborated:

> It did not really [meet my expectations]. Some of the food was not fresh. Some were not really fresh foods. Most of the foods was like not too nice to eat. [S]ometimes when I go in there, sometimes when I go in there, I will get what I go for. Most times I go there they don't have some of the things I want. What they have I will usually buy like corn, they have like corn flour, corn meal and different root and brown rice and different things like that. I would pick those things up because I do use those things. I like brown rice, so I will pick that up, and I like black beans and different things. Those things that I need.

In addition to being surprised by the lack of consistent and fresh produce, participants cited several other specific reasons they were disappointed by their experience as a co-op member. These reasons included: (1) staff turnover at the store and the fact that the staff were not residents of the ENY community; (2) the store always appearing '*empty*' because the space '*was too big*'; (3) a lack of response by the store staff to stock requested items that the community would deem more enticing and/or culturally appropriate; (4) the staff's inability to utilize members for work shifts; and (5) a lack of leadership at the co-op board-level. Regarding the latter concern, one member noted:

> I had [received] emails about the board meetings. So, I joined to come to the meetings. And when I came, they weren't on time. No board member was there on time. That disappointed me because, in my church, my pastor teaches us that you start a meeting on time, and you end a meeting at the time you said you gonna end the meeting. If you had to extend it then you ask the persons at the meeting, 'Can you do that?' So, when they didn't show up on time, I was very disappointed. It wasn't all the board members there at the meeting, so I felt that people just took positions just to have a position and not to really want to be active in building the co-op.

On the other hand, members did also respond to questions about whether or not there were ways in which the food cooperative did meet their expectations. A member noted that the co-op met his expectations in the sense that he felt it was a community-driven initiative:

> The one way that it sorta caught my expectations was by holding monthly meetings to discuss what was happening with the store. I definitely like that process where everybody that is a member has a voice, that you can just walk into the room every month with your opinions about what you think is working or not working, make suggestions, and come up with ways that create a better model so that the store continues to exist.

Two of the other members noted that they really liked the fact that the store carried books on nutrition and healthy eating as well as food items. They liked that the store had a holistic approach to health. Finally, members had a very positive view of the ancillary services that were provided at the store (the health screenings and the cooking/nutrition workshops). When asked if she ever took advantage of the health screenings that the co-op offered, one member said:

> Yes, I did, and it was actually toward the end, but yes, we had . . . [someone] in store taking your blood pressure, checking your cholesterol, and I thought that was nice . . . that it was so convenient to come in the store, you didn't have to wait for a particular fair to come out into the community. You walk into the store, and you had someone there. . . . [They were] very professional. Matter of fact, I asked if I could do some things. Even with the workshops, could I be a part of the workshops, and I was told sure just come and tell us what you want to do. So, I was happy how persons were so open to helping develop the food cooperative.

Another member said that he thought these ancillary services were:

> one of the greatest things that [the co-op] did. To try and include people who were even non-members of the community or who were even non-members of the co-op to attend these free seminars. I saw a lot of teenagers, a lot of young people interested in educating themselves about what they eat, and where the food comes from. And I thought that was great. I did participate in a few of those myself and I think that is probably the best thing that they ever did. . . . I attended one of the cooking ones, on using the salts and the sugars. There was another one about grains and beans and how to prepare them and how to use them in different ways. . . . It was very positive, and I also liked the way that they had someone screening people for high blood pressure and cholesterol right there. It was very nice.

Store Structure, Pricing, and Shopping Habits

Members were also asked to reflect on whether they thought the cooperative should have structured itself as a 'health food store' with a strict emphasis on organic products versus a store that offers both organic and conventional items with a 'healthy' and 'local' bent. Although there were divergent opinions about exactly what types of items the co-op should have carried (i.e., less packaged, more bulk, etc.), there was consensus that the store structure struck the right balance by offering both organic and conventional items. One member said:

> I think as we build up the membership, we could have introduced more organic and we could teach people about organic, but just to have more variety we could have more conventional. I don't have a problem with that.

Another member spoke to the same issue:

> I think the co-op had a good balance on that. They were aware of who their customers were going to be. They did try and make that accessible for everybody. Unfortunately, they did have to pay a high price to begin with, so the markup has to be high. Or at least, not high, it does reflect the original price. But I was comfortable with the mix of products. They did have some conventional products, not a lot, but I thought it was a good mix of what they had.

The members also noted that their shopping patterns at the co-op were sporadic, and they typically spent less than $50 per shopping trip at the store. They also said that, despite their intentions when going into the store, they usually ended up buying more nonperishables because the selection and/or quality of the fresh produce was poor:

> I bought the books, the grains, the brown rice, the peas. The oats. I bought the veggie wash to wash the vegetables, some boxed cereal. The honey. Canned goods. Those are basically what I purchased. . . . I mean there was one time that the food co-op offered some greens during a holiday season, and I must have bought up all of those [laughs]. . . . And it gave me a good feeling [because] I thought 'oh this is going to continue' and when I went again it was like, 'no we get it like that sometimes.' So, I was kinda disappointed.

> For me, no. For me [pricing] wasn't a barrier. . . . To me, [the difficulty] was more obtaining the good quality produce and fruits that were not available at some times during the co-op's existence.

None of the members said the prices of the food items at the store were a barrier for them personally and they generally thought they were comparable to the same items at other stores carrying similar products, if not even a little cheaper. However, the members did think that pricing was a barrier for other ENY residents. One member said, 'People that I talked to about [the store], sometimes they would say 'oh the price is a little high' and things like that. The following is an exchange between the Interviewer and another member on the subject:

Interviewer: And something you said there just makes me want to ask you a follow up question that isn't necessarily on my list here, but did you have any success that you know of in convincing any of your peer group, family, church friends or whoever to join?

Member: I know I had success in getting people to go to the store, but not necessarily becoming members. I think one of the things that stopped many of them was that they didn't find the prices accessible to them based on their budget. The food was great, but it wasn't as accessible as we thought it would be.

Interviewer: In your sense, people would go, but the pricing was a barrier?
Member: That is correct.

Community Perceptions of the Store
In fact, the members that were interviewed believed that the community-maintained misperceptions about the store led, in many ways, to the store's inability to sustain itself. Specifically,

members noted that the fact that the store often looked empty. One member described the store as, 'just another storefront. It wasn't attractive in the front that you would want to come in'. Another member said she didn't think many people in ENY even knew about the store, which she thought could have benefitted from more marketing:

> When I saw that it opened, I said that is very good. It is a good thing for the neighborhood. But after a while it wasn't, you know. The neighborhood maybe didn't even know about it. . . . When I said to my friend 'I am going up here to get to the co-op to get some food'; [he] said 'what are you talking about'. I say 'yes, come with me and see'. He says, 'you joking, I never see that place up there'.

Another member who tried to get people to join had difficulty:

> [I'd] take some flyers [to] go put them [up] in the church . . . and people would say, 'oh I gotta join; oh, how is it?' and I would say, 'you know, well, you gotta join'. . . . That was always my response. . . . They are so busy that they don't think of it, until they see me or see a flyer. So that is where I could have played a part to stay on their case. Come on join the food co-op. Did you join? We just have to be led. You can't just put it out there. You have to lead, like telemarketers, you have to lead people.

More than anything else, the members said that they thought the larger community really didn't understand the concept of a food cooperative, and that more education from the start of the initiative might have gone a long way in addressing what they identified as community misperceptions about the store. While one member said, 'I don't think a lot of people really understand what [the ENY Co-op] was really, really about. I don't think so', another member elaborated further on the topic:

> I heard people when we had our annual event, I actually heard residents say things like, 'Well I'll be damned if I am going to pay to shop some place and I am gonna work to shop some place.' And they actually made comments like, 'Oh, that is like work-fare', referring to the wel-fare to work program. . . . So I think that there was a cultural and practical disconnect between the concept underlying how a co-op is established and run and how it succeeds and what the community viewed, as to what the co-op has to offer and what they needed to do to be a part of that process. I don't think they got it. On any level.

Still another member spoke to the community's perceptions of the store:

> The other perception that I always heard at community board meetings is the reaction that you have to pay to shop there. And people did not understand the concept. They didn't see it an investment into their nutrition habits. They didn't understand it as an investment in their own well-being and their life; they just thought that they had to pay in order to shop there, so they compared it to other clubs where you buy in bulk. They didn't quite understand the co-op movement and I think that is one of the things that kept them [from joining]. Also, the work requirements. You bundle that up with having to pay, having to work, just so I can buy a box of cookies. And that just did not sit well with people.

This same member also added that the lack of understanding about what a co-op is, and what it can offer a member, might have impacted how the residents in ENY viewed both the types of products the store carried and how they were priced:

> I thought that they did put a big emphasis on carrying mostly things that were organic or not having preservatives, or bad preservatives, that are more wholesome. More nutritional. But they were mostly packaged goods, there were not really fresh stuff you could take home yourself and

prepare yourself in different ways. And because of that, the aspect of the product being packaged, it did end up costing more. It was not alternative for people in the neighborhood just walking by and wanted to come into the store. To people that are uneducated, it just looks like the same thing they buy at the corner store. It is a different box, a different color, but a lot more money. They will not read the ingredients on the boxes; they will not educate themselves as to what is it that they are buying.

Recommendations

When asked what, if anything, they believed the ENY food cooperative could have done that might have helped it to become sustainable over the long run, the members provided several suggestions. One member said that she thought it took too long to get the food stamp program in place, which was an important factor for the population living in the area. Several members also reiterated that they thought much more could have been done regarding advertising/marketing the co-op among local residents. During an exchange, one member said:

Member: Reach out . . . [to the] churches, . . . there are so many churches right on that block. It could have been people going out and talking to the churches.

Interviewer: Okay, so you are saying that you think churches would have been an effective place to reach?
Member: Oh, sure!

Interviewer: But from what you know it didn't really happen?
Member: No. Not at all.

Another member suggested the value of having a *'champion'* from the community who could have promoted the efforts of the food cooperative:

> When you have more than half the population on Medicaid and you know, high rates of disability and that sort of thing, really is [the co-op] the first thing on my mind? Probably not. But I mean, I like Charles Barron [a local elected official] and if he shops there, maybe I should shop there. You know what I mean?

Finally, while the members expressed disappointment but saw the food co-op not as a failure, but a first step. They said in the end that they saw it as a small success, a *'beginning'*, for the community:

> I think that it was a wonderful experience in the neighborhood, and I really feel in my heart so disappointed that it didn't kick up off the ground and I just hope that we have another opportunity, because East New York is a growing community, and we have a lot of residents in this community that I am sure could benefit from it. And so, I just hope that if there is anything that can be done that, we are able to build another food co-op because I always tell people, 'You know, [the] Park Slope [Food Co-op] didn't start off to where it is now'.

> Yes, the only other thing is that I did see eye to eye with the coordinators and the founders of the co-op. I did like where they were going, I did like their ideals, and where they were going with the co-op. And the only [thing] that needed to be worked out was the implementation. You know, these are all great ideas, but look at where we are and the kind of people we are working with, and how we need to educate them. You know not necessarily to make a profit, but just [to] get the broader community healthy and motivated. I think that the implementation of that just didn't work out.

> I think the effort in and of itself; I can't see it as a failure. It is a stepping stone if nothing else, because if that wasn't established then we couldn't have further conversation. But I don't know, I

think that the relationship with the East New York Farms was great. You know, sort of taking produce from local gardens and selling it. I thought that was very [good], not just right from the food supply standpoint, but just from civic engagement and integration with the community. At least it assured that a small constituency, albeit [one that was] far more aware of food issues, was tied in and bought into the concept.

CONCLUSION

Program planning, implementation, and careful process evaluation are the building blocks necessary for rigorous outcome and impact evaluation described in the next chapter (Chapter 12). In fact, it might be argued that the program planning of effectiveness trials is the most time-consuming part of program projects because it requires the careful selection of key stakeholders and an in-depth knowledge of the targeted community, their needs, and expected behaviors to form a viable plan. For food environment interventions, the indispensable element of a public-private partnerships makes program planning more difficult, because it requires that the funders, food store operators, community members, and evaluators are all present early enough in the planning process to write a rigorous program plan. Food environment intervention projects are also often impeded by the divisive agendas brought forth by stakeholders when planning the intervention that is the 'right fit' for the community. For example, stakeholders may need to balance the desires for the community to control the types of products sold in the new food store, with experienced operators and funders desires to make profits, in a retail business where profit margins are low. Finally, local food environment program planning requires the identification of funds, which can be scarce and competitive. Any food environment modification is expensive and HFFI funds may not cover the whole implementation phase which includes the costs for evaluation. Therefore, program planners are likely to be working with many different government agencies, foundations, and private funders for years before one project plan can be implemented. The realistic length of these projects and need for a steadfast group of stakeholders cannot be over emphasized.

Food environment interventions are very different than typical public health interventions that focus on health education or other individual-level modifiable factors. Food environment change takes place within the food system, hence LFE effectiveness trials are like pragmatic trials used in health care. The shift from efficacy trials to effectiveness trials allows stakeholders to concentrate on one underserved area at a time without the need to plan for programs that would be easily disseminated to other areas as well. Whereas it may be considered that the introduction of a supermarket would be the best food environment intervention in an underserved community and would be easily disseminated to other areas, there may be reasons why a smaller, more culturally sensitive store that has more flexibility in offering products may be a better fit for some communities. The effectiveness trials allow program planners to develop core components of the intervention, and with process evaluation, measure their impact to improve components that are less effective, fortifying the success of the program for that community.

Finally, the use of both quantitative and qualitative methods in process evaluation gives stakeholders the ability to understand the successes and failures of the program from many different perspectives. Even with the most detailed needs assessment, there will be some unknown factors that program planners do not understand about the community or the retail business that is likely to impact the program's success. With the use of qualitative methods in particular, evaluators can conduct focus groups and key stakeholder one-on-one interviews to gain information from people uniquely qualified to report on the program as users of the new store, store operators, or others with intimate knowledge of the program implementation. All this information is necessary to interpret the short-term outcomes and longer-term impacts of the food store implementation discussed in the next chapter.

CRITICAL THINKING QUESTIONS AND ACTIVITIES

1. Identify a Low-Income/Low-Access area near you. Identify the key stakeholders and an approach for beginning a collaborative public-private partnership to address the absence of food stores in the area.
2. Draw a logic model for a local food environment program project to support a program plan aim to address the needs of the underserved area.
3. Identify both economic and health factors that you might expect to be impacted by the implementation of the new food store or other planned modification to the food environment. Describe how these measures will be evaluated as part of the program plan.
4. Identify the behavioral theories that would be useful in developing a program plan aimed to evaluate the impact of the new store on diet. Use the behavioral theories to create a timeline on when to expect observable behavior changes in food purchases and eating to happen in relation to the changed food environment.
5. List at least three items that you would want to include in your process evaluation to evaluate the program's fidelity. Also describe how and when those measurements would be taken.
6. Review the information collected from the ENY Food Co-op process evaluation, then describe how that underserved community might approach modification to the current program plan or develop a new plan for implementing a program that addresses healthy eating in ENY based on the lessons learned.
7. Compare the findings presented from the ENY process evaluation to the ENY needs assessment presented in Chapter 10. Then describe the components of the planned program project, which is based on the needs assessment, that were met or unmet during the implementation of the program project.

REFERENCES

1. Lang B, Harries C, Manon M, et al. *The Healthy Food Financing Handbook: From Advocacy to Implementation*. Philadelphia, PA: The Food Trust; 2013.
2. National Center for Chronic Disease Prevention and Health Promotion. Program Planning and Implementation. In: Centers for Disease Control and Prevention, ed. Atlanta, GA; 2021.
3. Singh M. Why a Philadelphia Grocery Chain Is Thriving in Food Deserts. 2015; www.npr.org/sections/thesalt/2015/05/14/406476968/why-one-grocery-chain-is-thriving-in-philadelphias-food-deserts. Accessed December 17, 2020.
4. Baranowski T, Cullen K, Nicklas T, Thompson D, Baranowski J. Are current health behavior change models helpful in guiding prevention of weight gain efforts? *Obesity Research*. 2003;11:23S–43S.
5. Armitage CJ, Conner M. Social cognitive models and health behavior: A structured review. *Psychology & Health*. 2000;15:173–189.
6. Whetter AC, Goldberg J, King AC, Sigman-Grant M, Baer R, Crayton E, Devine C. How and why do individuals make food and physical activity choices? *Nutrition Reviews*. 2009;59:11S–20S.
7. Baranowski T, Perry C, Parcel GS. How individuals, environments and health behaviors interact: Social cognitive theory. In: Glanz K, Rimer B, Viswanath K, eds. *Health Behavior and Health Education: Theory, Research and Practice*. Vol. 3. San Francisco, CA: Jossey-Bass; 2002:246–249.
8. Contento I, Balch GI, Bronner YL, et al. The effectiveness of nutrition education and implementation for nutrition education policy, programs and research: Review of the research. *Journal of Nutrition Education*. 1995;27:284–418.
9. MacIntyre S, Ellaway A. Ecological approaches: Rediscovering the role of the physical and social environment. In: Berkman LF, Kawachi I, Glymour M, eds. *Social Epidemiology*. Vol. 2. London, England: Oxford University Press; 2000:332–348.
10. Jacobs JA, Jones E, Gabella BA, Spring B, Brownson RC. Tools for implementing an evidence-base approach in public health practice. *Preventing Chronic Diseases*. 2012;9:1–9.

11. Center for Community Health and Development. The Community Tool Box. 2021; https://ctb.ku.edu/en. Accessed March 21, 2021.

12. Centers for Disease Control and Prevention. Evaluation planning: What is it and how do you do it? *What Do We Know About*. www.cdc.gov/healthcommunication/pdf/evaluationplanning.pdf. Accessed May 31, 2021.

13. Wagner MG, Rhee Y, Honrath K, Bolodgett Salafia EH, Terbizan D. Nutrition education effective in increasing fruit and vegetable consumption among overweight and obese adults. *Appetite*. 2016;100:94–101.

14. Dudley DA, Cotton WG, Peralta LR. Teaching approaches and strategies that promote healthy eating in primary school children: A systematic review and meta-analysis. *International Journal of Behavioral Nutrition and Physical Activity*. 2015;12:1–12.

15. Evans CE, Christian MS, Cleghorn CL, Greenwood DC, Cade JE. Systematic review and meta-analysis of school based interventions to improve daily fruit and vegetable intake in children aged 5 to 12 years. *American Journal of Clinical Nutrition*. 2012;96:889–901.

16. Andreyeva T, Luedicke J. Incentivizing fruit and vegetable purchases among participants in the Special Supplement Nutrition Program for women, infants and children. *Public Health Nutrition*. 2015;18:33–41.

17. An R, Sturm R. A cash-back rebate program for healthy food purchases in South Africa: Selection and program effects in self-reported diet patterns. *American Journal of Health Behavior*. 2017;41:152–162.

18. Moses H, Matheson DH, Cairns-Smith S, George BP, Palisch C, Dorsey ER. The anatomy of medical research: US and international comparisons. *JAMA*. 2015;313:174–189.

19. Morris ZS, Wooding S, Grant J. The answer is 17 years, what is the questions: Understanding time lags in translational research. *Journal of Royal Society of Medicine*. 2011;104:510–520.

20. Bauer MS, Damschroder L, Hagedorn H, Smith J, Kilbourne AM. An introduction to implementation science for non-specialists. *BMC Psychology*. 2015;3:1–12.

21. Hendricks Brown C, Curran G, Palinkas LA, et al. An overview of research and evaluation designs for dissemination and implementation. *Annual Review of Public Health*. 2017;38:1–22.

22. McGill E, Marks D, Er V, Penney T, Petticrew M, Egan M. Qualitative process evaluation from a complex systems perspective: A systematic review and framework for public health evaluators. *PLoS Medicine*. 2020;17:1–27.

23. French C, Pinnock H, Forbes G, Skene I, Taylor SJ. Process evaluation within pragmatic randomised controlled trials: What is it, who is it done, and can we find it? – a systematic review. *Trials*. 2020;21:1–16.

24. Moore GF, Audrey S, Barker M, Bond L, Bonell C, Hardeman W. Process evaluation of complex interventions: Medical Research Council guidance. *British Medical Journal*. 2015;350:1–12.

25. Craig P, Dieppe P, Macintyre S, Michie S, Nazareth I, Petticrew M. Developing and evaluating complex interventions: The new Medical Research Council guidance. *British Medical Journal*. 2008;337:1–14.

26. Saunders RP, Evans MH, Joshi P. Developing a process-evaluation plan for assessing health promotion program implementation: A how-to guide. *Health Promotion and Practice*. 2005;6:134–147.

27. Grant A, Treweek S, Dreischulte T, Foy R, Guthrie B. Process evaluations for cluster-randomised trials of complex interventions: A proposed framework for design and reporting. *Trials*. 2013;14:1–10.

28. Linnan L, Steckler A. Process evaluation for public health interventions and research: An overview. In: Steckler A, Linnan L, eds. *Process Evaluation for Public Health Interventions and Research*. San Francisco: Jossey-Bass; 2002:1–23.

29. Morland K. An evaluation of a neighborhood-level intervention to a local food environment. *American Journal of Preventive Medicine*. 2010;39:e31–e38.

30. Morland KB. Personal Communication ENY Residents. In: 2006.

31. Bell J. *Evaluation Brief: Measuring Implementation Fidelity*. Arlington, VA: James Bell Associates; 2009.

32. Munoz-Plaza CE. *ENY Food Co-Op Process Evaluation Report: Member Interviews*. CMP Consulting; November 13, 2009.

12 Introduction to Summative Evaluation for Food Store Implementation Programs

CONTENTS

INTRODUCTION

This chapter aims to provide readers with an approach for evaluating the short- and long-term impacts of food store implementation projects called *summative evaluation*. Simply put, summative evaluation are methods used to measure the effectiveness of an intervention. Unlike formative evaluations, such as process evaluation that measures the degree to which the program was implemented as planned or a needs assessment that identifies a community's deficiency, summative evaluation measures the effectiveness of the intervention on immediate factors, referred to as outcomes, as well as factors that may take longer to occur, called *impacts*. The value of summative evaluation is that results can be used to improve the current program and/or inform similar programs with lessons learned. Like other evidence-based recommendations, summative program evaluations provide systematic evidence for understanding how local food environment programs influence desired impacts and outcomes within specific underserved areas and allows advocates to compare and contrast areas identifying common facilitators and barriers within the food retail system in underserved areas.

Just like the formative stage of program planning, stakeholders can utilize both quantitative and qualitative methods to evaluate a program's effectiveness using original data gained from the community that is targeted for the intervention. Secondary data (information that is collected for a different purpose) may be economical, but because the information has not been collected for the purpose of answering the research questions posed by the program planners, may lack the specificity needed to make causal inferences in this stage of the evaluation. It is imperative that summative program evaluation is rigorous. The program

DOI: 10.1201/9781003029151-15

evaluation for these studies are not efficacy trials, as described in Chapter 11, they are effectiveness trials. However, this distinction does not lessen the need for the research methods to be held to the same standard as an efficacy trial.

Within this chapter, we present both quantitative and qualitative methods for summative program evaluation useful for food store programs. This chapter is an introduction to these methods, but it is beyond the scope of this book to prepare readers to conduct summative evaluation without further training and/or the necessary experience on the evaluation team. The intention is to present research questions that program planners are likely to be asking when modifying local food environments and provide a road map to the evaluation methods for answering those question. Just like the team building that is necessary for the planning and implementation of a program project, the program evaluation also requires a team with expertise in behavioral science; qualitative and quantitative methods; and biostatistics.

As stated earlier, summative evaluation aims to answer questions about the effectiveness of the program on factors that are believed to occur relatively quickly and those that take longer to happen. Outcome evaluation aims to evaluate the factors that may occur in the short term, whereas impact evaluation aims to capture the influence of the program that may occur months or years after implementation.[1] Table 12.1 lists a number of outcomes and impacts constructs that program planners may be expecting to assess from the implementation of a new food store or modifications of an existing one. These constructs are presented as quantitative or

TABLE 12.1
Outcome and Impact Measures in Food Environment Studies

Type of Evaluation Measure	Quantitative Constructs	Qualitative Constructs
Outcome		
	Knowledge of the new store	Satisfaction with the new stores
	Knowledge of the product available in the new store	Meeting expectations for types of foods offered and prices
	Knowledge of the prices of products in the new store	Feelings about customer service within the store
	Perception of the new store and products	Use of store compared to previous food shopping habits
	Attitudes about the new store, its location, and aesthetics	Beliefs about other community members adoption of the store
	New employment opportunities	Attitudes about the store owner hiring from within the community
		Descriptions of the use of new food store and other food retailers
		Transportation and other logistics involved in using the new store compared to the previous retailers
Impact		
	Food purchases of healthy foods	Reasons for purchasing food products
	Food consumption of healthy foods	Descriptions of food preparation and social dynamics of sharing food
	Diet-related diseases (e.g., obesity, hypertension, diabetes)	Feelings about diet-related disease risk
	Economic growth of the underserved area	Attitudes about other new retailers in the area
	Gentrification	

qualitative concepts based on how readily each method may address the issue. For example, one outcome question that program planners may be interested to assess is: Do people in the community know the store is there? This can be answered using a quantitative survey and does not require randomizing people to an experimental or placebo group. All the outcome measures are time dependent, meaning that the proportion of the community that has knowledge of the new store may increase over time as more community members use the store and talk about it with friends and family. Understanding why people in the community use the store, or don't use the store, as well as their feelings of satisfaction with different aspects of the store can be gained with qualitative methods. Why community members do not know about the store can be gained with qualitative measures as well as other outcomes of interest listed on Table 12.1.

The impact measures listed in Table 12.1 are expected to take longer to occur. Again, based on the Transtheoretical Model described in Chapter 11, members of the community need to move through pre-contemplative and contemplative stages before shopping at the store. Also, first-time shopping at the store does not guarantee immediate repeated shopping. One quantitative impact measure may be purchasing healthy foods available at the store, for instance. The qualitative impact evaluation allows program planner to understand why those foods were purchased and not others. Similarly, it cannot be assumed that all food purchased will be eaten by the food shopper. Since a food shopper is usually purchasing food for a family, there are food preferences within the family as well as food sharing practices. Qualitative methods allow program planners to understand these dimensions of eating within the targeted community. Finally in addition to the impact on community members food purchases, diet, or diet-related disease, the HFFI initiatives are part of a government effort to support the economic growth of underserved areas under the guise that an influx of capital to an area will lead to additional private investment. Therefore, in addition to the individual impact measures, program planners may be interested in the impact of the new food store on the underserved area by measuring the number and types of new services and retailers in the community over time. These are impact measures because they will likely take years to observe. There is also a concern that increasing the economic vitality of an underserved area may lead to gentrification, which is a worthy impact measure, especially if the intervention has a part in displacing members of the targeted community.

QUANTITATIVE SUMMATIVE EVALUATION METHODS

The approach for program evaluation relies on quantitative principals similar to any nutrition intervention.[2] As in efficacy studies, program planners are concerned with random and systematic error in effectiveness evaluation because these errors have the potential to distort investigators' estimate of the true impact of a new store on the targeted community. A true impact is the real 'direction and size' of the program effect on the outcome or impact measure, such as change of diet. Because of logistics, all studies are conducted using samples, and hence these samples aim to represent the population from which the sample was drawn. The research questions and hypotheses are derived from how program planners believe the new food retailing will impact the whole population, not the sample. Therefore, the most fundamental component of summative program evaluation is to evenly sample community members for the evaluation. This and other issues can influence the interpretation and internal validity of evaluation findings. The most significant components of quantitative summative evaluation methods include the following and are described in detail in the next section: (a) study design, (b) follow-up time, (c) dose of the intervention, and (d) systematic bias.

But before we launch into the components of quantitative program evaluation, we must first recognize that there are many different questions and hypotheses that may be important to program planners. For example, in Table 12.2, questions and alterative hypotheses related to

TABLE 12.2
Research Questions and Hypotheses in Quantitative LFE Summative Research

	Research Question	Alternative Hypothesis
Availability	Will the availability of a greater variety of fresh produce increase fresh produce **purchases** among the community?	The availability of a greater variety of fresh produce will increase fresh produce **purchases** among the community.
	Will the availability of a greater variety of fresh produce increase fresh produce **consumption** among the community?	The availability of a greater variety of fresh produce will increase fresh produce **consumption** among the community.
	Will the availability of a greater variety of fresh produce **cause weight loss** among the community?	The availability of a greater variety of fresh produce will **cause weight loss** among the community.
Affordability	Will the affordability of fresh produce increase fresh produce **purchases** among the community?	The affordability of fresh produce will increase fresh produce **purchases** among the community.
	Will the affordability of fresh produce increase fresh produce **consumption** among the community?	The affordability of fresh produce will increase fresh produce **consumption** among the community.
	Will the affordability of fresh produce **cause weight loss** among the community?	The affordability of fresh produce will **cause weight loss** among the community.
Quality	Will the quality of fresh produce increase fresh produce **purchases** among the community?	The quality of fresh produce will increase fresh produce **purchases** among the community.
	Will the quality of fresh produce increase fresh produce **consumption** among the community?	The quality of fresh produce will increase fresh produce **consumption** among the community.
	Will the quality of fresh produce **cause weight loss** among the community?	The quality of fresh produce will **cause weight loss** among the community.

the impact of a new store's variety, lower cost, and higher quality of fresh produce are posed in relation to the impact of purchases and consumption of produce as well as health of the community. Each research question is analyzed separately during data analysis, and therefore program planners need to specify every question they are interested in evaluating in the program plan. This ensures that the evaluation methods are specific to the questions. For data analysis, research questions are transformed into hypotheses to conduct statistical testing. The transformation of each research question to an alternative hypothesis is shown on Table 12.2. Hypothesis testing aims to reject the 'null hypothesis' associated with each 'alternative hypothesis'. A null hypothesis is the opposite of the alternative hypothesis and typically indicates that there is no relationship between the independent and dependent variables. For example, the null hypothesis for the first research question listed on Table 12.2 is: the availability of a greater variety of fresh produce in the food store will *not* increase fresh produce purchases among community members. We use p-values to determine the statistical significance of the measures of effect during data analysis. Typically, we rely on a p-value of 0.05 or lower as the benchmark for rejecting the null hypothesis; for a p-value greater than 0.05, the null hypothesis would not be rejected. It is a common mistake to assume the failure to reject a null hypothesis (e.g., the p-value is greater than 0.05) means the null hypothesis is true. There are many reasons that we may fail to reject the null hypothesis for each research question that have nothing to do with the true relationship between the independent and dependent variables being analyzed in our research questions. For example, the independent variable is the intervention, and the dependent variables are the factors expected to be influenced by the intervention and described as purchases, consumption, and weight loss in the examples in Table 12.2. The reasons we may fail to reject the null hypothesis relate to how the summative evaluation is conducted. Even in randomized controlled trials (RCT), evaluators have the potential to introduce systematic bias into the summative evaluations, including selection bias, misclassification, and confounding. Systematic bias tends to attenuate the size of the true effects and obstructs the ability to detect true statistically significant findings. These methodological considerations are presented in the next section.

STUDY DESIGN

The choice of a study design is one of the first decisions program planners will make in setting up the summative evaluation plan. Choices of study designs range from observational studies with follow-up time, such as a prospective cohort, to observational studies with no follow-up time, such as cross-sectional studies. Cross-sectional studies are not appropriate for summative program evaluation due to the inability to detect causation with this study design. In prospective cohort studies, the evaluators do not control anything the study participants do and instead records observed behaviors over time. For example, a prospective cohort would be a study where evaluators waited to see who would shop at a new supermarket, then measured the use of the store at multiple time points. Conversely, a study design where the evaluator controls the study participants use of the new market is called a *randomized control trial* (RCT).[3] In implementation and dissemination science, these study designs are widely used to determine the program's effectiveness in real-world settings and are called *pragmatic trials*. There are choices of the type of pragmatic trial including within-site, between-site, crossover, and others that are all RTCs.[4] Although there are choices, pragmatic trials aiming to measure the effectiveness of a food store implementation on an outcome or impact factor using within-site designs are ideal. In addition to where study participants are recruited from, pragmatic trials randomly assign each study participant to the treatment or placebo group. Once the study sample is established, half of the residents would be randomly selected by the evaluator to shop at the new food store and are called the *experimental group*. The other half is assigned to shop at the grocery store where they shopped prior to the arrival of the new store. This is called *usual care* in health care studies where the treatment cannot be removed completely. In food environment studies, the treatment of obtaining food cannot be removed. This is the comparison group, also known as the placebo group. In real-world settings, it may appear challenging or even unfeasible to control where study participants shop, especially if the evaluation requires a long follow-up period of several months. However, randomizing food store usage is a necessary feature of the study design to control confounders and low dose of the exposure, factors that will make detecting an effect during data analysis difficult to achieve. This type of rigorous evaluation will likely require incentives, such as paying for groceries at the assigned markets.

However, pragmatic trials are not always experimental, meaning the evaluators control the use of the store. In fact, some argue that the random assignment of study participants in effectiveness trials is unnecessary and compromises the ability to measure the true uptake of the intervention in real time.[4] This argument is pertinent depending on the research question. If the research question is 'How is a new store adopted as a primary food store by residents?' then randomization would compromise the ability to evaluate the sequence of events that led residents to adopt the store. However, if the question is 'How does a new store effect the intake of fresh produce by residents?' then pragmatic trials benefit from randomizing study participants assignment to the store. If both questions are of interest to program planners, then two study samples may be necessary. This is because self-selected use of the store will introduce selection bias for the second research question, 'How does a new store effect the intake of fresh produce by residents?' People self-selecting the store may be more health conscious, interested in new products, or may be wealthier than those that do not select the store. Therefore, these people using the store do not reflect the whole targeted community. Why is this a problem? It is expected that some residents of the community will not select the store, and some will. It is a problem because the purpose of the program evaluation is to identify facilitators and barriers within the new food retail system that influence purchases and intake of healthy foods for the whole underserved community. When all the people in the community are not represented in both the experimental and placebo groups, findings will only reflect the facilitators and barriers of the self-selected group.

Another aspect of the study design that bears on who is eligible for the evaluation is the choice of a within-site versus a between-site pragmatic trial. Recalling Figure 11.2, the aim is to gain information on *'Did it work?'* on the specific underserved community the program that planners have targeted. A between-site pragmatic trial assumes the people living in the two different sites are the same and would respond similarly to the changed food environment. The between-site design compares the behaviors of the underserved community targeted by the program planners and compares behaviors to a similar underserved community. The between-site design pragmatic trial assumes that the only difference between the two communities is the type of food stores. This assumption contrasts with the philosophy behind effectiveness trials that acknowledges a response to an intervention will not be the same in all locations, even if two communities share the description of underserved. The use of a between-site design has the potential to introduce unmeasured confounders that are likely to attenuate measures of effect. As measures of effect become attenuated, they are also less likely to reach statistical significance.[2,3] This is why a within-site pragmatic trial is ideal.

FOLLOW-UP TIME

Pragmatic trials also require an amount of follow-up time and can range from days to months. The amount of time between the pre-intervention and post-intervention assessments needs to be grounded in behavioral theory such that the study has a feasible amount of follow-up time to observe the behavioral or health change hypothesized by the program planners. Longer periods of follow-up may warrant intermediate assessment points between the pre- and post-measurements. Using the example of obesity, the two groups would need to be followed for a period long enough to see obesity incidence change in the placebo and experimental groups, which is likely to be several months or years. Behavioral changes, such as changes in diet, are thought to occur more quickly after the introduction of a new food store; however behavioral theories on the adoption of the new store and selection of new food items are needed to inform the length of follow-op necessary to answer these research questions. Depending on the length of follow-up time, investigators may decide to add additional follow-up points between the pre- and post-measures to gain short-term outcomes and remain in contact with the study participants to avoid attrition.

If the study duration is not long enough for the outcome to occur, then the evaluation will produce a null finding. Again, this is when the behavioral theories are helpful in planning the necessary duration to detect true effects. Studies published without adequate follow-up time may report null findings that are not statistically significant due to this study design flaw.[3]

DOSE OF FOOD STORE EXPOSURE

The length of follow-up described in the previous paragraphs is presented in terms of how long it will take for the independent variable to occur for each research question. In addition to the length of time, the amount of shopping at the store is also conceptually a factor that will cause the desired behavior change. In general, when we think about an independent variable (e.g., a new food store) causing a behavior change (e.g., increased intake of fresh produce), we measure the dose as an indication of causality. We assume a linear trend between the dose of the exposure and the behavior, with an expectation that a lower dose of the independent variable is associated with a smaller change in behavior, and a higher dose is associated with a greater change. This relationship between the independent and dependent variables follows a linear stepwise pattern, whereby the dose of the independent variable incrementally increases the behavior change[3] and is often measured with a p-value for trend. Using this concept, evaluators need to hypothesize what dose of food shopping will produce any amount of the outcome (dependent variable) and if a linear trend is expected to occur. For example, for the first research question on Table 12.2, dose would be determined by: (a) the amount of food purchased at the store relative to all foods consumed; (b) the frequency (how often) the store is utilized; and (c) the duration (number of weeks, months, or years) of store use. A rigorous effectiveness trial would require that all foods and beverages consumed over the study period are purchased from the new store for the experimental group, and all the foods and beverages consumed over the study period for the placebo group are purchased from the placebo store to isolate the effect of the new store. If this is not feasible, these same dose measures would need to be collected for purchases of foods at all stores so the proportion of food purchases from the new food store can be calculated at the time of data analysis.

There are potential problems related to dose. If the dose is too small (e.g., short duration, small amount of food purchases), it will cause the evaluators to produce attenuated measures of effects that are unlikely to reach statistical significance.[3] This is where the health behavior models need to be considered again. The Transtheoretical model explained previously, described how a person might decide to adopt a new food store as their permanent grocery store. For impact research questions, the stores have been assigned; therefore, evaluators must consider the behaviors involved when food shopping in the assigned stores. The five steps of the Transtheoretical model reoccur for all shopping decisions where products, brands, and prices are new. Therefore, an investigator interested in measuring the effect of the new store on intake of fresh produce needs to consider how long it will take study participants to move from pre-contemplation to maintenance for each fresh produce type, using the longest period to determine the length of follow-up for the study. Again, an underestimated dose of exposure to the store at any stage of the behavioral model will hamper the ability to detect the true effect of the store on produce consumption. Also, subjects will be familiar with some produce at the new store because those products were stocked where they shopped previously. These types of fruits and vegetables may be adopted at the new store more readily. Other types of produce may be unfamiliar, seasonal, or expensive and therefore purchased less frequently or take longer to adopt. For these food items, participants may spend longer periods of time in pre-contemplative and contemplative stages. Therefore, measuring the uptake of specific food items allows researchers to evaluate the effectiveness of the new food store on variety of products, which may be useful in the 'making a program work' stage of implementation. Without measuring specific types of food purchased and/or allowing subjects a follow-up period long enough to adopt new products, investigators run the risk of not being able to detect true change in produce consumption.

TYPES OF SYSTEMATIC BIAS

Unlike random error, which is understood as variability within the independent or dependent variables that cannot be explained, sometimes characterized as occurring by chance,[5] systematic error is known as a bias introduced by researchers and study participants.[6] Unlike random error that can be reduced by increasing the sample size, systematic error is introduced into program evaluation through bias in the selection of people into the evaluation; measurement error, known as information bias; and confounding by other related covariates.

Selection Bias

In addition to the study design, follow-up time, and dose as described earlier, who is selected to be in the evaluation needs to represent the targeted community in an effectiveness trial.

Eligibility criteria is determined at the onset of a study when selecting participants and used to ensure the study population represents the larger community, and the sample pertains to the research question. Study samples are randomly sampled from the community in order to be representative. Other issues of eligibility pertain to research question specificity. For example, a study about childhood obesity would have eligibility criteria on the age of the participants, selecting only children. If a trial aims to measure food purchases, the primary food shopper of a household may be an eligibility requirement because they are most knowledgeable about food purchases for their family. If the studies do not have eligibility criteria, the information the evaluators aim to gain may be inaccurate, irrelevant to the research questions, or even impossible to gain. If, for example, any member of a family is eligible, then any member of the family would be randomized to shop at the new store (e.g., adults, teenagers, children, older adults) with many of these groups of people having no ability to shop. By restricting enrollment to primary food shoppers, the evaluation results are specific to changes in food shopping patterns for the person who most often brings food into a household. In addition, study participants in a RCT with hypotheses regarding disease impact are typically required to be 'disease free' of the hypothesized diseases at the start of the study.[3] This is because in these studies, evaluators are aiming to establish a causal relationship between the independent variable (e.g., new food store) and the hypothesized disease (e.g., obesity). For example, if some people in the study population are already obese at the start of the study, then the new food store could not have caused obesity to occur for those individuals.[3] Other issues with deriving a study population pertain to the method for sampling. Using a 'convenient sample', defined as a sample of people at one location (e.g., people outside of a food store), is likely to have the same effect as not randomizing the use of food stores, which is to introduce selection bias into the study whereby the study participants do not reflect the community. This type of bias will distort the ability to detect the effect of the new food store on diet or other impact measures and will decrease the internal validity of the result for the targeted community.

Information Bias

In addition to selecting people to represent the community, there is much concern about how the independent and dependent variables are collected and coded. Measurement errors create misclassification that can be observed for all types of data collected. For example, biases in effectiveness trials may be due to the misclassification of the independent variable.[3] The independent variable in these studies is the food environment intervention (e.g., the new store). For example, even once randomized, a person may underestimate the frequency of use of a food store, and therefore their dose will be underestimated. There are no objective measures for assessing the use of food stores or the purchases of foods within stores; therefore local food environment projects are immensely susceptible to misclassification of the independent variable. Investigators using RCTs typically measure compliance of their randomization protocols.[3] For example, compliance would be measured when evaluating the effect of a new drug on a health outcome. The compliance measures would document if the assigned medications were obtained by study participants (e.g., prescription filled), if the protocol for taking the medications were followed (e.g., once a day at bedtime) and/or if the medications were finished as directed (e.g., thirty-day prescription is refilled). For rigorous RCTs in food environment evaluation, investigators need to employ similar compliance measures to monitor: (a) the amount of food purchased at the store relative to all foods consumed; (b) the frequency (how often) the store is utilized; and (c) the duration (number of weeks, months, or years) of store use. Without compliance measures, it is difficult for investigators to evaluate how the use of the new food store has impacted diet or other impact measures. If all study subjects underreport or overreport their dose of food store use, nondifferential misclassification will occur, which will attenuate the effect measure and make statistically significance findings more difficult to detect.[3] On the other hand, if one group has more misclassification of the dose than the other group (e.g., the placebo group had more self-reported error of store use than the experimental group), differential misclassification has occurred. In this case, the effect of the bias is unpredictable and can as easily attenuate the finding as erroneously produce false positive or negative effects. In addition, for RCTs, if the randomization of the two groups is broken (meaning for instance, that a person in the experimental group sometimes uses their old grocery store during the study period), misclassification has entered the study, making the results unreliable, even if an intent to treat analysis has been conducted.[3]

In addition to the measurement of the independent variable, the measurement of the dependent variable (e.g., fruit and vegetable consumption) can also be misclassified. Because an impact variable such as adiposity can be quantified with objective measurements (e.g., scales), there is less concern that this independent variable might be misclassified. But for self-reported dependent variable such as changes in diet, misclassification is a concern. For example, like the independent variable, if all study subjects underreport or overreport their dose of store dietary intake (e.g., underreport intake of sugar sweetened beverages, or overreport intake of fresh produce), like the misclassification of the independent variable, nondifferential misclassification will occur, which will attenuate the effect measure and make statistically significance findings more difficult to detect.[3] Similarly, if one group has more misclassification of the dose of the diet than the other group (e.g., the experimental group reported more intake of fresh produce than they had really eaten than the placebo group), differential misclassification has occurred. As with the misclassification of the independent variable, the effect of the bias is unpredictable and can as easily attenuate the finding as erroneously produce false positive or negative effects.

Some of the misclassification of diet may be due to study participants providing socially desirable responses, forgetting about foods consumed, poor estimations of serving sizes, or frequency of consumption. In addition, all of the validated dietary assessment tools do not have the same sensitivity and specificity for accurately measuring all foods and nutrients.[7] The validated measurement tools of diet that allow investigators to control for calories include food records, twenty-four-hour recalls, and food frequency questionnaires. Most of these dietary assessment tools are described in detail in Chapter 9. Briefly described here, food frequency questionnaires are a self-reported method of surveying diet in a population over a long period of time, usually one year. Intake of groups of foods are recorded by frequency of intake (e.g., once a day, once a week), and this method is valid for surveillance and ranking groups of people by food intake.[7] But this method is an imprecise measure of diet in a randomized controlled trial. Since individual foods are not assessed, it is assumed that diet does not vary over time, and portion sizes are often excluded from these measures or hard to interpret. With food records, participants write down all the foods and beverages they consume in a twenty-four-hour period and typically repeat it for a minimum of seven days. This process is known to cause fatigue by the third or fourth day and has potential to underreport intake due to missing items. There is also a concern with this method in a study design where the exposure assignment is not blinded. The experimental group may be better at recording their diet due to the exposure to the new store. A blinded RCT is when the study subject does not know if they have been assigned to the experimental or placebo group. Therefore, the only validated measurement of diet that would be appropriate for a randomized controlled pragmatic trial are interview-administered twenty-four-hour recalls. The validated twenty-four-hour recall protocol typically used to assess usual intake of foods and nutrients is to conduct three interviews within a seven-day period, ideally catching one weekend day.[7] The recalls are to be captured without prior notice. Interviewers document all foods, beverages, and supplements consumed by the participant during the twenty-four hours leading up to the interview. Intake is averaged for the three-day period, which provides the evaluator an estimate of intake for all foods, food groups, beverages, macro- and micronutrients, and supplements for that week for each study participant. The twenty-four-hour recalls are the gold standard for measuring usual diet, but they are also the most expensive option for dietary assessment. Interviewers need to be hired and trained to probe for all foods/beverages consumed. It also takes forty-five minutes to an hour to administer.

Confounding

Confounders are variables that are associated with both the independent and dependent variables and are a causal factor of the dependent variable.[6,8] With RCTs, it is widely accepted that the randomization of subjects to the experimental or placebo group also randomizes any confounding factors, thereby eliminating the influence of these causal risk factors on the relationship between the independent and dependent variables.[3,9] In lab settings, randomization controls confounders. However, effectiveness trials are by definition conducted within community settings; even with the randomization of the exposure, potential confounding factors may be introduced into these studies. If data are not collected on these covariates, they are called *unmeasured confounders* and cannot be adjusted during data analysis, hence biasing the effect measures.[3,9]

The problem with confounding also may occur in multiple component program plans. Since program planning for food environment studies typically have long-term goals for a change in consumption of healthy foods, effective programs typically recognize eating is a complicated behavior that is influenced by many factors. It is therefore reasonable for program planners to consider the interdependencies between individual, social, and environmental influence on eating and capitalize on them during program planning to reinforce stimuli at multiple levels to produce a change in diet. The problem with the approach is the ability to disentangle the program components during data analysis. Unless the stimuli were introduced into the study in a time series design, the intervention components are completely confounded, and the independent effect of the new store cannot be evaluated. A time-series design introduces more than one intervention into the study (e.g., new food store and health education) but staggers the exposures so the independent effect on the primary exposure can be measured (e.g., the new store) and then the joint effect, by introducing the second exposure at a later time during follow-up. However, even if a time-series approach has been implemented, without behavioral theory to understand how long each phase of the experiment should last before introducing the next component the study may remain confounded due to short steps that do not allow the study participants enough time to move through the stages of change for each component.

QUALITATIVE SUMMATIVE EVALUATION METHODS

Qualitative research employs a naturalistic approach to data collection that can inject stakeholders' voices into the research by uncovering participants' unique perspectives, attitudes, and life experiences about a specific area of inquiry.[10–12] There are numerous qualitative research paradigms that can guide this type of research. For instance, phenomenological research, developed from the field of philosophy, often relies on in-depth interviews and focuses closely on individuals and their life experiences by studying their perspectives, reactions, and feelings.[11] This approach could be useful for outcome evaluations whereby evaluators are beginning to understand how the community is accepting the new food store and products. Grounded theory is another common qualitative paradigm[13,14] that could be used when evaluators are aiming to explain a process or interaction and develop a theory specific to the group being studied by looking for common patterns and themes in the data. Because the theory developed is 'grounded' in the data collected for the specific groups, it is representative of the place and people being evaluated but may not be generalizable to other communities. This method is appropriate for effectiveness trials that are aiming to 'see how it works' in a specific community. Ethnography is rooted in cultural anthropology and places a large emphasis on direct field observation with the goal of telling the story of a culture through the lens of its own people, organizations, and institutions.[15] As a final example, case studies offer a very in-depth analysis of a specific context, such as an individual, service, or program.[16] All of the effectiveness trials for food environment interventions can be viewed as case studies where themes, grounded theories, and common experiences describe the specific underserved community, but not all underserved communities.

Qualitative researchers use a number of methods for data collection, including observation, focus groups, and key informant interviews.[17] Focus groups and individual interviews typically follow a semi-structured protocol of questions and prompts, giving interviewers and focus group facilitators unique leeway to follow new and relevant lines of inquiry with participants during data collection.[11,18] Qualitative data analysis typically involves researchers conducting repeated readings of their transcripts and/or field notes, whereby they assign labels or codes to their narrative data, subsequently organizing their coded data into hierarchical themes and subthemes.[19–22] Methods for increasing the rigor and trustworthiness of the data include using a team-coding approach (e.g., multiple coders who can work to resolve coding and analysis discrepancies).[23–25] Paying close attention to sampling approaches[26,27] and data saturation[28–31] are also important aspects of successful qualitative research. Data are often presented in manuscripts as quotes, rather than quantified, in order to capture the rich detail and contextualized meaning of the data. Ultimately, qualitative results are interpreted as an in-depth understanding of the questions posed to the specific community and are not generalizable to other similar communities.

Mixed methods research is a relatively new approach that combines quantitative and qualitative methods.[32] As with qualitative paradigms, there are a variety of common mixed-methods study designs that can be used,[20,33–36] including convergent designs where qualitative and quantitative data are collected at the same time; explanatory sequential designs where qualitative data collection occurs after quantitative data collection; and exploratory sequential design, where qualitative data is collected first, followed by quantitative data (often used in survey design and development).[33]

In pragmatic trials and complex health systems research, qualitative methods can be used effectively to shed light on quantitative findings in mixed methods design. For instance, quantitative results may highlight a gap in services or care but not explain why those gaps exist in a particular setting or offer recommendations for overcoming identified environmental-, individual-, or system-level barriers.[37] Qualitative methods can offer a deeper understanding of why a gap or a challenge may be occurring and the underlying feelings and perceptions of the stakeholders within that system. It is believed that with the triangulation of data, a fuller understanding of complex interactions between people and places can be understood.[38] Mixed methods are particularly useful in effectiveness trials because the findings are dependent on the environment where they are being tested. While it is accepted in dissemination research that the intervention is targeted to a specific area or group, the program plan for the specific community has core components. Without understanding why specific core components succeeded or failed, program planners cannot improve those portions of the food retail system for that community.[39,40] The use of qualitative approaches allows evaluators to glean insight into the nonlinear interactions between players within the complex food system, which may not be apparent from the quantitative data or from previous local food environment interventions.

CASE STUDY: FOOD ENVIRONMENT PROGRAM OUTCOME – HHFI PROJECTS

One of the most immediate outcomes from local food environment interventions is the presence of the new store or new offerings at the food store. Like the ENY Food Co-op described in Chapter 11, the new food store was the main outcome planned by the stakeholders for the program project. Similarly, in Chapters 4–8, each state healthy food initiative resulted in outcomes for new food stores, changes to existing ones, or modification to the larger food system as described in Chapter 8. Because the HFFI Program has been implemented at the federal level, other outcomes are documented across the United States from this funding. The planned 'outcome' from HFFI funding is not as clear because the federal funds were broadened to support a wider array of projects within the food system and also support them at all stages of development. Two rounds of funding have been allocated through the USDA HFFI at the time this book was written. In 2019, 23 U.S. programs were awarded funds for financial or technical assistance in the amount of $1.4 million (see Table 12.3) to support healthy food projects in underserved areas. Most of these projects were not aimed to be an outcome of a food store; rather, many projects supported the development of the planned program, which in this text would fall into program planning (Chapter 11). For example, Apple Street Market Co-operative received funds for remodeling and architectural design; and the Asian Pacific Self-Development and Residential Association received technical assistance for developing a business plan for a co-operative grocery store. At the completion of either of these programs, the local community would not see a greater access to healthy foods. However, in 2020, an additional $3 million was allocated to support twenty additional programs that resulted in the outcome of new or improved access to healthy food for residents of underserved areas (Table 12.4). For example, AEDS Little Africa Market and Food Business Incubator developed a food co-op and Fresh Start Farms Food Hub updated a mobile market. Other examples of outcome measures from these HFFI projects may be new job opportunities, the greater availability of specific fresh produce, and a lower cost of food items.

CASE STUDY FOOD ENVIRONMENT PROGRAM IMPACT: PHILADELPHIA, PA

The impact of any local food environment change has not been well studied. As stated earlier in this book, it could be argued that impact studies (evaluating the long-term effects of food environment changes) are unnecessary because, the outcome of better access to healthy foods is the main target for local food environment program plans. Whereas this may be well founded, as described in Chapter 9, investigators have developed a body of mainly cross-sectional studies to demonstrate an aggregate association between food store presence and impact measures such as diet and obesity. These studies were conducted as part of the needs assessment to support the political movement for HFFI funding.

Now, we are at a crossroads to decide if evaluating the impact of the HFFI projects described in the previous tables is necessary. Is it necessary to know if the reopening of the Major Market in Zuni New Mexico has caused residents to purchase more healthy food items and eat better? Because of the large number of cross-sectional studies that have been conducted to evaluate local food environments and diet, for instance, and the uncertainty that this body of research has left food environment activists with, there is an argument to be made to revisit these questions with more rigorous study methods. The 'rigor' is in the methods described throughout Chapters 10–12, beginning with the development of a steering committee and needs assessment to determine the best intervention for the community, then utilize mixed methods to identify a program plan, including the expected outcome and impact, conduct process evaluation, and finally perform summative evaluation based on behavioral models. These studies do not currently exist in the field of food environment research. Instead, investigators have used other methods to come to conclusions about the health impacts of new food stores.

We will use the studies that have been conducted in Pennsylvania as an example of how limited impact research is in this field. As recently stated, when aiming to conduct program evaluation on one food system, we typically would not select an area as large as a city.

TABLE 12.3

Healthy Food Financing Initiative: 2019 Targeted Small Grant Awards

Location	Project Title	Project Description	Award Amount ($)	Award Type
Cincinnati, OH	Apple Street Market Cooperative	Predevelopment needs including financial modeling, market study, architectural design, and technology	80,000	Financial Assistance
Crow Reservation, MT	Apsaalooke Abundance is Here	Feasibility study for a mobile market or other food retail outlet	n/a	Technical Assistance
Stockton, CA	Asian Pacific Self-Development and Residential Association	Feasibility study for a cooperative grocery store, business planning, and resident training	n/a	Technical Assistance
Willow, AK	Black Bear Farms	Establishment of a permanent retail store	200,000	Financial Assistance
Detroit, MI	Detroit Black Community Food Security Network	Project management support for a food commons development project that includes a retail grocery space and incubator kitchen spaces	n/a	Technical Assistance
Cleveland, OH	Environmental Health Watch	Conduct market analysis, strategic planning, consumer surveys, and community engagement for a cooperatively owned supermarket	76,600	Financial Assistance
Erie, PA	Erie Downtown Development Corporation	Development of a management and operations plan for a public market, food hall, and commercial incubator kitchen	n/a	Technical Assistance
Brooklyn, NY	Farragut Food Club	Business model development and evaluation plan for new online channels for accessing more affordable and convenient food	n/a	Technical Assistance
Rochester, NY	Foodlink, Inc.	Feasibility studies a full-service grocery store	n/a	Technical Assistance
Chicago, IL	Forty Acres Fresh Market	Development of a specialty grocery store	185,000	Financial Assistance
Macon, GA	Georgia Wellness and Fitness Festival, Inc.	Support hiring farmers market consultant to provide training and assist in planning a mobile farmers market	n/a	Technical Assistance
Pine Ridge, SD	GF Buche Co.	Reopening of a grocery store	100,000	Financial Assistance
Fargo, SD	Great Plains Food Bank	Feasibility and market study to examine the opportunities and sustainability for mobile markets in the state	n/a	Technical Assistance
Dona Ana County, NM, and El Paso, TX	La Semilla Food Center	Consolidate mobile retail efforts at three locations and establish a micro-retail market as a permanent home base	250,000	Financial Assistance
Lake Village, AK	City of Lake Village – Economic Development Commission	Market study that includes retail assessment, competition analysis, and consumer-needs analysis	n/a	Technical Assistance
Louisville, KY	Louisville Association for Community Economics (LACE)	Community engagement, ownership campaign, and business planning	n/a	Technical Assistance

(Continued)

TABLE 12.3 (Continued)
Healthy Food Financing Initiative: 2019 Targeted Small Grant Awards

Location	Organization	Description	Amount	Type
St. Louis, MO	Operation Food Search	Market analysis study and business plan development	n/a	Technical Assistance
Todd County, SD	REDCO Food Sovereignty Initiative	Expansion of a successful farmers market and economic feasibility and impact of year-round mobile market	150,000	Financial Assistance
Sumter, SC	Rogers Vegetable Farm	Development of a mobile market	110,000	Financial Assistance
Roanoke, VA	Roanoke College	Feasibility study, site planning, and capitalization planning for a grocery store	n/a	Technical Assistance
New Bern, NC	Veterans Employment Base Camp and Organic Garden	Development of a market complex that offers fresh and staple foods for sale, a community kitchen and café, and youth programming, training, and employment opportunities	33,000	Financial Assistance
Charleston, WV	West Virginia Food & Farm Coalition	Development of WV Grocer Lab to support coordinated retail development	215,400	Financial Assistance
Denver, CO	Westwood Food Cooperative	Predevelopment needs including updating the project's feasibility study and business plan	n/a	Technical Assistance

Source: www.investinginfood.com/impact/2019-impact-awardees/.

TABLE 12.4
Healthy Food Financing Initiative: 2020 Targeted Small Grant Awards

Location	Project Title	Project Description	Award Amount ($)	Award Type
St. Paul, MN	AEDS Little Africa Market and Food Business Incubator	Development of a cooperative market with retail food sales, a commercial kitchen and bakery, a new office headquarters, and community meeting and gathering spaces	200,000	Financial Assistance
Charles Town, WV	Bushel & Peck Food Hub	Expansion of wholesale aggregation operations and direct-to-consumer curbside sales for locally sourced retail grocery	125,000	Financial Assistance
Santa Rosa, CA	California Indian Traditional Food Incubator	Development for a California Indian Traditional Foods Incubator with resilient solar power	189,859	Financial Assistance
Honolulu, HI	Farm Link Hawai'i	Expansion of online local food hub marketplace to serve more SNAP customers	160,000	Financial Assistance
Laramie, WY	Feeding Laramie Valley on the Move	Development of a mobile market and food cooperative partnership	110,000	Financial Assistance
Albany, GA	Food for Less Albany	Development of a full-service independent grocery store	150,000	Financial Assistance
Tacoma, WA	Fresh Express Mobile Market	Reopen a mobile market as a retail model that accepts SNAP and offers 1:1 matching discount for SNAP purchases	53,597	Financial Assistance
Manchester, NH	Fresh Start Farms Food Hub	Update a mobile market to sell staple foods, open a retail site at the food hub, expand sales into local former stores, and support marketing through a community food ambassador program	100,000	Financial Assistance
Marks, MS	Jeffcoat's Family Market	Renovate and fit out a city-acquired new site for a full-service independent grocery store and partnership development with Farm Workers Opportunities food hub	200,000	Financial Assistance
Lexington, KY	Julietta Market	Development of a nonprofit multi-vendor public market that offers retail sales, shared kitchen space, and aggregation facilities	140,030	Financial Assistance
Zuni, NM	Major Market	Reopening of an independent grocery store with inventory, storage, and broadband	200,000	Financial Assistance
Saint Louis, MO	MARSH Community Grocery	Development of a storefront grocery	116,455	Financial Assistance
Marty, SD	Marty Food Lockers	Pilot a community-based drop-off program as part of five independent grocery stores near or on Indian Reservations	150,000	Financial Assistance
Drew, MS, and Shaw, MS	Mississippi Delta Online Grocery Delivery Program	Development of an online grocery delivery program which aggregates individual grocery orders from a retail partner	170,000	Financial Assistance
Flint, MI	North Flint Food Market	Development of a full-service community-owned food cooperative	200,000	Financial Assistance
Oshkosh, WI	Oshkosh Food Co-Op	Development of a full-service community-owned food cooperative	145,000	Financial Assistance
Philadelphia, PA	Philly Foodworks	Development of an on-site retail location within a food hub	131,600	Financial Assistance
New Orleans, LA	Sankofa Fresh Stop Market	Development of a Fresh Stop Market	200,000	Financial Assistance
Winston-Salem, NC	SHARE Cooperative's Harvest Market	Development of a full-service community-owned food cooperative	200,000	Financial Assistance
Portland, OR	Village Market	Renovation of a nonprofit grocery store's produce department	65,422	Financial Assistance

Source: www.investinginfood.com/impact/.

However, Pennsylvania has been at the forefront of local food environment changes with support beginning with the FFFI over twenty years ago. Therefore, it is also one area of the United States that has been under the microscope for impact changes. Fifteen studies have been conducted in Philadelphia between 2008 and 2020 that have investigated local food environments in Philadelphia.[41–55] Some of these studies have used qualitative methods that aimed to understand the behavior of food shopping,[42,48] while others have quantitatively measured the content of foods within stores.[43,46,50] Researchers have also assessed residents' perceptions of local food availability,[41,45,49,51,53] but few have aimed to measure the impact of the local food environment on residents' intake of healthy foods in Philadelphia. One study measured the effect of providing a $2 bonus coupon for every $5 spent on fruits and vegetables at twenty-two farmers markets located in low-income areas of Philadelphia.[55] However, in this context, the investigators hypothesized the cost of foods to be the barrier to healthy eating, not availability.

Only two studies aimed to measure the impact of the availability of food on diet. Neither investigator used a randomized controlled trial. Cannuscio et al. conducted a cross-sectional study that characterized the local food environments of a thirty-block area of Philadelphia and surveyed residents.[43] Within this study, 373 food stores were audited using the NEMS-S assessment tool, which scores stores based on the availability of healthy food options – higher scores indicating a greater variety of healthy food choices. Investigators found that for 78.6% of residents surveyed, corner stores or convenience stores were closest to their homes, but residents did not use those retailers for food shopping. Instead, 94% of the food shopping for the study population took place at supermarkets, and the researchers found that supermarkets had the highest NEMS-S score compared to all other types of food vendors. The study population of 514 people was gained with a door-to-door sampling method within the thirty-block area where the food stores were audited. The study population was predominately Black Americans (73%), female (66%), and families with children (48%). However, the choice of a cross-sectional design does not allow investigators to infer any causality between the availability of healthy foods and food shopping.

Cummins et al.[44] used a longitudinal cohort design and targeted two neighborhoods that were located 3 miles apart where the closest supermarket was located 1.5 miles away. These authors used random-digit dialing to collect survey data from residents in 2006 and gained a study population of roughly 700 people for each neighborhood with a 47% retention by the end of the study. Regular intake of fruits and vegetables was evaluated using the Block food-frequency questionnaire. The study populations' diets were re-evaluated in 2010, six months after a new supermarket opened in one of the neighborhoods. Investigators observed no difference in fruit and vegetable consumption between the before and after assessment of diet among the residents who acquired a supermarket. Although the authors followed subjects for four years, the study design suggests a hypothesis that a new food store will impact residents' diet within six months (the time between when the new food store opened and the end of follow-up). Therefore, this hypothesis implies subjects will move from pre-contemplation to maintenance in six months, and the effect of maintenance will increase intake of fruits and vegetables. There was, and remains, no empirical evidence to inform the plausibility of the length of the follow-up time. The authors measured usage in their study and found that only 26.7% of study participants adopted the new store as their primary food store. Also, the authors found that the new grocery store increased awareness of food access. These findings suggests that most subjects were in the contemplative or pre-contemplative stages of adopting the new store at the end of the study. Nevertheless, all the study subjects were grouped together in the data analyses, creating misclassification of the dose of the independent variable. The study is further limited by the choice of the measurement tool for assessing change in dietary intake. As said previously, food frequency questionnaires allow researchers to adequately rank populations into categories of low- and high-intake of foods and nutrients based on the frequency of intake of groups of foods, but poorly assesses daily intake for individual foods and nutrients.[7]

Consequently, this measurement tool would not be sensitive enough to detect additional daily or weekly servings of fresh produce. A third limitation is the choice of the comparison group. The authors have assumed that two neighboring communities are the same, except for the new food store and that random digit dialing has eliminated confounding from their study. Since this is not an RCT where the study subjects have been randomly assigned to the new food store, the authors cannot assume confounders have been randomly distributed between the two neighborhoods, which has resulted in reporting findings with uncontrolled confounders, leaving readers to consider other variables related to diet and neighborhoods that may be masking the true effect of the new food store on residents' consumption of fruits and vegetables.

Overall, this body of research in Philadelphia leaves readers with little empirical evidence to draw any conclusion about the impact that changes to the food environments in Philadelphia have had on residents. This is due primarily to the fact there are few studies conducted and those conducted lack rigor.

CONCLUSION

Pennsylvania is an area of the United States where the Fresh Food Financing Initiative (FFFI) was initiated, and it may be surprising that so few studies have been conducted to measure the effectiveness of the program. But there needs to be a distinction between the effectiveness trials and the FFFI program that The Food Trust, the Reinvestment Fund, and the Pennsylvania Department of Community and Economic Development implemented. The FFFI purpose was to provide the necessary capital to support new food retail enterprises. Evaluators of the FFFI have documented the program to have secured over $417 million to improve food environments in Pennsylvania. These funds have supported eighty-eight food retailers in underserved areas, created 5,000 jobs and developed 1.67 million square feet of food retail space.[56] The long-term impact of any specific FFFI funded store, such as Kennie's Market, would require program planning, including an effectiveness trial in order to understand the impact the store has on customers diets or health. This would require a separate program project with a unique set of inputs and outputs, and based on implementation and dissemination science would need to be conducted separately for each FFFI project.

Who should be responsible for evaluating the long-term impact of a food environment program such as Kennie's Market? Kennie's Market is a family- and employee-owned food store. This private-public partnership, which allowed this food store to receive funds, does not include technical assistance for program evaluation. The owners of Kennie's market are trained to evaluate fluctuations in sales, which impacts the sustainability of their business. But the owners have no training, and perhaps no interest, in evaluating how their food products effect customers eating behaviors and health. These are not the markers of success of the program for business owners; the marker is that the business profits are increasing.

The absence of long-term impact studies from program implementations, such as Kennie's market and the other FFFI and HFFI funded programs, is not evidence that these programs have not influenced the diets, health, or any other impact measure for the underserved community. There simply is little empirical evidence for understanding how these program projects have affected people and places. As said earlier, some argue that the long-term impact evaluations are unnecessary. The goal of the FFFI, along with other state and federal initiatives, is to reduce the disparity in access to healthy foods. For the state initiatives, that goal has been met in many different areas across the United States, and the HFFI is continuing this effort. However, the benefit for conducting impact evaluations for food environment projects is the ability to develop empirical evidence that quantifies and qualifies aspects of the different program projects that are more successful at bringing about economic and health changes among community members and the underserved areas. These lessons learned can then be incorporated into future food environment programs, thereby increasing the effectiveness of these programs over time. For HFFI, the programs are just beginning to be implemented, and frankly, this is a prime opportunity for people trained in program planning to make a public-private partnership with HFFI awardees to begin documenting the outcomes and impact of these food retail changes.

The federal government's determination to continue support for underserved areas with capital was reiterated with the announcement from the Biden administration on June 14, 2021, that $1.2 billion in funds have been allocated to 863 CDFIs for the purpose of improving the infrastructure of underserved communities such as food stores.[57] As these new programs develop from the funds authorized from the Consolidated Appropriated Act, 2021 (Pub. L 116260) and the existing HFFI funds are distributed through the three federal departments, public-private partnerships are called upon to work together to develop program plans. Program plans are mutually beneficial for public-private ventures because effectiveness trials allow store owners to gain information on the food products that are desired by the community they serve as well as understand barriers residents might have for adopting the store as a primary grocery store. This information will increase sales. For consumers who have been trained to shop for food outside of their neighborhoods, a voice in the program planning builds confidence by residents that the food store will address their perceived food access problems. This will also generate customer loyalty.

Program plans for these food environment ventures are living document with objectives that may take five years or longer to carry out. According to the Bureau of Labor, 50% of small businesses fail by the end of the fifth year.[58] Therefore, these ventures are risky and require that the stakeholders are committed to the project with time, necessary skill sets, and resources for the planned duration of the program. The turnover of program leaders hampers the ability for the program to reach benchmarks of success.[59] The program plans also need to contain realistic objectives and timelines with milestones flexible enough to pivot when parts of the program plans are unsuccessful. These changes need to be agreed upon among all members of the public-private program planning team. The hypothesized short-term outcomes and long-term impacts need to also be realistic and supported by business plans, behavioral theories, and the experience of the program planning team. Finally, the evaluation of outcomes and impact need to be imbedded in process evaluation that documents how the implementation was delivered and received. Mixed methods allow stakeholders to identify facilitators and barriers, while also gaining perspectives on why the successes and failures occurred. Most importantly, the public-private partnership is composed of people with unique skill sets. For example, the food store owner understands the grocery store retail business and should be relied upon for their expertise regarding stocking and pricing foods; marketing and promoting products; and staffing and financing the store. Similarly, residents understand the needs of the community; academics understand the methods necessary for rigorous program evaluation; and CDFI personnel understand the capital available for food environment projects through federal, state, and private mechanisms. These unique partnerships are needed for successful food environment program interventions.

CRITICAL THINKING QUESTIONS AND ACTIVITIES

1. Determine the timeline necessary to observe a behavioral change for the program plan prepared in Chapter 11. Draw a timeline noting key implementation milestones and expected outcomes and impacts. Support your timeline with behavioral theories.
2. Describe your targeted population and how you will enroll a study population, design your evaluation, and follow study participants.
3. Describe how you will measure the use of the food store by study participants.
4. Describe how you will measure the main impact and name some of the potential confounders.
5. Describe how qualitative methods can be used to triangulate data collected.

REFERENCES

1. Centers for Disease Control and Prevention. Evaluation planning: What is it and how do you do it? *What Do We Know About.* www.cdc.gov/healthcommunication/pdf/evaluationplanning.pdf. Accessed May 31, 2021.
2. Drummond KE, Murphy-Reyes A. *Nutrition Research: Concepts and Applications.* Burlington, MA: Jones & Bartlett Learning; 2018.
3. Rothman KJ, Greenland S. *Modern Epidemiology.* 2nd ed. Philadelphia, PA: Lippincott-Raven; 1998.
4. Hendricks Brown C, Curran G, Palinkas LA, et al. An overview of research and evaluation designs for dissemination and implementation. *Annual Review of Public Health.* 2017;38:1–22.
5. Rothman KJ. Random error and the role of statistics. In: *Epidemiology: An Introduction.* 2nd ed. New York: Oxford Press; 2012.
6. Rothman KJ. Dealing with biases. In: *Epidemiology: An Introduction.* 2nd ed. New York: Oxford Press; 2012.
7. Willett WC. *Nutritional Epidemiology.* New York, NY: Oxford University Press; 2013.
8. Rothman KJ. Controlling confounding by stratifying data. In: *Epidemiology: An Introduction.* 2nd ed. New York: Oxford Press; 2012.
9. Rothman KJ. Epidemiology in clinical settings. In: *Epidemiology: An Introduction.* 2nd ed. New York: Oxford Press; 2012.
10. Denzin N, Lincoln Y. *The SAGE Handbook of Qualitative Research.* 4th ed. Thousand Oaks, CA: Sage Publications; 2011.
11. Denzin N, Lincoln Y. *Collecting and Interpreting Qualitative Materials.* Thousand Oaks, CA: Sage Publications; 2008.
12. Padgett D. *Qualitative Methods in Social Work Research.* 3rd ed. Thousand Oaks, CA: Sage Publications; 2016.
13. Glaser B, Strauss A. *The Discovery of Grounded Theory: Strategies for Qualitative Research.* Chicago, IL: Aldine Publishing Company; 1967.
14. Strauss A, Corbin J. *Grounded Theory in Practice.* Thousand Oaks, CA: Sage Publications; 1997.
15. Grills S. *Doing Ethnographic Research: Fieldwork Settings.* Thousand Oaks, CA: Sage Publications; 1998.
16. Stake R. *The Art of Case Study Research.* Thousand Oaks, CA: Sage Publications; 1995.
17. Sofaer S. Qualitative research methods. *International Journal for Quality in Health Care.* 2002; 14:329–336.
18. Dicicco-Bloom B, Crabtree BF. The qualitative research interview. *Medical Education.* 2006;40:314–321.
19. Patton MQ. *Qualitative Evaluation and Research Methods.* 2nd ed. Newbury Park, CA: Sage Publications; 1990.
20. Miles M, Huberman A, Saldana J. *Qualitative Data Analysis: A Methods Sourcebook.* Thousand Oaks, CA: Sage Publications; 2014.
21. Ryan GW, Bernard HR. Techniques to identify themes. *Field Methods.* 2003;15:85–109.
22. Denzin N, Lincoln Y. *Collecting and Interpreting Qualitative Materials.* Thousand Oaks, CA: Sage Publications; 1998.
23. MacQueen KM, McLellan E, Kay K, Milstein B. Codebook development for team-based qualitative analysis. *CAM Journal.* 1998;10:31–36.
24. Fernald DH, Duclos CW. Enhance your team-based qualitative research. *Annals of Family Medicine.* 2005;3:360–364.
25. Berends L, Johnston J. Using multiple coders to enhance qualitative analysis: The case of interviews with consumers of drug treatment. *Addiction Research & Theory.* 2005;13:373–381.
26. Palinkas L, Horwitz S, Green C, Wisdom J, Duan N, Hoagwood K. Purposeful sampling for qualitative data collection and analysis in mixed methods implementation research. *Administration and Policy in Mental Health and Mental Health Services Research.* 2015;42:533–544.
27. Onwuegbuzie A. Sampling design in qualitative research: Making the sampling process more public. *The Qualitative Report.* 2012;12:238–254.
28. Guest G, Bunce A, Johnson L. How many interviews are enough? *Field Methods.* 2016;18:59–82.

29. Saunders B, Sim J, Kingstone T, et al. Saturation in qualitative research: Exploring its conceptu-alization and operationalization. *Quality and Quantity*. 2018;52:1893–1907.

30. Francis JJ, Johnston M, Robertson C, et al. What is an adequate sample size? Operationalizing data saturation for theory-based interview studies. *Psychol Health*. 2010;25:1229–1245.

31. Hennink MM, Kaiser BN, Weber MB. What influences saturation? Estimating sample sizes in focus group research. *Qualitative Health Research*. 2019;29:1483–1496.

32. Southam-Gerow MA, Dorsey S. Qualitative and mixed methods research in dissemination and implementation science: Introduction to the special issue. *Journal of Clinical Child & Adolescent Psychology*. 2014;43:845–850.

33. Creswell J, Plano CV. *Designing and Conducting Mixed Methods Research*. 2nd ed. Thousand Oaks, CA: Sage Publications; 2011.

34. Curry L, Krumholz H, O'Cathain A, Plano CV, Cherline E, Bradley E. Mixed methods in biomedical and health services research. *Circulation: Cardiovascular Quality and Outcome*. 2013;6:119–123.

35. Greysen S, Allen R, Lucas G, Wang E, Rosenthal M. Understanding transitions in care from hospital to homeless shelter: A mixed method, community based participatory approach. *Journal of General Internal Medicine*. 2012;27:1484–1491.

36. Tashakkori A, Teddie C. *Mixed Methodology: Combining Qualitative and Quantitative Approaches*. Thousand Oaks, CA: Sage Publications; 1998.

37. Munoz-Plaza C, Parry C, Hahn E, et al. Integrating qualitative research methods into care improvement efforts with a learning health system: Addressing antibiotic overuse. *Health Research Policy and Systems*. 2016;14:1–10.

38. Kettles AM, Creswell JW, Zhang W. Mixed methods research in mental health nursing. *Journal of Psychiatric and Mental Health Nursing*. 2011;18:535–542.

39. Glasgow RE, Vinson C, Chambers D. National Institutes of Health approaches to dissemination and implementation science: Current and future directions. *American Journal of Public Health*. 2012;102:1274–1281.

40. Albright K, Gechter K, Kempe A. Importance of mixed methods in pragmatic trials and dis-semination and implementation research. *Academic Pediatrics*. 2013;13:400–407.

41. Alber JM, Green SH, Glanz K. Perceived and observed food environments, eating behaviors, and BMI. *Am J Prev Med*. 2018;54(3):423–429.

42. Cannuscio C, Hillier A, Karpyn A, Glanz K. The social dynamics of healthy food shopping and store choice in an urban environment. *Soc Sci Med*. 2014;122:13–20.

43. Cannuscio CC, Tappe K, Hillier A, Buttenheim A, Karpyn A, Glanz K. Urban food environ-ments and residents' shopping behaviors. *Am J Prev Med*. 2013;45(5):606–614.

44. Cummins S, Flint E, Matthews SA. New neighborhood grocery store increased awareness of food access but did not alter dietary habits or obesity. *Health Aff (Millwood)*. 2014;33(2):283–291.

45. Flint E, Cummins S, Matthews S. Do perceptions of the neighbourhood food environment pre-dict fruit and vegetable intake in low-income neighbourhoods? *Health Place*. 2013;24:11–15.

46. Giang T, Karpyn A, Laurison HB, Hillier A, Perry RD. Closing the grocery gap in underserved communities: The creation of the Pennsylvania fresh food financing initiative. *J Public Health Manag Pract*. 2008;14(3):272–279.

47. Hirsch J, Hillier A. Exploring the role of the food environment on food shopping patterns in Philadelphia, PA, USA: A semiquantitative comparison of two matched neighborhood groups. *Int J Environ Res Public Health*. 2013;10(1):295–313.

48. Lucan S, Barg F, Karasz A, Palmer C, Long J. Concepts of healthy diet among urban, low-income, African Americans. *J Community Health*. 2012;37(4):754–762.

49. Lucan S, Hillier A, Schechter C, Glanz K. Objective and self-reported factors associated with food-environment perceptions and fruit-and-vegetable consumption: A multilevel analysis. *Prev Chronic Dis*. 2014;11:E47.

50. Lucan SC, Karpyn A, Sherman S. Storing empty calories and chronic disease risk: Snack-food products, nutritive content, and manufacturers in Philadelphia corner stores. *J Urban Health*. 2010;87(3):394–409.

51. Lucan SC, Mitra N. Perceptions of the food environment are associated with fast-food (not fruit-and-vegetable) consumption: Findings from multi-level models. *Int J Public Health*. 2012;57(3):599–608.

52. Lucan SC, Varona M, Maroko AR, Bumol J, Torrens L, Wylie-Rosett J. Assessing mobile food vendors (a.k.a. street food vendors) – methods, challenges, and lessons learned for future food-environment research. *Public Health*. 2013;127(8):766–776.

53. Mayer VL, Hillier A, Bachhuber MA, Long JA. Food insecurity, neighborhood food access, and food assistance in Philadelphia. *J Urban Health*. 2014;91(6):1087–1097.

54. Peng K, Rodriguez DA, Peterson M, et al. GIS-based home neighborhood food outlet counts, street connectivity, and frequency of use of neighborhood restaurants and food stores. *J Urban Health*. 2020;97(2):213–225.

55. Young CR, Aquilante JL, Solomon S, et al. Improving fruit and vegetable consumption among low-income customers at farmers markets: Philly Food Bucks, Philadelphia, Pennsylvania, 2011. *Prev Chronic Dis*. 2013;10:E166.

56. Lang B, Harries C, Manon M, et al. *The Healthy Food Financing Handbook: From Advocacy to Implementation*. Philadelphia, PA: The Food Trust; 2013.

57. U.S. Department of the Treasury. *U.S. Treasury Awards $1.25 Billion to Support Economic Relief in Communities Affected by COVID-19*. June 15, 2021.

58. Carter T. The true failure rate of small businesses. *Entreprenuer*. 2021; www.entreprenuer.com/amphtml/361350. Accessed July 3, 2021.

59. Morland K. An evaluation of a neighborhood-level intervention to a local food environment. *American Journal of Preventive Medicine*. 2010;39:e31–e38.

Afterword

Since the first edition of this book, much has changed. National conversations about equity have become more sophisticated, and the attention paid to the social determinants of health as a key underpinning of disease has increased greatly. We hope this new edition clearly expresses these contextual developments and their implications for understanding the impact of healthy food access. Further, we especially hope that the text captures the sense that food access in America should be taken seriously. One of the most significant advancements was the Obama administration's acknowledgment that disparities in access to healthy food is parallel to the disparities in housing, education, and job opportunities experienced by community members living in underserved areas – a connection that had not been previously made by legislators. In doing so, a floodgate has opened for capital investment from the CDFI Fund for food retailers, funding that had previously been targeted for other retail sectors. Now, CDFIs are charged with identifying food retailers and supporting their development in underserved communities.

The connection the Obama administration made between local food environment disparities and underserved communities has linked poor access to food with the discriminatory banking practices used by traditional banks. The terminology of underserved communities is used in the federal government for identifying areas of the United States that have been subjected to redlining. The framing of this second edition is intended to help readers understand how these banking practices have undermined communities with opportunities and basic needs for generations, stemming from policies and societal norms dating back to the colonization of the United States.

With this edition, we aim to change the conversation about local food environments. Disparities in access to food retailers in the United States is no longer in question. Further, the importance of the issue has been supported through the CDFI Fund from the Obama, Trump, and Biden administrations. Over the past two decades, local food environment research has drawn interest and collaboration from many academic disciplines, including public health, nutrition, community health, health behavior, city and urban planning, geography, community medicine, and policy. An unnecessary disagreement about the benefits of correcting disparities in access to healthy food has emerged within these academic disciplines. The disagreement is unnecessary because all of the academics are working toward the greater good of communities, and now the federal HFFI has made possible what seemed like a hope and a prayer twenty years ago: the needed capital that is drawing food retailers to underserved communities. It might be said, 'the ship has sailed'. Formative research has influenced public policy and now it is time for food environment academics to work with HFFI awardees, through CDFIs or other means, to begin gaining impact information about the new food retailers or other changes to the food system that brings healthy food to underserved communities. To this end, we have provided a framework in this second edition for program evaluation utilizing effectiveness trials and mixed-methods research. These methods are founded on the understanding that the ways in which food access influences community health is as diverse as communities themselves. We also encourage impact and outcome evaluation to incorporate a range of measures and rethink the mechanisms by which food equity restores health. Public health researchers and advocates are further encouraged to abandon more highly restrictive constructs, such as obesity or dietary metrics alone, and become more open to multiple outcomes and impact measures, and models that collectively measure the interdependencies of new retailers on the economic, human development, mental, emotional, social, and familial factors that impact residents of underserved communities. Further, measures of community food access and healthy food availability require thoughtful consideration where, not unlike studies of educational equity, attention to understanding the types of opportunities and resources offered directly, or indirectly by the food access operation are critical to making a reasonable determination as to the value of the investment.

What is next for the local food environment movement? The advances from the federal government to utilize the CDFI Fund to support food retail development is laudable. However, there are components within the infrastructure of the CDFI Fund that determine the disbursement of capital to healthy food retailers that can be enhanced. Three examples are described here.

First, the importance of preventing food retail dollar leakage cannot be overstated. The HFFI program would be strengthened by supporting local enterprises by balancing funding from purveyors that are outside of the community such as large grocery chains, with local businesses, thereby increasing local taxes, jobs, and the wealth of residents. The Biden administration and the 117th Congress offer CDFIs the chance to engage on a wider range of issues than in previous years. In addition to policy priorities related to access to capital and community development finance, today the CDFI industry is called on to engage on a broader agenda that includes racial justice, infrastructure investments, climate resiliency, and more. Moving forward, there is an opportunity to support the important work of the approximately 1,200 CDFIs operating nationwide, with food retail projects that support food retail businesses owned by underserved community members and/or coordinating the supply chain to incorporate local small farmers and other local businesses with the corporate food store operations.

Second, CDFIs are defined as 'private financial institutions that are 100% dedicated to delivering responsible, affordable lending to help low-income, low-wealth, and other disadvantaged people and communities join the economic mainstream';[1] and are in contrast to 'traditional' banks, which are financial institutions that accept deposits from the public and make loans and have a fiduciary responsibility of generating profits to satisfy their shareholders. As with traditional banks, the leadership of CDFIs may not reflect the community it serves in terms of race or other factors. In fact, an 'asset gap' has been identified where CDFIs led by Black, Indigenous, and People of Color (BIPOC) have a lower average-asset size when compared to their White-led counterparts. BIPOC-led institutions hold approximately 12% of all total CDFI assets while White-led CDFIs hold 75% of all assets reported – that's more than six times the amount held by BIPOC-led CDFIs.[2] We need to advocate for more private investment in CDFIs led by BIPOC. Interested partners, including corporations, philanthropic organizations, banks, and others, can provide further investment in various CDFI efforts and funds.

Third, there is a need for additional support for smaller CDFIs and organizations seeking to become CDFIs, as they have fewer resources to go toward CDFI certification or grant-writing. Now is an exciting time to think through how smaller CDFIs can support food suppliers, producers, and retailers with HFFI funding.

In addition to the suggested improvements in the CDFI Fund to support the HFFI, one of the existing federal agencies that is well positioned to further align with the HFFI program is the National Institutes of Health (NIH). Although NIH is contributing to the HFFI through the Community Economic Development Program within the Office of Community Services to support the implementation of food retail projects, underserved communities would benefit with a further alignment by NIH to support program evaluation. Whereas one of the agency's goals is 'to expand the knowledge base in medical and associated sciences in order to enhance the Nation's economic well-being and ensure a continued high return on the public investment in research',[3] the progress of NIH-funded research on local food environments has remained stagnant and narrowly focused on diet and obesity. This agency's goal can support new HFFI program evaluation by shifting the focus of local food environment funded research. The large emphasis on diet and obesity can be exchanged with a call for impact measures on the 'economic well-being' of underserved communities who have received HFFI program projects with new requests for proposals and program announcements. This will offer the necessary funding to support program evaluation of HFFI projects to ensure a high return on the public investment of the HFFI Program as well as the research that supports it.

FINAL WORD

As individuals, we can join together with our allies, including existing coalitions and associations, to improve our local food environments through grassroots organizing and advocacy. By identifying the specific, measurable, and attainable outcomes, we can create the change we want to see in these communities. Small groups of people can make a difference, especially when larger task forces are formed. For example, the history of agencies like The Food Trust which, at the time the FFFI work started, consisted of a small group of eight people. The formation of food access task forces, backed by data about the problem and invitation to the food retail industry to discuss their needs and priorities, reset conversations away from blame and adversarial dialogue to solutions. We encourage more such dialogue.

While this text is domestic in nature, we encourage its application to international problems of food access. The Sustainable Development Goals (SDG) recognize hunger as a top priority, while at the same time call for public-private partnerships to address international challenges (SDG #17). Again, reciprocal dialogue, and broader coalition-type approaches such as those described in this text are also encouraged globally. This textbook was designed for undergraduate and graduate students, although we recognize its potential appeal to a wider audience with differing levels of policy proficiency and expectations for the ways in which food access efforts should and can bridge important gaps across America. Therefore, we hope that this book can serve as a resource to students, community organizers, policymakers, and others working to increase access to affordable, healthy food in this country. Above all we call for advocates to continue to prioritize food access and find ways to work together to improve HFFI funded programs and provide the necessary impact evaluation that will continue to support the legislation.

ADDITIONAL RESOURCES

For additional resources, please refer to some of the following organizations:

- **PolicyLink**: For a resource guide on how to build an equitable food system, www.policylink.org/our-work/community/food-systems and a toolkit on equity advocacy and development: www.policylink.org/taxonomy/term/313

- **Opportunity Finance Network**: To find a CDFI near you, https://ofn.org/cdfi-locator

- **Reinvestment Fund**: Capacity building and financing resources to build a more equitable food system that supports the health and economic vibrancy of all Americans, www.investinginfood.com/

- **The Food Trust**: To find information on how to build political support for a grocery store in your community, http://thefoodtrust.org/uploads/media_items/hffhandbookfinal.original.pdf

- **Centers for Disease Control and Prevention**: To learn more about the Polaris Policy Process and advocate for better policy, www.cdc.gov/policy/polaris/policyprocess/index.html#:~:text=CDC's%20Policy%20Process%20provides%20a,results%20in%20implementing%20a%20policy

- **National Black Bank Foundation**: For nonprofit support to Black-owned banks through legal, regulatory, strategic, and technical advice and assistance, NBBFoundation.org

REFERENCES

1. Opportunity Finance Network. What is a CDFI? 2021; https://ofn.org/what-cdfi.
2. Hope Policy Institute. Closing the CDFI Asset Gap Blog Post. 2020; http://hopepolicy.org/blog/closing-the-cdfi-asset-gap/.
3. National Institutes of Health. About NIH. www.nih.gov.

Abbreviations

ARIC	Atherosclerosis Risk in Communities Study
ASA24	Automated Self-Administered Twenty-Four-Hour Recall
BIPOC	Black, Indigenous, and People of Color
CAFO	Confined Animal Feel Operations
CARDIA	Coronary Artery Risk Development in Young Adults Study
CDBG	Community Development Block Grant
CDC	Centers for Disease Control and Prevention
CDCs	Community Development Corporations
CDFI	Community Development Financing Institution
CED-HFFI	Community Economic Development-Healthy Food Financing Initiative
CEF	Colorado Enterprise Fund
CFPCGP	Community Food Projects Competitive Grants Program
CGIAR	Consultive Group on International Agriculture Research
CHFA	Colorado Housing and Financing Authority
CI	Confidence Interval
CO4F	Colorado Fresh Food Financing Fund
CPA	Certified Public Accountant
CRA	Community Reinvestment Act of 1977
CSA	Community Supported Agriculture
CSFP	Commodity Supplement Food Program
DEGC	Detroit Economic Growth Corporation
DFFAI	Detroit Fresh Food Access Initiative
EBT	Electronic Benefit Transfer
EC	Enterprise Communities
ENY	East New York (Brooklyn)
ENY-FPC	East New York Food Policy Council
EPA	Environmental Protection Agency
ERS	Economic Research Service
EZ	Empowerment Zone
FARA	Food Access Research Atlas
FHA	Federal Housing Administration
FFFI	Fresh Food Financing Initiative
FFQ	Food Frequency Questionnaire
FFRI	Fresh Food Retailer Initiative (New Orleans)
FLSA	Fair Labor Standards Act
FPAC	Food Policy Advisory Committee (New Orleans)
FRESH	Food Retail Expansion to Support Health
FSRA	Farm Systems Reform Act
GIS	Geographic Information System
GMO	Genetically Modified Organism
HFFI	Healthy Food Financing Initiative
HFFI-TSG	America's Healthy Food Financing Targeted Small Grants Program
HFHC	Healthy Food, Healthy Communities Fund
HHS	Department of Health and Human Service
HOLC	Homeowners' Loan Corporation
HOPE	Hope Enterprise Corporation
HUD	Department of Housing and Urban Development

IARC	International Agency for Research on Cancer
KM	Kilometer
LFE	Local Food Environment
LIIF	Low Income Investment Fund
LILA	Low Income and Low Access
LSA	Limited Supermarket Analysis
MGFF	Michigan Good Food Fund
NAICS	North American Industry Classification System
NAWS	National Agricultural Workers Survey
NCI	National Cancer Institute
NDRS	Nutrition Data System for Research
NEMS	Nutrition Environment Measures Survey
NEMS-S	Nutrition Environment Measures Survey – short form
NIEHS	National Institute of Environmental Health Sciences
NICHD	National Institute of Child Health and Human Development
NMTC	New Markets Tax Credit
NSLP	National School Lunch Program
NYC	New York City
OSHA	Occupational Safety and Health Administration
OZ	Opportunity Zones
P.U.M.A.	Progressive Urban Management Associates
PZ	Promise Zones
QALICB	Qualified Active Low-Income Community Businesses
RC	Renewal Communities
RFA	Request for Application
RR	Relative Risk
RWJF	Robert Wood Johnson Foundation
SFSP	Summer Food Service Program
SNAP	Supplemental Nutrition Assistance Program
SNI	Supermarket Need Index
TEFAP	The Emergency Food Assistance Program
UNIA	Universal Negro Improvement Association
UNOP	Unified New Orleans Plan
U.S.	United States
USDA	United States Department of Agriculture
WIC	Women, Infants and Children Program

Index

Note: Page numbers in **bold** indicate tables and those in *italics* indicate figures.